P9-DCI-815

NEWBORNS AT RISK

Medical Care and
Psychoeducational Intervention

Second Edition

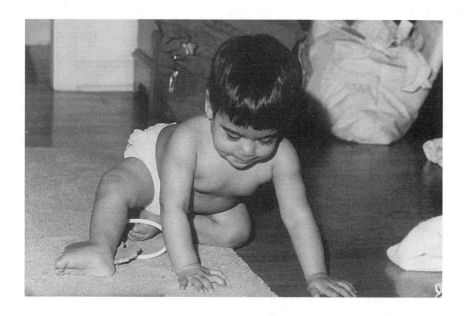

NEWBORNS AT RISK

Medical Care and Psychoeducational Intervention

Second Edition

Gail L. Ensher, EdD
Associate Professor and Coordinator
Graduate Study in Early Childhood Special Education
School of Education
Syracuse University
Syracuse, New York

David A. Clark, MD
Professor and Vice Chair
Head, Division of Neonatology
Department of Pediatrics
Louisiana State University Medical School
New Orleans, Louisiana

AN ASPEN PUBLICATION®
Aspen Publishers, Inc.
Gaithersburg, Maryland
1994

Library of Congress Cataloging-in-Publication Data

Ensher, Gail, L.
Newborns at risk : medical care and psychoeducational intervention /
Gail L. Ensher, David A. Clark. — 2nd ed.
p.   cm.
Includes bibliographical references and index.
ISBN 0-8342-0555-6
1. Infants (Newborn)—Diseases—Treatment. 2. Child development.
3. Sick children—Education. I. Clark, David A. (David Albert)
II. Title.
RJ254.E57   1994
618.92′01—dc20
94-9872
CIP

Copyright © 1994 by Aspen Publishers, Inc.
All rights reserved.

Aspen Publishers, Inc., grants permission for photocopying for limited personal or
internal use. This consent does not extend to other kinds of copying, such as copying for
general distribution, for advertising or promotional purposes, for creating new collective
works, or for resale. For information, address Aspen Publishers, Inc., Permissions
Department, 200 Orchard Ridge Drive, Suite 200, Gaithersburg, Maryland 20878.

The authors have made every effort to ensure the accuracy of the information herein, particularly with regard to drug selection and dose. However, appropriate information sources should
be consulted, especially for new or unfamiliar drugs or procedures. It is the responsibility of
every practitioner to evaluate the appropriateness of a particular opinion in the context of actual
clinical situations and with due consideration to new developments. Authors, editors, and the
publisher cannot be held responsible for any typographical or other errors found in this book.

Editorial Services: Ruth Bloom

Library of Congress Catalog Card Number: 94-9872
ISBN: 0-8342-0555-6

Printed in Canada

1   2   3   4   5

*We dedicate this work to
Kimberly Elizabeth, Lindsey Michelle,
Darlene, Kim, Jenny, and Mindy*

Table of Contents

    Newborn** **170**
    Gail L. Ensher, David A. Clark, and Linda M. Yarwood

    Prenatal Exposure to Drugs, Alcohol, and Cigarette
        Smoking 170
    Influence of Prescribed Drugs 181
    Breast-Feeding and Drugs 185

Chapter 14—Ethical Issues and the High Risk Infant **190**
    Historical Perspectives 190
    Basic Principles 191
    Prenatal Problems 192
    Intrauterine Therapy 193
    Withholding and Withdrawing Life Support 193
    Anencephalic and Fetal Transplant Donations 195
    Maternal versus Fetal Rights 196

**Chapter 15—Assessing Infants and Preschool Children within a
    Family Context** **199**
    Screening, Diagnosis, and Issues of Prediction 200
    Applications 210
    Best Practice: Interaction of Family, Child, Professionals,
        and Community 222

**PART III—INTERVENTION: PROCESS AND PRACTICAL
    APPLICATION** **225**

Chapter 16—Intervening in Intensive Care Nurseries **227**
    Mary Jo Hayes and Gail L. Ensher

    Goals of Intervention in the Neonatal Unit 227
    The Vulnerable Brain 229
    Infant Behavior 230
    Intervention with Newborns 233
    Intervention with Parents 243

Chapter 17—One Nursery: A Scenario of Change **249**
    *Anne C. Mastropaolo, Larry Consenstein, and
    James J. Pergolizzi, III*

    Pain 249
    Development of the Neonatal Intensive Care Unit
        (NICU) 252
    Lessons Learned 255
    Family-Centered Care and Discharge Planning 258

Contributors

Dianne S. Apter, MA
Director
Early Childhood Direction Center
Syracuse University
Syracuse, New York

Larry Consenstein, MD
Neonatologist and Director
St. Joseph's Neonatal Intensive Care Nursery
Syracuse, New York

Andrea M. DeSantis, PT
Physical Therapist
Margaret L. Williams Developmental
    Evaluation Center
Syracuse, New York

Helen Harrison, MS
Teacher
Jowonio School
Syracuse, New York

Mary Jo Hayes, PT
Physical Therapist
Valley Memorial Hospital
Livermore, California

Anne C. Mastropaolo, BS
Physical Therapist
St. Joseph's Neonatal Intensive Care Nursery
Syracuse, New York

Margaret P. Ninno, CAS
Teacher/Coordinator
Birth to 2 Year Services
Early Education Program
Main Street School
North Syracuse, New York

James J. Pergolizzi III, MD
Neonatologist
St. Joseph's Neonatal Intensive Care Nursery
Syracuse, New York

Mary Elizabeth Redmond, BS
Infant Program Coordinator
Jowonio School
Syracuse, New York

Nan S. Songer, BS Ed
Family Specialist
Early Childhood Direction Center
Syracuse University
Syracuse, New York

Linda M. Yarwood, MS
Teacher/Service Coordinator
Head Start Program
Syracuse, New York

MAJOR CONTRIBUTORS TO PHOTOGRAPHY

David A. Clark, MD
Professor and Vice Chair
Head, Division of Neonatology
Department of Pediatrics
Louisiana State University Medical School
New Orleans, Louisiana

Debra A. DeSocio, MS
Early Education Program
Main Street School
Syracuse, New York

Susan E. Gelling, MS
Jowonio School
Syracuse, New York

Alix Lawson-Board
Newhouse School of Public Communications
Syracuse University
Syracuse, New York

Andréjs Ozolins, BA
Cortland, New York

Preface

The first edition of this book evolved from very special interests and experiences during the course of a 3-year contract awarded in August 1979 to Syracuse University's School of Education by the New York State Office of Mental Retardation and Developmental Disabilities. The project was funded with the specific goal of delivering home-based intervention services to markedly premature and other high risk infants discharged from intensive care nurseries in the metropolitan area of Syracuse, New York. During this 3-year course of collaboration, students and professionals working with young children and their families, representing multiple disciplines, raised many questions and sought much information about these new and challenging populations who were entering their educational and programmatic settings. The first edition of *Newborns at Risk* was written with the hope and intent of addressing some of these needs.

Since 1986, there have been major, dramatic changes in neonatology, the clinical fields, and early childhood special education. New technologies are saving newborns on the edge of viability. Public Laws 99–457 and 102–119 have been passed, introducing new concepts, new methods of carrying out our interventions, new ways of cooperating and collaborating with families and with other professionals, and new challenges. New ethical issues confront physicians in their everyday work. Likewise, the dilemmas of substance abuse, the epidemic of human immunodeficiency virus (HIV), and the other social/medical problems of inadequate prenatal care are yet to be adequately addressed by all relevant professionals in this country. These topics and more are the substance of this second edition.

The book is organized into three parts, each covering different aspects of medical care and psychoeducational intervention with high risk and disabled infants and their families.

Part I—*From Conception to Discovery of the World*—deals with a brief history and a discussion of contemporary perspectives and future initiatives; information about high risk pregnancies, perinatal events, major problems of the newborn, infant development and follow-up studies; and descriptions of neonatal care in selected developing countries.

Part II—*Clinical Issues: Problems, Identification, Assessment, and Prognosis*—focuses on major medical insults of the newborn, including neurological problems, jaundice, respiratory distress, nutrition and metabolism, problems of physical development, infection, effects of parental substance use and abuse on the newborn, ethical issues, and new developments in the assessment of infants and young children.

Part III—*Intervention: Process and Practical Application*—discusses working with newborns and families in neonatal intensive care settings, issues relating to families and their environments, interventions for young children with sensori-motor and regulatory problems, and new themes and research in early education. The final two chapters of this section consider the mandate and challenge of new collaborations and partnerships with families and among professional disciplines that have emerged with the passage of Public Laws 99–457 and 102–119.

Gail L. Ensher
David A. Clark

Acknowledgments

This book would not have been written without the help of many people. Our first and greatest appreciation goes to our own families: to Kimberly Elizabeth, Lindsey Michelle, Darlene, Jenny, Kim, and Mindy, who have taught us the real meaning of parenting, child development, and patience, of love and understanding, and to our own parents, who have given so unstintingly of themselves in support of our endeavors over the years.

Several colleagues have made a special difference in our professional lives. These people include the late Burton Blatt, Walter Meyer, and Margaret Williams, who were always present to offer wisdom and encouragement to go on, as well as Eric Gardner, Ernest Kraybill, Jacqueline Meyer, and Albert Murphy, who have been faithful mentors, friends, and examples of the very best in our respective fields.

A number of people have contributed to the writing of this book. We owe a sincere debt to those families who have opened their homes, allowed us to visit week after week, and written personal accounts of their lives. They are Henry and Effie Buie, Gary and Margaret Brockway, Pamela and William Corrigan, Michael and Beth Daly, Fred and Sarah Edelman, Linda and Patrick Fullan, Nicholas and Carol Marsella, and Robert and Ann Pratt. Professional colleagues and students also have contributed substantially by writing portions of chapters or entire chapters. In this regard, we are grateful to Dianne Apter, Larry Consenstein, Andrea DeSantis, Helen (Nita) Harrison, Mary Jo Hayes, Anne Mastropaolo, Margaret Ninno, James Pergolizzi, Mary Elizabeth Redmond, Nan Songer, and Linda Yarwood. We deeply appreciate the time and effort of those who have been responsible for preparing other aspects of this book: for the beautiful pictures taken by Ellen Barnes, Leslie Buecheler, Joy Casey, Larry Consenstein, Andrea DeSantis, Debra DeSocio, Martin Elks, Susan Gelling, Karen Holl, Julie Garrity, Christine Garneau, Peter Knoblock, Alix Lawson-Board, Linda Louko, Sondra

Nelson, Andrejs Ozolins, Marie Sarno, and Kathleen and Ronald Wilson, and for the endless typing of this manuscript in its various stages by Sharon Bedell, Donna Fecteau, and Ana Sison.

Finally, we thank all of those graduate students and families of infants and young children who have listened to our thoughts and ideas along the way and who were genuinely responsible for the conception of the first edition and an impetus for the writing of the second edition.

Part I

From Conception to Discovery of the World

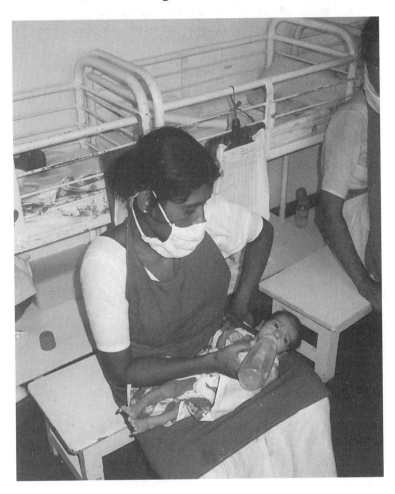

Every year, approximately 4 million infants are born in the United States. National surveys have indicated a decline, over the past 10 to 12 years, in the proportion of young, unmarried women receiving adequate prenatal care, especially in underrepresented and least educated ethnic groups. Likewise, the incidence of premature births in this country has remained a disturbing 7.6 percent, again reflecting larger numbers of families from "less advantaged" homes. Such trends are troubling in light of known evidence that the well-being of newborns begins long before birth and is intimately related to the welfare and nutrition of mothers and fathers. Research in the field of neonatology over the past 20 years has been responsible for vast improvements in mortality rates and has perceptively enhanced prospects for normal developmental outcome, even among extremely low birthweight populations. Yet, progress toward the prevention of developmental problems could be advanced even further were this country to address seriously some of the overwhelming social problems that continue to plague many families.

Chapter 1

The High Risk Infant: The Past, Contemporary Perspectives, and Future Initiatives

Today, our respective fields of health, clinical practice, and education hold much promise for the high risk and disabled infant and young child. The newest technologies in neonatology have vastly improved both the rates of survival and the incidence of developmental and behavioral problems. Babies of 25 to 26 weeks gestation, weighing 500 to 750 grams, no longer are viewed as incapable of sustaining life. Moreover, even those newborns who have borne the impact of major insults and neurologic impairment now have the benefit of the earliest intervention with the passage of Public Law (PL) 99–457. Families, too, have achieved a new and higher priority in the scheme of policymaking and implementation. The new legislation reaffirms in detail the centrality of the family, with its concerns and agendas, in the process and product of early intervention programing. Professionals, as never before, are being called on to bring together their individual and collective expertise and experience in forward-looking paradigms of collaboration. In addition, the focus of contemporary research in developmental pediatrics and early childhood special education likewise has changed. Building on insights from the past (Sameroff, 1981; Sameroff & Chandler, 1975), experts in their respective fields are now asking questions that are more specific, set within a naturalistic context, and examined along a continuum of outcomes. For example, general issues surrounding the efficacy of early intervention in neonatal intensive care units and educational infant and preschool programs have been laid to rest. Current thinking is centered clearly on inquiries about what kinds of programing, within what time frames, with what kinds of children and families, are most effective.

As our perspectives have broadened, so have the multifaceted social, health, and economic problems of our time. In the decade ahead, for example, we surely will need to address the effects of escalating numbers of newborns delivered to families who have abused drugs and alcohol and thus compromised the health and development of their children. The implications of service for such multirisk families, infants, and young children are vast in terms of their complexities and pervasiveness within our contemporary and ethnically diverse cultures. Experts in educational, medical, and human service fields universally are concerned about the rapidly rising numbers of mothers and young children now being identified who are testing seropositive for human immunodeficiency virus (HIV). Hospitals and intermediate care facilities in major cities across the United States are overwhelmed with the magnitude of this problem and are poorly equipped to cope with the compelling developmental, nurturing, and educational needs of the afflicted populations. Even though new technologies proliferate in this country, those who most require services, beginning with quality prenatal follow-up, often are least able to gain access to the health care system. Too frequently, these consumers are an "absent" group, until they again surface in crisis in the midst of neonatal intensive care and early intervention programs. Also, it is highly likely that the widespread neglect and abuse of infants and young children—often those who are premature and disabled—are symptomatic of the social ills in this country that continue unchecked despite preventive programs.

Realistically, we do not need a superficial regeneration of enthusiasm for early childhood special education, but rather the assurance that present high interest and the genuine promise of PL 99–457 will fulfill our most pressing obligations through research, training, and service. The charge is a formidable one. Six elements are essential to its fulfillment:

1. more naturalistic measures of child and family growth
2. defined yet holistic programing
3. understanding of the full parameters of risk
4. inclusive perspectives of community-based early intervention
5. strategies for evaluating program effectiveness
6. creative solutions that involve families at the heart of our medical and service delivery systems.

VULNERABILITY AND RISK IN NEWBORNS

The *neonatal period* includes the first 4 weeks of life and, despite recent scientific progress, remains the time of greatest mortality in childhood, with the risk highest within the first 24 hours of life. The *perinatal period* is a broader term used to designate the time extending from week 12 of gestation through the neonatal period. The high incidence of death and disease during the perinatal period makes it essential to identify those at risk as early and rapidly as possible and to initiate intervention whenever feasible. The goal, therefore, becomes not only a reduction in mortality, but also a decrease in the incidence of disabling conditions.

Some Historical Considerations in Neonatal Care

As defined by the late Alexander Schaffer, *neonatology* is the "art and science of diagnosis and treatment of disorders of the newborn infant" (Schaffer, 1960). Pierre Budin, a French obstetrician, was the first individual recognized as having articulated and published a set of guidelines for medical care of the newborn. In 1892, he established "a special department for weaklings" in a Parisian maternity hospital (Budin, 1907). He used the weight of 2,500 grams or less (454 grams = 1 pound) as a definition for prematurity. This statement subsequently was adopted by the American Academy of Pediatrics in 1935 and the World Health Organization in 1950.

Advances from 1892 to 1950 focused primarily on prevention of infection and on early nutrition for sick newborns. Dr. Julius Hess established the first premature infant center in Chicago just after World War I. Meanwhile, significant strides in understanding the growth, nutrition, physiology, and pathology of newborns were made by European researchers in Finland, Germany, and France. Unfortunately, as a consequence of two world wars and the economic depression of the 1930s, much of this information was slow to be transmitted to the United States.

A major contributor to the field of neonatology in this country was Ethel Dunham. After an appointment in the Department of Pediatrics at Yale University, she worked as the director of the Division of Research in Child Development of the Children's Bureau in Washington, D.C. Between 1919 and 1940, she compiled information on premature infants and subsequently published that material as a book entitled *Premature Infants: A Manual for Physicians* (Dunham, 1955). This work not only provided guidelines but also generated interest in the care of newborns.

By the 1950s, much research on the physiology and treatment of the neonate was being initiated. Concurrent with these developments, major changes were occurring in adult medicine, especially in the fields of cardiology and hematology. The American Cancer Society and the American Heart Association were founded during this time, and funding for research was allocated to diseases that affected adults.

Thus, it was not until the 1960s that more government and business funds finally were made available for research on the problems and care of the newborn. Since that time, there has been rapid growth both in the understanding of newborns and in the status of current technology. Prematurity during this era was redefined to include criteria of birthweight, as well as indications of physical and neurologic maturity. As a result of these changes in classification, morbidity associated with variations of intrauterine growth then could be identified more precisely and addressed within that time frame. In addition, there have been technological advances with smaller and more accurate pieces of equipment to monitor and treat the newborn—a byproduct of research carried out during the early space exploration programs of the National Aeronautics and Space Administration (NASA).

Throughout the 1960s, numerous studies were done to analyze various causes of neonatal mortality and morbidity. In states such as Wisconsin and Massachusetts, regional perinatal centers were developed to provide for the unique needs of the obstetrical patient with medical complications and the sick newborn. The reduction in mortality demonstrated by these facilities became the impetus for the establishment of perinatal centers across the country.

Organization of Perinatal Care

Careful delineation of risk factors that could be life-threatening in mothers or that might result in problems in newborns helped immeasurably to determine the developmental periods when medical intervention would be most beneficial. Medical facilities within given geographic regions varied markedly in their ability to offer perinatal care, with differences reflecting population density of the area, size and financial health of the institution; experience and skill of the medical and nursing staff; proximity to larger facilities; and available equipment. Consequently, institutions within specific localities joined together to afford optimal care.

In the United States, three basic levels of treatment have emerged. A Level One service is the community hospital that generally has fewer deliveries and is designed primarily for the mother and baby with no risk factors. These institutions must, however, have available the equipment and personnel for competent emergency service and newborn resuscitation and stabilization prior to transport of the mother or child when the need arises.

A Level Two facility is the hospital that has larger maternity and nursery services. These institutions usually are located in urban and suburban areas and are capable of giving service to selected mothers and newborns with problems. However, there is considerable diversity among such institutions, depending on resources and the skills of the personnel.

The Level Three facility can handle the full range of complications of pregnancy and sick newborns. Most but not all of these facilities are associated with medical schools. They provide for the care of mothers with complex pregnancies and of newborns with severe respiratory distress, cardiac diseases, and various surgical problems. Consultation of subspecialists in various areas of pediatrics must be readily accessible.

Many Level Three facilities have been designated as regional perinatal centers, and thus they have responsibility for developing systems of patient transport, setting the standard for care within a given location, and improving the level of service in the smaller referring institutions by outreach education. The impact of this approach has led to a decrease of nearly 60 to 70 percent in infant mortality over the last 25 years (Bucciarelli, 1994). There also has been a concomitant decrease in the percentage of infants with residual disabilities.

Stresses of Medical Care

While new scientific approaches have altered dramatically what can be done for sick infants, many tensions surrounding the care of these newborns have surfaced. Some of these are social issues, such as the increased number of pregnancies in adolescence, legalization of abortions, the working mother, and the dissolution of families. Added to these considerations are the often unrealistic expectations that parents have for healthy children.

One significant problem for both the family and society is the cost of this highly technical care. A baby born 12 weeks prematurely with no medical complications is usually hospitalized for a minimum of 2 months, and the infant with complications may be hospitalized 6 months or longer. The cost per day ranges between $500 and $1,000 and for a sick newborn, may approach several thousands of dollars. Thus, hospital bills of $50,000 or more for a critically ill, small newborn are not uncommon. Annually, the estimated cost for neonatal intensive care in this country is approximately $4 billion. For the most part, this expenditure is being borne by state financial aid and by private insurance companies.

Although social and financial pressures are considerable, the increasing legal and ethical obligations for newborn care are even greater. Who decides what technology should be used and for how long in the case of an individual baby with little or no hope of survival, let alone meaningful existence? In the past, three infants who received national publicity have brought to light some of these specific concerns: Baby John Doe, Baby Jane Doe, and Baby Faye. Baby John Doe was an infant with Down syndrome, born in the Midwest; a portion of his esophagus was missing. Although this condition was surgically correctable, the family and medical staff chose not to intervene and the baby died. While this was a common practice 30 years ago, it is highly unlikely that such a child would not have surgery today.

A second child, Baby Jane Doe, was a little girl born in New York with hydrocephalus and a large open myelomeningocele. While prognosis for long-term survival for a baby having these conditions is very tenuous, the typical care is supportive. Care includes the closing of the myelomeningocele and decompression of the abnormally large head filled with excessive cerebrospinal fluid. The parents and medical staff elected not to pursue this route; yet the baby did not expire as rapidly as predicted by the medical staff. This information subsequently was given to a "right-to-life" lawyer, who pursued a court order for certain medical services. Baby Jane Doe then became a "test case" in the much larger national conflict. Subsequent events were very costly financially and emotionally to the family, medical staff, and institution in which the child was receiving care. Considerable debate followed, with the former Surgeon General, C. Everett Koop, taking a leading role in the courts, which ruled that neonates with disabilities will receive extensive care.

Superimposed on these two cases was the widely publicized baboon heart transplant in Baby Faye in California in 1984. The infant had a form of congenital heart disease for which no existing surgical technology other than a transplant was available. The medical staff responsible for her care presented an overly optimistic picture of the potential for success of the procedure and, in fact, predicted less than 48 hours before she died that this child might live to 21 years. Surgical and medical complications and her body's rejection of the baboon heart initially were concealed, resulting in subsequent criticism of the physician staff for an overzealous and highly experimental approach in this child.

Taken together, these three cases barely scratch the surface of moral and legal dilemmas facing the families and the nurses and other medical professionals in intensive care nurseries. The majority of neonatologists are overwhelmingly committed to the ancient principle of medicine that human life is worth saving. Toward that end, the regionalization of perinatal care and technology has improved the survival and outcome of babies within the last 30 years. Issues now confronting intensive care nurseries are less technical and more ethical, as neonatologists seek to define those fine lines between saving a life, prolonging death, and enhancing the quality of life.

Defining the Parameters of Risk

Concepts of vulnerability and risk in infants and young children for years have formed the fabric of research and service in early childhood special education and continue to do so today. Professionals in education, psychology, pediatrics, child development, and other related clinical fields remain focused on work with children at high risk for impairment and developmental delay—categories that are consistently expanding with the benefit of new medical knowledge, mounting social dilemmas, and widespread epidemics of infectious disease. Basically, however, despite the larger or smaller parameters of child and family, factors of risk have been attributed to one or a combination of three main influences:

1. biological conditions that have been associated consistently with neurological or physical damage and developmental delay (e.g., Down syndrome, fragile X chromosome, and hydrocephalus)
2. other medical conditions such as maternal (and thus neonatal) substance abuse or severe respiratory distress requiring extensive ventilator support, which frequently are related to later developmental and behavioral difficulties

3. environmental influences (often multifaceted) that may have an adverse impact on early development and later school performance (e.g., restricted or aberrant patterns of interaction between family and child).

Such categories are by no means mutually exclusive but invariably interact to promote additional developmental problems beyond the initial insult. Indeed, in the ways that disabled and high risk infants are perceived, there may be individual differences so ordinary or so subtle as to conceal or minimize the probable magnitude of their real effect.

In large measure, educational programs for infants and young children, until recently, have been organized around the premise that discrete deficits could be identified in the early months after birth and that appropriate treatment would prevent or ameliorate these deficits. This has proven to be an unworkable assumption. Developmental screening techniques for assessing newborns still are, at best, gross in estimating current functioning, and they largely have fallen short of the goal of predicting the greatest need or future potential. The large number of children leaving intensive care nurseries who have eluded early identification but have later manifested moderate to severe disabilities confirms that, even in the face of significant impairment, evidence most often is tentative and outcome is uncertain. Any valid risk indices appropriate to the newborn period must encompass biomedical criteria relative to both the child and the environmental conditions in the family and the community. In the long run, there is no substitute for astute clinical acumen in the early identification process. Criteria carefully drawn but applied without attention to individual child and family characteristics may prove to be of little benefit, leading to neglected opportunities and eventual untoward developmental consequences.

Finally, because potentially disabling conditions are not discerned readily in many preterm and other high risk infants, professionals need to conceptualize a network of services for all youngsters suspected of serious developmental insult or delay. Specifically, with the prominence of neonatal medicine and the heightened focus on infants as a national priority, early identification of children and families who meet certain eligibility criteria should become a routine and financially recognized practice, even in economically stressful times. However, the strategy is not without problems. Attempts at implementation in the past have been disappointing due to errors of overreferral or inadequate detection of disabling conditions. Accurate screening during the newborn period and subsequent early months of life is a considerable undertaking, which requires multiple samplings of behavior that are based on a broad spectrum of risk parameters and measures of child development and are taken over an extended period of time. This prevention approach thus allows for the monitoring of behavioral and developmental milestones without recourse to labeling or the early stigmatizing of child and family. Among populations at risk, the main goal is to determine which infants and families are in greatest jeopardy. With research and commitment to a new philosophy and new legislation, many medical and educational centers now are combining resources to achieve this purpose.

INFANT AND EARLY CHILDHOOD SPECIAL EDUCATION REVISITED

Past and Present Approaches

Early childhood special education over the past 30 years has witnessed noteworthy changes in focus and format. In large part, these changes are a reflection of contemporary society and the evolution of major socioeconomic, political, and philosophical forces impacting on life in the American family.

The decade of the 1960s saw the rise of idealism and "unprecedented interest" in preschool, compensatory education, which culminated in the national adoption of Project Head Start and the War on Poverty (Winschel, 1970; Zigler & Valentine, 1979). Invested with a faith that the cycle of social and intellectual delays often observed among the economically disadvantaged youngsters could be prevented, Project Head Start served 500,000 impoverished children during its first year. The decade from 1960 to 1970 also laid claim to numerous federally supported demonstration projects for 2- to 5-year-old children (Blatt & Garfunkel, 1969; Hodges, McCandless, & Spicker, 1967; Karnes, 1969; Klaus & Gray, 1968; Levenstein, 1970; Weikart, 1967). Like Project Head Start, these programs were rooted in the concept of the educability or modifiability of intelligence and a firm belief that intervention could make a difference in producing long-term gains and circumventing later school failure. Contrary to high hopes and widespread conviction, this prophecy remained largely unfulfilled, and the efficacy of education in the early years was opened to scrutiny, doubt, and controversy. Analyses ranging from unrealistic predictions to errors of interpretation and methodological problems were prevalent in searching for answers.

Years later, with experience and hindsight to our advantage, researchers and service providers have acknowledged the folly of our assumptions and our limited vision of the requisites for effecting enduring change within vulnerable families. The national debate on compensatory education proceeded and, at least in the short term, the unbridled idealism and promising expectations of the decade were tempered in response to the doubting and dissident.

The period that followed the late 1960s and early 1970s gave pause for reflection and re-examination of program goals and target populations. These years also were a boon to intervention with infants and young children of low income and disadvantaged families. The hope in the hearts and minds of many was that earlier stimulation, for longer periods, with active parent participation, might yield the enduring developmental gains that had not been witnessed with the older preschool child. Educators sought answers both within and outside the home, and research took form in several models of intervention. Underlying all of these early projects was the overriding goal of identifying those conditions most instrumental in the development of the young child. In retrospect, one must ask whether the concept and mode of implementation were sufficiently bold to counter the prevailing biological and environmental influences for a sizeable proportion of our population. The burning controversies of effectiveness remained. But despite the new wave of funding, overwhelming investments of interest and time, public sympathy, and program expansion, interventions for the most part continued to be "broad band," nonspecific, and "directed at infants with widely differing risk conditions" (Keogh & Kopp, 1978, p. 533).

Programs for the severely disabled received impetus during this time from parents, with the passage of PL 94–142, and slowly there emerged a concurrent focus on the multiply disabled infant. These developments, however, were little solace to the educator plagued with the ambiguity and imprecision of the art. The pioneering work of Provence and Lipton (1962) and others on evaluation and follow-up of infants in institutions seemed to offer ample rationale for preventing custodial care and its adverse developmental consequence. Also, burgeoning contemporary programs such as those initiated for preschool children with Down syndrome at the Experimental Education Unit of the University of Washington's Child Development and Retardation Center (Hayden & Dmitriev, 1975; Hayden & Haring, 1976) reported convincing, short-term progress.

In the early 1980s, the literature was replete with labels of dysfunction, short-term solutions, inadequately explained contradictions, and lingering issues unresolved. Rapid changes in society, political paradoxes, newborn technologies, complex family problems, and economic constraints made it nearly impossible for educational systems to keep pace with demands. Moreover, in 1986, Amendments to the Education of the Handicapped Act (PL 99–457) ushered in the most sweeping and bold legislation enacted in the history of education of high risk and disabled young children in the United States (Meisels, 1989). The full implementation of this law is yet to be met in the decade of the 1990s. *The Twelfth Annual Report to Congress* by the U.S. Department of Education spelled out the parameters of this legislation which addresses the needs of young high risk and disabled children through two programs. The first is the Handicapped Infants and Toddlers Program (Part H of PL 99–457). This program

> . . . . offers funds to assist States in planning, developing, and implementing an interagency system of early intervention services for handicapped infants, toddlers and their families. Systems are to be statewide, comprehensive, coordinated and multidisciplinary. (U.S. Department of Education, 1990, p. 47)

The second program promulgated by PL 99-457 (Section 619 of Part B) for 3- to 5-year-old children assures "a free appropriate public education for all children" (U.S. Department of Education, 1990, p. 47) within this age group. The *Twelfth Annual Report to Congress* further noted: "the same regulations that govern the provision of special education and related services to school age children apply to children age 3–5" (p. 47).

Research and Service Delivery in the Decade Ahead

Over the past three decades, the fields of early childhood development, developmental and behavioral pediatrics, and human development have seen many changes in methods of study, target populations, assessment techniques, and strategies for intervention, as well as in the theoretical constructs for understanding infant development. By the same token, many of the same basic questions raised by pioneers in early intervention research have persisted as variations on a central theme. We have erred at both ends of the continuum in our quest for data and explanation, examining minute pieces of behavior only to lose sight of the larger picture or conceptualizing global issues to the neglect of the finer subtleties of individual difference. Still, the rationale for continued research and the interest among professionals have not been diminished by such obstacles. If anything, they have been intensified.

In a sense, we again stand at a turning point, with opportunities for setting new directions and priorities in research and the delivery of services to the very young who have suffered medical and environmental insult. Future research must be unfettered by conventions of the past. The minimal requirements of the task call for research that:

- coordinates findings from biomedical, educational, and clinical fields
- is carried out in diverse ecological environments of hospital, home, school, and community
- adopts strategies of periodic follow-up of high risk children at least into their elementary school years
- involves families, as well as the child, as part of the core of research models
- invests energy in developing prevention models in medical care and psychoeducational intervention, as well as treatment and remediation approaches
- focuses on the social competence and behavioral dimensions of development in high risk and disabled children at a level equal to current high interest in the study of cognition, language, and motor skills.

BIBLIOGRAPHY

Blatt, B., & Garfunkel, F. (1969). *The educability of intelligence: Preschool intervention with disadvantaged children*. Washington, DC: The Council for Exceptional Children.

Bucciarelli, R.L. (1994). Neonatology in the United States: Scope and organization. In G.B. Avery, M.A. Fletcher, & M.G. MacDonald (Eds.), *Neonatology: Pathophysiology and management of the newborn* (4th ed.) (pp. 12–31). Philadelphia: J.B. Lippincott.

Budin, P. (1907). *The Nursling.* London: Caxton Publishing.

Dunham, E. (1955). *Premature Infants: A Manual for Physicians* (2nd Ed.). New York: Paul B. Hoeber.

Hayden, A.H., & Dmitriev, V. (1975). The multidisciplinary preschool program for Down's Syndrome children at the University of Washington model preschool center. In B.Z. Friedlander, G.M. Sterritt, & G.E. Kirk (Eds.), *Exceptional infant: Assessment and intervention* (Vol. 3, pp. 193–221). New York: Brunner/Mazel.

Hayden, A.H., & Haring, N.G. (1976). Early intervention for high risk infants and young children: Programs for Down's Syndrome children. In T.D. Tjossem (Ed.), *Intervention strategies for high risk infants and young children* (pp. 573–607). Baltimore: University Park Press.

Hodges, W.L., McCandless, B.R., & Spicker, H.H. (1967). *The development and evaluation of a diagnostically based curriculum for preschool psychosocially deprived children.* Washington, DC: U.S. Office of Education.

Karnes, M.B. (1969). *Research and development program on preschool disadvantaged children: Final report.* Washington, DC: U.S. Office of Education.

Keogh, B.K., & Kopp, C.B. (1978). From assessment to intervention: An elusive bridge. In F.D. Minifie & L.L. Lloyd (Eds.), *Communicative and cognitive abilities—Early behavioral assessment* (pp. 523–547). Baltimore: University Park Press.

Klaus, R.A., & Gray, S.W. (1968). The early training project for disadvantaged children: A report after five years. *Monographs of the Society for Research in Child Development, 33,* (4, Serial No. 126).

Levenstein, P. (1970). Cognitive growth in preschoolers through verbal interaction with mothers. *American Journal of Orthopsychiatry, 40,* 426–432.

Meisels, S.J. (1989). Meeting the mandate of Public Law 99–457: Early childhood intervention in the nineties. *American Journal of Orthopsychiatry, 59*(3), 451–460.

Provence, S., & Lipton, R.C. (1962). *Infants in institutions.* New York: International Universities Press.

Sameroff, A.J. (1981). Psychological needs of the mother in early mother-infant interactions. In G.B. Avery (Ed.), *Neonatology: Pathophysiology and management of the newborn* (2nd ed.) (pp. 303–321). Philadelphia: J.B. Lippincott.

Sameroff, A.J., & Chandler, M.J. (1975). Reproductive risk and the continuum of caretaking casualty. In F.D. Horowitz, M. Hetherington, S. Scarr-Salapatek, & M. Siegel (Eds.), *Review of child development research* (Vol. 4, pp. 187–244). Chicago: University of Chicago Press.

Schaffer, A. (1960). *Diseases of the newborn.* Philadelphia: W.B. Saunders.

U.S. Department of Education. (1990). *Twelfth annual report to Congress on the implementation of The Education of the Handicapped Act* (pp. 46–47). Washington, DC: Office of Special Education and Rehabilitative Services, Division of Innovation and Development.

Weikart, D.P. (1967). *Preschool intervention: A preliminary report of the Perry Preschool Project.* Ann Arbor, MI: Campus Publishers.

Winschel, J.F. (1970). In the dark . . . Reflections on compensatory education 1960–1970. In J. Hellmuth (Ed.), *Disadvantaged child—Compensatory education: A national debate* (Vol. 3, pp. 3–23). New York: Brunner/Mazel.

Zigler, E., & Valentine, J. (Eds.). (1979). *Project Head Start: A legacy of the war on poverty.* New York: The Free Press.

Chapter 2

Before Birth

FETAL-MATERNAL INTERACTION

The importance of prenatal life was best expressed by Samuel Taylor Coleridge when he wrote, "The history of man in the nine months preceding his birth would probably be far more interesting and attain events of greater moment than all the three score and ten years that follow it" (Coleridge, 1968). To paraphrase this quote, he correctly implied that the threat to intact physical and mental survival of a human being starts long before birth and is linked inextricably to the well-being of the mother. To understand the high risk infant, professionals must appreciate events prior to birth.

Conception

It is well recognized that the general health and nutrition of the mother may limit or enhance her ability to conceive and maintain a pregnancy (Campbell & Gillmer, 1983; Scholl, 1990). Over the past 30 years, multiple advances in medicine have allowed mothers with metabolic diseases such as diabetes mellitus to conceive and maintain pregnancies, resulting in viable newborns (Gilbert & Harmon, 1993). Similarly, infants born to mothers with chronic illnesses often are born prematurely and have altered physiology, which originates from the mother's illness. Exposure of the father or mother to heavy metals or anesthetic agents increases first trimester spontaneous abortions and causes a higher percentage of low birthweight infants (Joffe, 1979). In addition, parental use of cigarettes, alcohol, and recreational drugs and exposure to anesthetic agents are associated with a higher incidence of congenital anomalies (Ad Hoc Committee, 1974; Soyka & Joffe, 1980). The existence of a large number of couples seeking help becuase they are unable to conceive has led to a proliferation of specialists in infertility. Drugs used to promote ovulation frequently result in superovulation with multiple eggs released and, therefore, great potential for multiple gestation. A similar effect may be seen with women who have used birth control pills. When they stop using oral contraception because they wish to become pregnant, superovulation is more likely for several months. The result may be multiple gestation, the mother is unlikely to be able to carry the babies until term gestation and miscarries especially in a first pregnancy (Benirschke, 1992).

Table 2–1 documents the significant number of previously unrecognized early fetal losses. A very sensitive assay test (radioimmunoassay) for detection of the human chorionic gonadotropin (hCG) has been developed. This hormone is produced by early fetal membranes (chorion) and is the chemical measured in the typical urine test for pregnancy; a large quantity of hCG in the urine indicates a pregnancy. The radioimmunoassay allows for detection of hCG in blood in very small quantities. Using this assay, researchers have monitored monthly a population of women of childbearing age; they found that 50 percent more pregnancies were identified by this method than by any other technique (Simpson, 1980). These additional pregnancies ended spontaneously in the first 4 to 6 weeks of gestation.

Fetal Wastage

The human gestational period (estimated days of confinement) is approximately 40 weeks. An infant is considered to be full term within the range of 37 to 42 weeks. The first trimester of pregnancy is an especially hazardous time. The egg must be fertilized, implanted in the uterine wall, and develop into an embryo, and the placental tissue must be rapidly established to maintain fetal growth. Failure of the placenta to develop leads to fetal wastage, i.e., early spontaneous abortion. Some miscarriages during the first trimester are associated with chromosomal abnormalities (Kerr, 1976). The first trimester of pregnancy also is a time in which the embryo and fetus grow rapidly, with many crucial cell divisions occurring. Drugs, maternal infections, and other agents that may cause malformations exert the greatest effect during this period (Kurczynski, 1992; Schardlein, 1985).

Table 2–1 Outcome per 1,000 pregnancies

Number	Outcome
320	Early unrecognized fetal loss
100	Fetal wastage
8	Perinatal loss
10	Neonatal death
562	

However, despite known associations for some spontaneous abortions, the vast majority have no identifiable medical cause.

Placenta

The placenta has three crucial functions (Kaufmann & Scheffen, 1992). The first is to provide for transfer of essential nutrients from the mother's blood to the fetus. In general, the concentrations of glucose, fats, and other nutrients are higher in maternal circulation than in the baby's blood. The placenta also provides a means of elimination of waste products from fetal blood (Mead Johnson Symposium on Perinatal and Developmental Medicine, 1981). Since the fetus has a very high metabolic rate, calories are burned quickly; waste products such as carbon dioxide are transferred across the placenta and excreted by the mother's lungs. Breakdown products of protein, such as urea, are excreted by the maternal kidneys, and bilirubin, formed from the breakdown of the red blood cell hemoglobin, is cleared by the mother's liver. The placenta is living tissue and, as such, synthesizes hormones that are important for the growth of the placenta and the fetus. In this capacity, it assumes its third role, as an endocrine organ.

All basic nutrients necessary for fetal growth must be transferred from the mother to the baby (Sibley & Boyd, 1992). These include simple sugars, proteins, fats, minerals, vitamins, and water. In the human placenta, there are initially only thin layers of cells in the connective tissue between the maternal and fetal blood circulations. As the pregnancy proceeds, the placenta increases in both weight and diameter, forming a larger surface area for transfer of nutrients to the fetus and excretion of waste products from the fetus.

On the maternal side, many factors influence the rate at which nutrients cross the placenta. The first of these is the mother's blood supply to the placenta. Diseases such as hypertension or severe diabetes may limit blood flow to the placenta, thereby decreasing fetal nutrients and potentially restricting elimination of fetal waste products. If this condition is severe enough, it may lead to spontaneous abortion. Malformations of the placenta may cause inefficient mixing of maternal blood, offering a poor gradient for nutrient release to the fetus (Benirschke & Kaufmann, 1991). Similarly, the surface area of membrane across which nutrient diffusion occurs may be limited in situations such as multiple gestation. Because the tissues between the fetus and mother have a high protein and fat content, the transfer of compounds across these membranes may be restricted by the molecular size, fat, and protein solubility and the electrical charge of their ions. Glucose has a specific transport system and some stereospecific forms of amino acids may be transferred preferentially. Deficiencies in amounts of protein, fat, and glucose transferred across the placenta result in retarded fetal growth.

Another very important placental function is the protection of the fetus from maternal rejection. Since one-half of the fetal genes are from the father, some proteins produced by the baby's cells would be recognized as tissue foreign to the mother. In situations such as heart and kidney transplantation, the foreign proteins of the transplanted organ may result in rejection of the organ by the recipient. The placenta creates a barrier that is in part physical and perhaps immunologic; this barrier minimizes the mixing of fetal and maternal blood and blocks the mother's immune response, thus allowing her to tolerate the proliferation of foreign proteins (Anderson, 1971).

Furthermore, the placenta functions as an endocrine organ during pregnancy, producing many hormones such as hCG, placental lactogen, progesterone, and estrogens (Siler-Khodr, 1992). These secretions aid in establishing the appropriate hormonal milieu for maintenance of the pregnancy. In addition, they encourage increased blood supply to the uterus and prevent the cyclic shedding of endometrium. Thus, all of these functions—nutritive, excretory, and endocrine (protective)—are vital to the developing baby.

Amniotic Fluid

The amniotic fluid surrounding the infant derives its name from the innermost layer of the membranes, the amnion. In early pregnancy, the fluid is derived primarily from this membrane, but in late gestation, the prominent sources of amniotic fluid are fetal urine and fetal pulmonary secretions. A small portion of the amniotic fluid arises from transudates across the immature fetal skin and umbilical cord (Plentl, 1966).

The amniotic fluid has numerous roles, the most important being mechanical protection of the infant against trauma (Harmon, 1993). The fluid also allows a gravity-free environment in which delicate structures such as the hands, feet, and face can grow without compression from the muscular uterus.

Circulation in the amniotic fluid has other functions. In the last trimester, the fetus may swallow as much as one pint of liquid daily (Ostergard, 1970). Because the amniotic fluid contains protein, there is an early induction of enzymes to digest protein in the fetal intestinal tract. An insufficiency of amniotic fluid may result if there are no kidneys or if the kidneys are not functioning properly in utero. This condition leads to compression of the fetus and to subsequent maldevelopment of the lungs. An excess of amniotic fluid suggests the possibility of obstruction of the fetal intestine or fetal neurologic disease, often manifested as poor sucking, as in the trisomy 21 syndrome. In addition, amniotic fluid samples may be taken to assess fetal maturity, to determine the chromosomal number and the sex of the fetus, to detect inherited metabolic abnormalities, and to assess fetal well-being.

HIGH RISK PREGNANCY

A high risk pregnancy implies jeopardy to both the mother and the fetus. If the mother has a serious health problem such as congenital heart disease, the pregnancy may be life-threatening to her. More typically, however, the term *high risk pregnancy* is used to imply some maternal problem that may result in perinatal morbidity or mortality. Approximately 15 to 20 percent of women account for over 50 percent of the fetal and neonatal deaths. For these reasons, physicians have suggested that careful attention to the needs of mothers would bring about the greatest impact on fetal and neonatal well-being (Committee on Perinatal Health, 1976).

Fetal Growth

The growth of the fetus is critically dependent on maternal nutrition before, as well as throughout, the pregnancy. Mothers with a prepregnancy weight of less than 100 pounds have more than twice as many infants of low birthweight than mothers with a prepregnancy weight of 120 pounds or greater (Eastman & Jackson, 1968). Moreover, women who lose weight or do not gain weight during pregnancy have a threefold increase in low birthweight infants, compared with those who gain 20 pounds or more during gestation. A normal weight gain generally can be accomplished by intake of approximately 300 additional calories per day (Emerson, Saxena, & Pomdexter, 1972). About one-third of the increase during pregnancy represents fetal weight; the placenta, amniotic fluid, and uterus each account for approximately 10 percent of the additional gain. An increase in fluid and blood volume of the mother contributes to another 15 percent of the increased weight; breast enlargement contributes approximately 5 percent, and the remaining 10 to 15 percent results from fats and other maternal stores held in reserve in anticipation of breastfeeding (Campbell & Gillmer, 1983).

In recent years, there have been many changes in our information concerning maternal and infant growth during pregnancy. The old concept that the fetus develops at the expense of the mother's nutrition has not proved to be valid. One study showed that when a mother's diet is magnesium deficient, the mother may show no ill effect, but the fetus usually is runted and very ill (Dancis, Springer, & Cohlan, 1971). No simple generalization can be made about all of the nutrients required by the fetus. Each nutrient seems to be handled individually, and fetal growth and welfare may be affected only minimally, if at all. Close spacing of pregnancies may deplete maternal body stores, resulting in a higher incidence of low birthweight babies in subsequent pregnancies. It is important to emphasize that the health of the fetus and mother depend, not simply on the quantity of food ingested, but also on adequate quality of the nutrients required for fetal growth.

Fetal development is assessed in many ways during pregnancy (Sparks & Cetin, 1992). The most obvious of these methods is the monitoring of progressive uterine enlargement. If uterine growth lags behind that expected by the date of the mother's last menses, fetal growth retardation due to fetal or maternal disease may be the cause. At the other end of the continuum, if the uterus is growing more rapidly than expected, excess amniotic fluid, an overgrown fetus, or multiple gestation may be responsible. The growth of the fetus can be documented readily with the use of ultrasound (Harrison, Golbus, & Filly, 1991). In this technique, sound waves allow visualization of the fetal head, and the transverse or biparietal diameter provides an estimate of fetal growth. The femur length of the fetus also can be measured as an estimate of fetal maturity. When the mother is known or suspected to be at risk for various illnesses, it is essential that monitoring be conducted routinely.

Fetal Maturity

Assessment of fetal maturity cannot be based only on estimated weight, head size, uterine size, or calculated date of delivery. X-ray examination of the fetal femur can be used as a rough estimate for fetuses older than 36 weeks gestation. Commonly, this technique has been abandoned because of potential hazards of fetal radiation. It is well recognized that the most important index of fetal maturity is the determination of the biochemical maturity of the lung (Veille, 1992). As the fetal lungs mature, an increased concentration of lecithin and other fats are shed from the fetal lung fluid via the trachea into the amniotic fluid. Sphingomyelin, another fat in the amniotic fluid, remains at a fairly constant level throughout pregnancy. Thus, the ratio of lecithin to sphingomyelin in amniotic fluid serves as an important index of fetal lung maturity. If the ratio is 2:1 or greater, the risk of premature lung disease (surfactant deficiency) is very low. This assessment of fetal lung maturity can be used to allow early appropriate delivery of an infant prior to term, if continuation of pregnancy is considered to be harmful to the mother or the fetus.

Maternal Characteristics and Conditions Affecting the Fetus

Numerous high risk maternal characteristics or conditions may lead to increased fetal mortality and neonatal morbidity or mortality. Some of these factors are social; others relate to specific anatomic variations in the mother. Some of these conditions are associated with reproductive history or medical problems, either pre-existing or acquired during the pregnancy (Creasy & Resnick, 1989). For years, there has been ample evidence that maternal age of less than 15 or greater than 40 years may result in vulnerability to the mother or newborn. Low socioeconomic groups also have a disproportionately greater number of low birthweight infants. In addition, unwed mothers frequently have severe social and emotional problems during pregnancy that may impinge on adequate nutrition and may limit obtaining prenatal care. By different mechanisms, obesity, malnutrition, and short stature of the mother may impact on fetal well-being and the ability of the mother to carry the pregnancy to term.

Physical problems are a primary concern among high risk pregnancies. Abnormalities of the maternal genital tract, such as incompetent cervix and malformation of the uterus, may prevent the pregnancy from reaching term. Mothers who have had two previous abortions, either induced or spontaneous, or those who have had a stillborn, premature, or overgrown infant are likely to repeat the experience, unless there is a determination of the etiology of the problem and appropriate intervention. Women with high blood pressure, severe renal disease, heart disease, diabetes, cancer, sickle cell disease, drug addiction or alcoholism, pulmonary disease, or various surgical problems are at great risk for pregnancy loss or may produce a premature or growth-retarded fetus (Lott, 1993). Early in pregnancy, drug exposure or transplacental infection may lead to fetal malformations. Severe anemia in the mother may result in poor fetal oxygenation and spontaneous abortion. Later, abnormal position or premature separation of the placenta may cause fetal demise or premature delivery. In addition, a prolonged gestation may result in severe fetal distress as a result of placental aging and, thus, inability of the placenta to provide appropriate nutrients and eliminate waste products. Toxemia of pregnancy, which is characterized by maternal edema, high blood pressure, and protein in the urine, threatens both fetal survival and maternal health.

The detrimental effect of maternal smoking is one of the more pressing problems of prenatal care (see Chapter 13). Multiple studies of pregnancy outcome for smoking mothers have shown a reduction in birthweight of the fetus of approximately 5 to 8 ounces, compared with the birthweights of fetuses of nonsmoking mothers. In addition, there is a 25 to 35 percent increase in perinatal mortality resulting directly from maternal cigarette smoking (Witter & King, 1980). Every effort should be made to discourage the mother from smoking before and during pregnancy. Although many factors are associated with compromised fetal growth and development, the picture is more optimistic than it may seem. Relatively few mothers are at risk for these adverse conditions or factors.

Primary Fetal Disease

Certainly, not every problem of the fetus or newborn can be attributed to poor maternal health or nutrition or adverse pregnancy factors. There are a number of significant fetal diseases (Gross & Sokol, 1989). Primary among these are conditions resulting from fetal genetic disorders (aberrant chromosomes or inherited diseases) or malformations with no known specific predisposition. More particularly, early embryonic and fetal development may be altered drastically by the presence of additional or the absence of essential genes or chromosomes.

The most common and obvious genetic abnormality is trisomy 21 (Down syndrome). Infants with this syndrome have a number of distinguishing physical and neurological features, as discussed in Chapter 11. There seems to be an increased incidence of neonates with Down syndrome born to mothers with advanced maternal age (older than 35 years), but no specific factor for this association has been identified (Dickerman & Park, 1991).

Other diseases with a specific genetic inheritance such as phenylketonuria (PKU) or galactosemia usually are not immediately evident in the newborn. With such disorders, damage to the central nervous system, which ultimately leads to mental retardation, arises from abnormal metabolism and the inability to clear toxic products from the body. Prior to birth, the placenta provides an efficient mechanism for clearing these materials. After delivery, however, the toxic chemicals begin to accumulate and, in the instance of phenylketonuria, can cause severe developmental delays in the absence of intervention and dietary control.

Finally, infants may have malformations leading to their demise that have either no genetic basis or a variable origin. These include intestinal anomalies, defects of the abdominal wall, and deformities of the lungs. Other malformations such as cleft palate may have a primary genetic disposition with increased expression due to environmental factors.

In conclusion, it is clear that all reasonable social and medical efforts need to be directed toward the prevention of these conditions. Through specific attention to these problems that affect the mother and child, it may be possible by the 21st century to reduce the current morbidity statistics by 25 to 30 percent. Such preventive efforts will require the coordination of many disciplines in health care settings, schools, and the home, in order to educate and monitor potential parents before conception and throughout gestation.

BIBLIOGRAPHY

Ad Hoc Committee on the Effect of Trace Anesthetics on the Health of Operating Room Personnel. (1974). *Anesthesiology, 41*, 321–340.

Anderson, J.M. (1971). Transplantation—Nature's success. *Lancet, 2*, 1077–1082.

Benirschke, K. (1992). Multiple pregnancy. In R.A. Polin & W.W. Fox (Eds.), *Fetal and neonatal physiology* (Vol. 1, pp. 97–106). Philadelphia: W.B. Saunders.

Benirschke, K., & Kaufmann, P. (1991). *The pathology of the human placenta* (2nd ed.). New York: Springer.

Campbell, D., & Gillmer, S. (1983). *Nutrition in pregnancy.* New York: Perinatal Press.

Coleridge, S.T. (1968). In M.B. Strauss (Ed.), *Familiar medical quotations* (p. 179). Boston: Little, Brown & Co.

Committee on Perinatal Health. (1976). *Toward improving the outcome of pregnancy: Recommendations for the regional development of maternal and perinatal health services.* White Plains, NY: National Foundation—March of Dimes.

Creasy, R., & Resnick, R. (1989). *Maternal-fetal medicine: Principles and practice* (2nd ed.). Philadelphia: W.B. Saunders.

Dancis, J., Springer, D., & Cohlan, S.Q. (1971). Fetal homeostatis in maternal malnutrition: II. Magnesium deprivation. *Pediatric Research, 5*, 131–136.

Dickerman, L.H., & Park, V.M. (1991). Cytogenetic and molecular aspects of genetic disease and prenatal diagnosis. In A.A. Fanaroff & R.J. Martin (Eds.), *Neonatal-perinatal medicine: Diseases of the fetus and infant* (5th ed.) (Vol. 1, pp. 57–79). St Louis: C.V. Mosby.

Eastman, N.J., & Jackson, E. (1968). Weight relationships in pregnancy. *Obstetrical and Gynecological Survey, 23*, 1003–1025.

Emerson, J.K., Saxena, B., & Pomdexter, E.L. (1972). Caloric cost of normal pregnancy. *Obstetrics and Gynecology, 40*, 786–794.

Gilbert, E., & Harmon, J. (1993). *High risk pregnancy and delivery* (2nd ed.). St. Louis: C.V. Mosby.

Gross, T.J., & Sokol, R.J. (1989). *Intrauterine growth retardation: A practical approach*. Chicago: Year Book Medical.

Harmon, J. (1993). High-risk pregnancy. In C. Kenner, A. Brueggeyemer, & L.P. Gunderson (Eds.), *Comprehensive neonatal nursing* (pp. 157–170). Philadelphia: W.B. Saunders.

Harrison, M.R., Golbus, M.S., & Filly, R.A. (1991). *The unborn patient: Prenatal diagnosis and treatment* (2nd ed.). Philadelphia: W.B. Saunders.

Joffe, J.M. (1979). Influence of drug exposure of the father on perinatal outcome. *Clinics in Perinatology, 6*, 21–36.

Kaufmann, P., & Scheffen, I. (1992). Placental development. In R.A. Polin & W.W. Fox (Eds.), *Fetal and neonatal physiology* (Vol. 1, pp. 47–56). Philadelphia: W.B. Saunders.

Kerr, M.G. (1976). Chromosome studies of spontaneous abortions. In J.J. Kellar (Ed.), *Modern trends in obstetrics and gynecology* (pp. 114–136). London: Butterworth.

Kurczynski, T.W. (1992). Congenital malformations. In A.A. Fanaroff & R.J. Martin (Eds.), *Neonatal-perinatal medicine: Diseases of the fetus and infant* (5th ed.) (Vol. 1, pp. 372–398). St. Louis: C.V. Mosby.

Lott, J.W. (1993). Fetal development: Environmental influences and critical periods. In C. Kenner, A. Brueggemeyer, & L.P. Gunderson (Eds.), *Comprehensive neonatal nursing* (pp. 133–156). Philadelphia: W.B. Saunders.

Mead Johnson Symposium on Perinatal and Developmental Medicine. (1981). *Placental Transport, 18*, 3–34.

Ostergard, D.R. (1970). The physiology and clinical importance of amniotic fluid: A review. *Obstetrical and Gynecological Survey, 25*, 297–319.

Plentl, A.A. (1966). Formation and circulation of amniotic fluid. *Clinical Obstetrics and Gynecology, 9*, 427–439.

Schardlein, J.L. (1985). *Chemically induced birth defects*. New York: Marcel Dekker.

Scholl, T.O. (1990). Weight gain during pregnancy in adolescence: Predictive ability of early weight gain. *Obstetrics and Gynecology, 75*, 948–952.

Sibley, C.P., & Boyd, R.D. (1992). Mechanisms of transfer across the human placenta. In R.A. Polin & W.W. Fox (Eds.), *Fetal and neonatal physiology* (Vol. 1, pp. 62–73). Philadelphia: W.B. Saunders.

Siler-Khodr, T.M. (1992). Endocrine and paracrine function of the human placenta. In R. A. Polin & W.W. Fox (Eds.), *Fetal and neonatal physiology* (Vol. 1, pp. 74–86). Philadelphia: W.B. Saunders.

Simpson, J.L. (1980). *Suboptimal outcome of pregnancy*. New York: March of Dimes Birth Defects Conference.

Soyka, L.F., & Joffe, J.M. (1980). Male mediated drug effects on offspring. In R.H. Schwarz & S.J. Yaffe (Eds.), *Progress in clinical and biological research: Drugs and chemical risks to the fetus and newborn* (pp. 49–66). New York: Allan R. Liss.

Sparks, J.W., & Cetin, I. (1992). Intrauterine growth and nutrition. In R.A. Polin & W.W. Fox (Eds.), *Fetal and neonatal physiology* (Vol. 1, pp. 179–197). Philadelphia: W.B. Saunders.

Veille, J.-C. (1992). Obstetric management of prematurity. In A.A. Fanaroff & R.J. Martin (Eds.), *Neonatal-perinatal medicine: Diseases of the fetus and infant* (5th ed.) (Vol. 1, pp. 205–220). St. Louis: C.V. Mosby.

Witter, F., & King, T.M. (1980). Cigarettes and pregnancy. In R.H. Schwarz & S.J. Yaffe (Eds.), *Progress in clinical and biological research: Drugs and chemical risks to the fetus and newborn* (pp. 83–92). New York: Allan R. Liss.

Chapter 3

Perinatal Events

While many high risk characteristics can be identified among pregnant women before labor begins, most adverse perinatal factors arise *intrapartum* without warning. Through careful monitoring of the fetus, perinatologists are attempting to identify some of these unforeseen problems in order to improve management of pregnancy and, therefore, medical and developmental outcome. This chapter deals with the events surrounding labor and delivery and the subsequent problems that may ensue for high risk infants as a result of complications during those processes.

LABOR AND DELIVERY

Labor is defined as the onset of regular uterine contractions (Creasy & Resnick, 1989; Friedman, 1981; Pritchard & MacDonald, 1985). At the least, it is a complex process; the physiologic and hormonal developments still are not fully understood. Furthermore, although we do not have information about all of the changes that finally initiate this sequence of events, sufficient technology is available to enhance or inhibit the process by the use of oxytocin or tocolytic agents, respectively (Hemminki & Starfield, 1978).

The initial stage of labor is called the *latent phase* because little of consequence seems to be happening. Subclinically, however, uterine contractions are becoming more coordinated and organized. The cervix has not yet begun to dilate, but its consistency changes in preparation for dilation and fetal descent. The latent phase for a first pregnancy averages approximately 6.5 hours and only rarely exceeds 20 hours. In the second or subsequent pregnancies, the average time of the latent phase is 4.8 hours and seldom exceeds 14 hours (Creasy & Resnick, 1989).

The *active phase* of labor starts when the cervix begins to dilate. This process takes place at 1.2 to 1.5 centimeters per hour and usually is completed at 9 to 10 centimeters within a 6-hour period. As the cervix expands, it also thins and retracts and fetal descent begins. This course reaches its maximum rate once the cervix is fully dilated and can be traced by examining the relationship of the leading edge of the fetus (usually the head) to the bony prominences on the maternal pelvis, called the *ischial spines*. Descent of the fetus is more rapid in the *multiparous* than in the *primiparous* (first delivery) mother, but in either case, it should exceed 1 to 2 centimeters per hour (Friedman, 1981; Pritchard & MacDonald, 1985).

Effect of Labor on the Fetus

The mechanical energy of the contracting uterus during labor constitutes a significant stress to the fetus. Prior to the rupture of the membranes, the amniotic fluid provides a cushion that helps to distribute the intrauterine pressure quite evenly across the fetus. In the second stage of labor, intrauterine pressure increases to approximately 5 to 8 times that in the resting phase. If the mother "bears down," pressure may rise to 12 to 15 times that in the quiet state (Sureau, 1974).

There is, of course, considerable variation from mother to mother regarding the intensity, frequency, and duration of uterine contractions. Once the membranes have been ruptured and the amniotic fluid escapes, however, the fetus typically orients in preparation for delivery. The fetal body part then nearest the cervix begins to descend into the maternal pelvis and is said to be *engaged*. In 90 percent of pregnancies, the head is the presenting body part. A *breech presentation* occurs if the buttocks or feet are engaged first. In either case, with the cushion of amniotic fluid lost, the greatest pressure then is exerted on the presenting part, which is located in the narrowest portion of the uterus, at its outlet toward the cervix (Lindgren, 1972). At this point in the delivery, problems may arise. In some newborns, especially the preterm baby (see Figures 3-1 and 3-2), pressure is transmitted to the skull and may be responsible for intracranial hemorrhage. Compression of the infant's head by uterine contractions also may result in a transient lowering

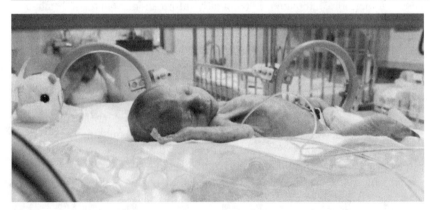

Figure 3–1 Very low birthweight infant (one of twins), born at 820 grams

of the fetal heart rate. This response does not seem to be deleterious if the duration is short and if there is a prompt return to normal heart rate once the contraction has ceased (Schifrin, 1982).

In addition to the changes described, uterine contractions also place pressure on the placenta and interfere with placental blood flow. This situation is important to the fetus since nutrients and waste products must be exchanged through the placenta. Thus, the oxygen content of the fetal blood is lower during labor and the content of carbon dioxide, a waste product, is higher. Because oxygen is crucial for normal tissue metabolism, and carbon dioxide interferes with metabolic processes (partly by lowering the blood pH), a prolonged labor can lead to severe metabolic stress for the infant (Sureau, 1974).

The trauma of labor for the fetus is difficult to quantitate. In general, the healthy newborn can tolerate this unavoidable stress. Consequently, the goal of modern obstetrics is identification of those fetuses with reduced tolerance, such as the preterm infant, who should be monitored carefully to avoid serious complications.

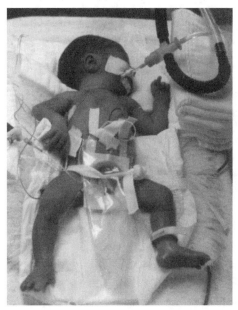

Figure 3–2 Steven at 28 weeks on ventilator in neonatal intensive care unit

Fetal Monitoring

As we have mentioned, the general health and development of the fetus is evaluated throughout pregnancy by measuring the progress of uterine growth (Tropper & Fox, 1982). While many maternal illnesses (e.g., diabetes or toxemia of pregnancy) may result in chronic fetal distress, unplanned events just prior to or during labor in otherwise healthy mothers can lead to acute fetal distress. These conditions include premature separation of the placenta (placental abruption), compression or prolapse of the umbilical cord through the cervix, or the acute onset of maternal illness such as pneumonia, which may impair maternal and thus fetal blood oxygenation. In each case, the well-being of the fetus is assessed during labor to determine whether the condition of an infant will warrant transfer to an intensive care nursery. Understandably, the decision to "rescue" the fetus from an adverse intrauterine environment becomes very difficult when the fetus is more than 10 weeks premature and the outcome is more tenuous (Polin & Franipane, 1986).

Obviously, the fetus cannot be monitored through direct access during labor. Its well-being must be ascertained indirectly by several techniques. The fetal heart rate pattern can be measured by an external monitor, or, once the membranes have been ruptured, a fetal scalp electrode can be used. Researchers using such methods have described several patterns of fetal heart rate abnormalities. In general, if the fetal heart rate slows and quickens in response to various stresses, there is assurance that the fetus is not compromised. On the other hand, fetal *tachycardia* (rapid heart rate) or *bradycardia* (low heart rate) indicates severe distress, requiring immediate intervention on behalf of the newborn (Hon & Koh, 1981).

In response to severe intrauterine stress, infants older than 34 weeks gestation may pass meconium (the contents of the fetal bowel) into the amniotic fluid (Holtzman, Banzhaf, Silver, & Hagerman, 1989; Kresch, Brion, & Fleischman, 1991). This material is sterile, viscous, and dark green, and contains many proteins as well as cellular debris from the developing fetal gastrointestinal tract. The release of meconium should prompt careful evaluation of fetal well-being even if the heart rate has been considered normal. Another method of monitoring the fetus once the membranes have been ruptured is to sample the fetal blood, usually from the scalp of the engaged head. The blood pH is measured to determine whether the newborn is compensating metabolically for the stress of labor (Miller, 1982). These strategies will not resolve all of the problems that may arise during labor and delivery. They do, however, offer guidelines for the modern obstetrician to use in pursuit of the best possible outcome for mother and child.

Birth Trauma

Just as labor is stressful, vaginal delivery is traumatic to nearly every baby (Mangurten, 1992). Virtually every healthy newborn will have molding of the head, commonly with edema of the scalp. Newborns also may acquire cephalhematomas, caused by bleeding under the outer surface of the bones of the lateral skull that have been scraped across the pelvic ischial spines. Cephalohematomas usually enlarge within several days after birth as additional fluid is drawn into the area in response to breakdown of the red blood cells. They then resolve slowly by calcifying around the outer edges until a firm mass is formed. As the infant's head grows during the first year, the skull remolds and the lump on the side of the head becomes less obvious and finally resolves (Brann & Schwartz, 1987).

Other injuries to the head are possible as a result of delivery; they include paralysis of the seventh cranial nerve, which is the *facial nerve*. This nerve may be damaged by pressure, especially with the application of forceps near the point where the nerve emerges from the skull at the edge where the jaw articulates with the skull. Such trauma frequently leads to paralysis of the involved muscles. Clinically, when the infant cries, the mouth is drawn to the normal side, and there tends to be drooping and loss of wrinkles on the affected side. The child also may have difficulty closing the eyelid on the affected side. The majority of facial palsies begin to diminish spontaneously within several days, but total recovery may require several weeks to months (Manning & Adour, 1972).

Any prominence from the head may be traumatized during delivery. The eyes and eyelids may become edematous with bruising; there may be hemorrhage in the sclera of the eye, and corneal abrasions can occur. In addition, the ears are prone to abrasions, hematomas, and occasional lacerations, which require cleansing and suture. The majority of these insults clear over the first several weeks with little residual effect.

Most serious are injuries that tend to occur in the area of the neck. For example, the lateral neck swelling seen in newborns may result from bleeding into the belly of the sternocleidomastoid muscle (Sanerkin & Edwards, 1966), which connects the sternum and the clavicle (cleido-) to the mastoid area of the skull. Contraction of this muscle allows for turning of the head. A hematoma in the muscle, as it resolves, frequently causes scarring and foreshortening of the muscle, leading to torticollis (stiffening of the neck). If this condition is not recognized early and appropriate physical therapy initiated, it becomes a severe problem.

The nerves of the neck are especially susceptible to impairment (Mangurten, 1992). The *brachial plexus* includes the nerves that extend from the neck to innervate the arm. *Erb's palsy* (paralysis of shoulder and upper arm) results from injury to the fifth and sixth cervical nerve roots. *Klumpke's paralysis* (paralysis of lower arm) results from injury to the eighth cervical and the first thoracic nerve roots (Eng, Koch, & Smokvina, 1978).

Such paralysis usually follows a prolonged and very difficult labor. Commonly, the infant is large and has had severe fetal distress, and the increased pressure applied to the head and shoulders to assist delivery may result in trauma. The principal treatment for these conditions is the maintenance of an appropriate range of motion for the affected joints. Treatment consists of partial immobilization, followed by an active physical therapy program by 7 to 10 days of age. If the nerve roots are intact, function may return within several days, as local edema and hemorrhage resolve. Although the rate of recovery varies with the degree of injury, most infants return to normal function within 3 to 6 months. Occasionally, however, an infant with severe injury may show continued improvement over a period of several years. In particular, paralysis of the lower arm has a poor prognosis, with the possibility that a claw deformity of the hand will develop (Behrman & Mangurten, 1977).

Several other nerves in the neck may be affected similarly. The *phrenic nerve*, which innervates the diaphragm, may be disrupted, resulting in a paralyzed diaphragm and asynchronous respiration. In addition, there may be trauma to the *recurrent laryngeal nerve*, leading to unilateral vocal cord paralysis, which is often associated with respiratory distress.

Other potential birth injuries include a fractured clavicle or extremity; rupture of the liver or spleen; hemorrhage into the adrenal gland; and, in a breech presentation, trauma to the genitalia. The prognosis in each of these events varies considerably. Fortunately, however, most of these conditions are treatable, with good return of function in a relatively short time. Whenever a form of birth trauma has been identified, it is important to examine the infant carefully for other injuries.

EVALUATION, STABILIZATION, AND TRANSITION

Apgar Score

Before 1953, there were no objective assessments at birth for the condition of the newborn. Subsequently, Virginia Apgar, an anesthesiologist, proposed a scoring system to rate five characteristics of the infant that were thought to correlate with recovery from intrauterine stress (Apgar, 1953). The five parameters are *heart rate, respiratory effort, muscle tone, reflex irritability,* and *color.* Each of these variables is scored on a scale of 0 to 2. A 0 is given for the complete absence of a response; for instance, no heart rate, no respiratory effort, and blue color (cyanosis). A 2 is given for the best response, such as a heart rate of greater than 100 beats per minute, a regular respiratory effort, and a totally pink color. These scores are assigned at 1 and 5 minutes.

Although there has been considerable debate about interpretation, many physicians agree that the 1-minute Apgar score is a relatively accurate reflection of the severity of intrauterine distress and is an indication of how well the infant has responded. The 5-minute Apgar score is thought to be more predictive of morbidity and mortality (Drage, Kennedy, & Schwarz, 1964). Over the last 30 years, some authors have attempted to modify the original evaluations by weighting the parameters that seem to be more important (i.e., heart rate and respiratory effort). By and large, those more precise evaluations are being used as research tools, rather than as aids to clinical practice.

There are serious difficulties with use of the Apgar score as a prediction of outcome. Many infants who are born with distress may not be evaluated accurately in the hectic activity of the resuscitation effort. Also, it is a common belief among obstetricians that pediatricians tend to give lower 1-minute and higher 5-minute Apgar scores than do obstetricians. Despite the simplicity of the measure, the Apgar score has been very helpful in offering a general description of the state of the newborn (Catlin et al., 1986). Yet, it is essential to remember that this score in no way replaces an accurate recording of the sequence of resuscitation and the timeliness of the infant's response, in order to assess accurately the degree of intrauterine asphyxia.

Resuscitation

Resuscitation is the process of stabilizing an individual in an acutely weakened condition that is life-threatening—in this instance, the neonate. The process has three phases, including the anticipation of problems, proper recognition, and appropriate treatment (American Academy of Pediatrics, 1992; Lamb & Rosner, 1987). As mentioned in Chapter 2, there are multiple prenatal and perinatal factors that may place an infant at risk (Ringer & Stark, 1989).

Approximately 90 percent of the newborns who have low Apgar scores could be predicted to have low scores prior to birth. In these situations, an appropriate resuscitation team should be available to address the specific needs of the baby. At birth, the neonate is very wet and loses heat rapidly. Therefore, the child needs to be quickly dried and placed under a radiant form of heat. The newborn should be stimulated to cry, not by hanging the infant by the ankles and slapping the buttocks, but by a gentle flicking of the feet or stimulation to the chest. A stethoscope should be used to assure that there is an adequate heart rate and respiratory effort. If there is a good respiratory effort with a heart rate greater than 100 beats per minute, a simple clearing of the airway with a bulb syringe to remove mucus generally is all that is necessary. On the other hand, if the respiratory effort is compromised, the child may require oxygen, occasionally including manual ventilation with a mask over the face. In the event that this attempt is unsuccessful, the infant may need intubation and manual ventilation via the trachea. If the heart rate begins to fall, cardiac massage often is necessary. The relatively few newborns who do not respond to this combination of efforts may show improvement with the addition of medications.

Some newborns have a low blood pressure and may respond to expansion of the blood volume with protein, blood, or a salt solution. Following this treatment, correction of the low blood pH with sodium bicarbonate, as long as respiration is being supported, may be beneficial. Additionally, a cardiac stimulant such as epinephrine (adrenaline) may be useful.

After resuscitation of a newborn who has suffered birth asphyxia, many biochemical alterations may occur. These changes may include continued acidosis (disturbance in the acid balance of the body), which needs correction. Because this is a very stressful period, available calories may have been consumed, and these infants thus are prone to *hypoglycemia* (deficiency of sugar in the blood). Potassium loss from cells may be excessive, with the blood calcium becoming inappropriately low 24 to 48 hours after birth.

Other sequelae of asphyxia that must be anticipated include the following:

- pulmonary problems, such as more severe respiratory distress, pulmonary hemorrhage, and acquired surfactant deficiency
- cardiovascular difficulties, such as congestive heart failure, and enlarged heart

- renal disorders such as blood or protein in the urine and failure to produce urine
- central nervous system problems, as evidenced by cerebral edema, hemorrhage, seizures, irritability, or tremulousness
- gastrointestinal conditions, such as poor intestinal motility, hemorrhage, and ulcers.

All of these consequences should be anticipated and recognized in a timely fashion so that prompt treatment can be given to ensure minimum future compromise.

Temperature Control

Prior to birth, the temperature of the fetus always is slightly more than 1°F greater than that of the mother. Heat in the fetus is a waste product and results from a metabolic rate that is very high in comparison with the mother's. Heat is transferred across the placenta to the mother and dissipated. This occurrence may explain why many women in their third trimester are very flushed. At the time of birth, there is an abrupt temperature decrease in the newborn as a result of evaporative heat loss. This temperature decrease is one of several mechanisms thought to be responsible for the initiation of respiration. Thus, infants who are placed in a warm water bath at birth may stop breathing and have a reduction in heart rate as a consequence of poor blood oxygenation.

In intensive care nurseries, temperature control is one of the most important therapies carried out by the medical and nursing staff. The goal is maintenance of newborns in their *neutral thermal environment,* which is defined as the point at which body temperature is normal and the baby is using the least amount of oxygen (oxygen consumption), thus reflecting a low, conservative caloric consumption (Brück, 1992).

There are two levels or types of heat loss. The *internal gradient* is a term used to describe how neonates fail to conserve heat. Babies who are premature or growth retarded have little subcutaneous fat as insulation, and internally generated heat is readily lost to the skin. These infants frequently have a large ratio of surface area to body mass and are less able to conserve heat (Brueggemeyer, 1990). The *external gradient* refers to the process whereby heat is dissipated from the skin surface. Radiant heat loss, which is the most common form for humans, refers to heat energy that escapes directly into the environment; e.g., the sun radiating heat over long distances. Evaporative heat loss is the amount of heat required to vaporize a specific amount of water. Generally, this factor is important for neonates primarily in the delivery room. Convective heat loss is the equivalent of a windchill factor; infants in a draft or those exposed to excessive manipulation are less able to maintain the unstirred layer of warm air close to the skin. Conductive loss refers to heat transferred from one solid body to another; e.g., from a baby to a cold blanket or cold stethoscope (LeBlanc, 1992).

All of these forms of heat loss are addressed in some way in an intensive care nursery (Perlstein, 1992). Two primary pieces of equipment are used—the radiant warmer and the incubator. The radiant warmer (see Figure 3–3) provides compensating radiant heat to maintain body temperature. This treatment is used more frequently with very ill neonates, who require ready access to therapeutic devices. The primary hazard of the radiant warmer is excessive fluid loss, frequently 50 percent greater than that of infants placed in an incubator (Williams & Oh, 1974).

The second device used to prevent heat loss is an incubator (see Figure 3–4). In the incubator, blankets, walls, and equipment are warmed to near the body temperature of the infant. Convective heat loss is minimized because the infant is shielded from drafts, and radiant heat loss is diminished because the inner surface of the incubator is warmed. As a consequence, the first gradient of radiant heat loss from the baby to the inner surface of the incubator reduces the neonate's heat loss.

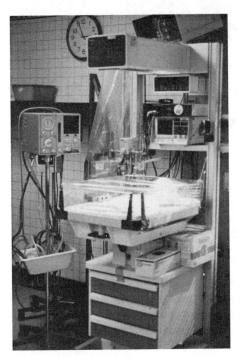

Figure 3–3 Radiant warmer

Failure to maintain a proper thermal environment may be fatal to the newborn. Studies published as late as 1964 reveal a 50 percent or greater increase in mortality in infants nursed at room temperature versus those fed in a warmed environment (Buetow & Klein, 1964; Day, Caliguiri, Kamenski, & Ehrlich, 1964). In addition, it is well known that children with respiratory distress frequently require additional oxygen because their rate of caloric expenditure is higher. Calories (from carbohydrate, fat, and protein) that have been used excessively to maintain body temperature, are therefore not available for tissue repair and growth. Such babies require longer stays in intensive care nurseries.

Physiology and Behavior during Transition

Transition from intrauterine to extrauterine existence is one of the most traumatic periods experienced in our lives. The baby is cut loose from his or her life support system and must make a very rapid transference to air breathing, which

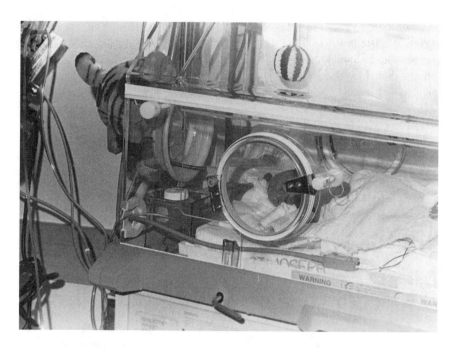

Figure 3–4 Incubator

requires major changes in the circulatory system. Virtually every body system now must adapt to this hostile environment. The lungs, which have been filled with fluid, must expel or absorb the fluid to allow adequate exchange of oxygen and carbon dioxide. The central nervous system now must deal with stimuli that have not been present or were muted within the uterus, including touch, smell, taste, vision, and hearing. The kidneys begin to concentrate and dilute the body's waste products in order to excrete them. The gastrointestinal system must digest food properly to provide appropriate nutrition for the baby, who is in a very rapid growth phase.

One of the most profound of these changes is the rapid transition of the circulatory system. Prior to birth, less than 5 percent of the blood pumped by the heart enters the lungs. Blood returning from the placenta has sufficient oxygen for fetal needs. As it enters the right side of the heart, this blood either may cross directly to the left side and travel to the body, or may be pumped by the right muscle chamber (ventricle) out toward the lungs. Most of this blood bypasses the lung through a vessel called the patent ductus arteriosus, connecting the pulmonary and systemic circulations. At birth, the lungs expand rapidly and blood flow must match the lung expansion if the baby is to survive. Resistance in the lung blood vessels drops precipitously over the first 24 to 48 hours, and thus there may be backflow of small amounts of blood from the systemic circulation toward the pulmonary circulation, which now has lower pressure. An increase in the blood oxygen level typically leads to contraction of muscles in the wall of the patent ductus arteriosus and histologic obliteration of this vessel, within 1 week after birth. However, in many preterm infants, this vessel does not close, and heart failure may result.

During the transition from intrauterine to extrauterine existence, there are three phases of newborn behavior. On delivery, if the infant is vigorous and reactive to the experience of being born, a characteristic series of changes in vital signs and clinical appearance take place. These include a first period of reactivity, a relatively unresponsive interval, and a second period of reactivity (see Table 3–1). The first reactive phase begins at birth or shortly thereafter and may last as long as 6 hours. The neonate is alert and exploratory, and responds quickly to various stimuli. The second phase is a sleep state, which may last from 3 to 6 hours. A second reactive phase follows, by which time the healthy infant has established

Table 3–1 Transitional Period Behavior of Newborn

	First Period of Reactivity (alerting, exploratory behavior)	Unresponsive Interval (sleep phase)	Second Period of Reactivity
Age	Birth to 1 hour	2–3 hours	3–4 hours
Color	Transient cyanosis, flushing	Pink	Swift color changes
Heart Rate	Tachycardia (180 beats per minute) decreasing over 15 minutes to 140 beats per minute	Slow 100–120 beats per minute	Wide swings in heart rate
Respiration	Flaring, grunting, retracting common in first 15 minutes, then rapid	Shallow, regular	Irregular brief apneic pauses
Activity	Intense activity—eyes open, sucking, spontaneous reflexes	Occasional brief startle during sleep	Variable
Tone	Increased tone, especially in upper extremities	Relaxed	Variable
Bowel	Sounds heard after 15 minutes	Frequent visible peristalsis	Frequent meconium passage

Sources: From "The Relation of Maternal Disease to Fetal and Neonatal Morbidity and Mortality" by M. Desmond et al., 1961, *Pediatric Clinics of North America*, 8, pp. 421-440. Copyright 1961 by W.B. Saunders Company; "The Clinical Behavior of the Newly Born: The Term Baby" by M. Desmond et al., 1963, *Journal of Pediatrics*, 62, pp. 307-325. Copyright 1963 by The C.V. Mosby Company; "The Transitional Care Nursery: A Mechanism for Preventive Medicine in the Newborn" by M. Desmond et al., 1966, *Pediatric Clinics of North America,* 13, pp. 651-668. Copyright 1966 by W.B. Saunders Company.

good control of respiration and circulation (Desmond, Franklin, Blattner, & Hill, 1961; Desmond et al., 1963).

During the first period of reactivity, changes

> ... include tachycardia, rapid respiration, transient rales, grunting, flaring and retractions, a falling body temperature, hypertonus and alerting exploratory behavior. . . . Bowel sounds become evident during the first 15 minutes, and oral mucus may be visible.

> After the first period of reactivity, heart and respiratory rates decline while diffuse motor activity reaches a peak and then diminishes. General responsiveness declines and the infant sleeps. After sleep, the infant enters a second period of reactivity. Oral mucus may again become evident, the infant becomes more responsive to exogenous and endogenous stimuli, and heart rates become labile. The bowel is cleared of meconium. In some infants the secondary reactivity period results in waves of heightened autonomic activity. Wide swings in heart rate (bradycardia to tachycardia) occur along with the passage of meconium stools, the handling of mucus, vasomotor instability, and irregular respiration with apneic pauses. (Desmond, Rudolph, & Phitaksphraiwan, 1966, pp. 655–656)

Not surprisingly, there is marked variability in the behavior of newborns during transition. Failure to respond in accordance with the described patterns does not suggest that the infant is brain damaged or even temporarily compromised. Labor and delivery pose an especially stressful time for the infant. In most cases, however, the anticipation of potential problems and their correction lead to a smooth transition of the fetus from intrauterine existence to existence in the hostile outer world.

BIBLIOGRAPHY

American Academy of Pediatrics, IN. (1992). *Neonatal resuscitation program.* Evansville.

Apgar, V.A. (1953). A proposal for a new method of evaluation of the newborn infant. *Anesthesia and Analgesia, 32,* 260–267.

Behrman, R.E., & Mangurten, H.H. (1977). Birth injuries in neonatal-perinatal medicine. In R.E. Behrman (Ed.), *Neonatal-perinatal medicine* (pp. 70–94). St. Louis: C.V. Mosby.

Brann, A.W., & Schwartz, J.F. (1987). Central nervous system disturbances. In A.A. Fanaroff & R.J. Martin (Eds.), *Neonatal-perinatal medicine: Diseases of the fetus and infant* (4th ed.) (pp. 495–553). St. Louis: C.V. Mosby.

Brück, K. (1992). Neonatal thermal regulation. In R.A. Polin & W.W. Fox (Eds.), *Fetal and neonatal physiology* (Vol. 1, pp. 488–515). Philadelphia: W.B. Saunders.

Brueggemeyer, A. (1990). Thermoregulation. In L.P. Gunderson & C. Kenner (Eds.), *Care of the 24–25 week gestational age infant: Small baby protocol* (pp. 23–38). Petaluma, CA: Neonatal Network.

Buetow, K.C., & Klein, S.W. (1964). Effect of maintenance of "normal" skin temperature on survival of infants of low birthweight. *Pediatrics, 34,* 163–170.

Catlin, E.A., Carpenter, M.W., Brann, B.S., Mayfield, S.R., Shaul, P.W., Goldstein, M., & Oh, W. (1986). The Apgar score revisited: Influences of gestational age. *Journal of Pediatrics, 109*(5), 865–868.

Creasy, R.K., & Resnik, R. (1989). *Maternal-fetal medicine: Principles and practice* (2nd ed.). Philadelphia: W.B. Saunders.

Day, R.L., Caliguiri, L., Kamenski, C., & Ehrlich, F. (1964). Body temperature and survival of premature infants. *Pediatrics, 34,* 171–181.

Desmond, M.M., Franklin, R.R., Blattner, R.J., & Hill, R.M. (1961). The relation of maternal disease to fetal and neonatal morbidity and mortality. *Pediatric Clinics of North America, 8,* 421–440.

Desmond, M.M., Franklin, R.R., Vallbona, C., Hill, R.M., Plumb, R., Arnold, H., & Watts, J. (1963). The clinical behavior of the newly born: The term baby: I. *Journal of Pediatrics, 62,* 307–325.

Desmond, M.M., Rudolph, A.J., & Phitaksphraiwan, P. (1966). The transitional care nursery: A mechanism for preventive medicine in the newborn. *Pediatric Clinics of North America, 13,* 651–668.

Drage, J.S., Kennedy, C., & Schwarz, R.K. (1964). The Apgar score as an index of neonatal mortality. *Obstetrics and Gynecology, 24,* 222–230.

Eng, G.D., Koch, B., & Smokvina, M.D. (1978). Brachial plexus palsy in neonates and children. *Archives of Physical Medicine and Rehabilitation, 59,* 458–464.

Friedman, E.A. (1981). The labor curve. *Clinics in Perinatology, 8,* 15–25.

Hemminki, E., & Starfield, B. (1978). Prevention and treatment of premature labour by drugs: Review of controlled clinical trials. *British Journal of Obstetrics and Gynaecology, 85,* 411–417.

Holtzman, R.B., Banzhaf, W.C., Silver, R.K., & Hagerman, J.R. (1989). Perinatal management of meconium staining of the amniotic fluid. *Clinics in Perinatology, 16*(4), 825–838.

Hon, E.H., & Koh, K.S. (1981). Management of labor and delivery in neonatology. In G.B. Avery (Ed.), *Neonatology: Pathophysiology and management of the newborn* (2nd ed.) (pp. 120–131). Philadelphia: J.B. Lippincott.

Kresch, M.J., Brion, L.P., & Fleischman, A.R. (1991). Delivery room management of meconium-stained neonates. *Journal of Perinatology, 11*(1), 46–48.

Lamb, F.S., & Rosner, M.S. (1987). Neonatal resuscitation. *Emergency Medicine Clinics of North America, 5*(3), 541–557.

LeBlanc, M. (1992). Neonatal heat transfer. In R.A. Polin & W.W. Fox (Eds.), *Fetal and neonatal physiology* (Vol. 1) (pp. 483–488). Philadelphia: W.B. Saunders.

Lindgren, L. (1972). The engagement of the foetal head in the uterus when the vertex presents. *Acta Obstetrica and Gynecology Scandinavia, 51,* 37–45.

Mangurten, H.H. (1992). Birth injuries. In A.A. Fanaroff & R.J. Martin (Eds.), *Neonatal-perinatal Medicine: Diseases of the fetus and infant* (5th ed.) (Vol. 1) (pp. 346–371). St. Louis: C.V. Mosby.

Manning, J., & Adour, K. (1972). Facial paralysis in children. *Pediatrics, 49,* 102–109.

Miller, F.C. (1982). Prediction of acid-base values from intrapartum fetal heart rate data and their correlation with scalp and funic values. *Clinics in Perinatology, 9,* 353–361.

Perlstein, P. H. (1992). Physical environment. In A.A. Fanaroff & R.J. Martin (Eds.), *Neonatal-perinatal medicine: Diseases of the fetus and infant* (5th ed.) (Vol. 1) (pp. 401–419). St. Louis: C.V. Mosby.

Polin, J. I., & Franipane, W. L. (1986). Current concepts in management of obstetric problems for pediatricians. *Pediatric Clinics of North America, 33*(3), 621–646.

Pritchard, J.A., & MacDonald, P.C. (1985). The physiology of labor. In J.A. Pritchard & P.C. MacDonald (Eds.), *Williams obstetrics* (pp. 295–321). Norwalk, CT: Appleton-Century-Crofts.

Ringer, S.A., & Stark, A.R. (1989). Management of neonatal emergencies in the delivery room. *Clinics in Perinatology, 16*, 23–41.

Sanerkin, N.G., & Edwards, P. (1966). Birth injury to the sternocleidomastoid muscle. *Journal of Bone and Joint Surgery, 48B*, 441–447.

Schifrin, B.S. (1982). The fetal monitoring polemic. *Clinics in Perinatology, 9*, 399–408.

Sureau, C. (1974). The stress of labor. In S. Aladjem & A. Brown (Eds.), *Clinical perinatology* (pp. 291–335). St. Louis: C.V. Mosby.

Tropper, P.J., & Fox, H.E. (1982). Evaluation of antepartum fetal well-being by measuring growth. *Clinics in Perinatology, 9*, 271–284.

Williams, P.R., & Oh, W. (1974). Effects of radiant warmer on insensible weight loss in newborn infants. *American Journal of Diseases of Children, 128*, 511–514.

Chapter 4

The Newborn

Prior to the early 1960s, newborns weighing less than 2,500 grams (5½ pounds) arbitrarily were classified as premature infants, whereas those weighing more than 2,500 grams were identified as full term. In 1961, the World Health Organization discarded this definition of preterm infants. Newborns weighing less than 2,500 grams subsequently were termed *low birthweight,* regardless of the duration of gestation. Following these changes, birthweight alone no longer was used as a measure of the maturity of the newborn. Subsequently, an independent assessment of growth (including weight, length, and head circumference) was considered in relation to determinations of gestational age (Colman & Rienzo, 1962; Warkany, Monroe, & Sutherland, 1961). Moreover, new information led to a characterization of infants on the basis of appropriateness of intrauterine growth for newborn gestational age. Today, according to present criteria, a *full-term infant* is considered to be 38 to 42 weeks gestation (37 to 41 weeks by World Health Organization standards). Babies born prior to this period are considered premature, and babies born after this time frame are judged *post-term.* The purpose of this chapter is to describe the aspects of *sizing* and *routine newborn care* and the implications of both for treatment and outcome of the neonate.

It should become obvious, as we progress through this discussion, that certain conditions are more likely than others to predispose infants toward a higher degree of risk and vulnerability. In terms of subsequent follow-up, we need to be alert to the needs of babies with such medical histories.

SIZING

Gestational Age Assessment

Historically, intrauterine assessment of gestational age has been difficult. X-rays for bone growth and sonograms for head development may be extremely inaccurate if the fetus is growth retarded. Although maternal dates are useful, irregular menstrual periods, hemorrhage, especially in the first trimester, and abnormal fetal size also may confuse the issue. More recently, first trimester obstetrical sonograms have become quite accurate for estimation of fetal age. In addition, several methods have been developed for assessment of gestational age on the basis of physical and neurologic characteristics of the newborn.

External Physical Characteristics

Many external physical characteristics of newborn infants progress in an orderly fashion during gestation (Farr, Kerridge, & Mitchell, 1966; Farr, Mitchell, & Neligan, 1966). Table 4–1 presents representative physical characteristics for neonates born at 28, 32, 36, and 40 weeks gestation. The first of these indicators is the vernix caseosa, a cheese-like material that initially appears at approximately 24 weeks gestation. It covers the body of the fetus and begins to diminish at approximately 36 weeks gestation. In the full-term infant, it is scant and found generally only in the creases of the body.

The skin of the extremely premature infant (28 weeks or less) is thin and translucent. Blood vessels are prominent and are most easily seen over the abdomen. With increasing gestation, vessels become less apparent as a result of deposition of fat and thickening of the skin. The *lanugo,* which is the fine hair of the fetus, covers the entire body as early as 22 weeks gestation. It begins to vanish from the face only 3 to 4 weeks prior to birth and still can be seen on the shoulders of most newborns.

The nipple and the surrounding tissue (areola) are not visible or are barely evident in the very premature infant. It is only at 34 weeks gestation that the areola begins to raise. In response to maternal hormones and with good nutrition, fat is deposited in the breast and, by term, a 5- to 6-millimeter nodule can be felt.

The ear in the full-term infant has a well-defined incurving of the outer edge. It is firm with developed cartilage and stands erect from the head. By comparison, the ear of the preterm infant between 28 and 32 weeks is flat, somewhat shapeless, and does not spring back when it is folded, because little cartilage is present.

Development of genitalia is another indicator of gestational age. The maturity of males, in part, can be traced by descent of the testes, which begin as intraabdominal organs, first appearing at the beginning of the inguinal canal at approximately 28 weeks gestation. The testes then descend into the scrotum and are pendulous at term. In response to this development, the scrotum manifests increased folds and becomes progressively more pigmented. In the female, deposition of fat again plays a role. In the premature infant of 32 weeks or less, the clitoris is very prominent, and the labia majora (outer lips) are small and widely separated. As the fetus approaches term, there is fatty deposition in the labia majora and, by term, the labia minora (inner lips) and clitoris are covered completely.

Table 4–1 Physical Characteristics for Gestational Age

Physical Finding	Gestational Age (weeks)			
	28	32	36	40
Vernix	Covers body	Covers body	Diminishing	Scant in creases
Skin	Thin, translucent prominent blood vessels	Thicker, blood vessels less apparent	Pink, few blood vessels apparent	Early desqua-mation
Lanugo	Covers body	Covers body	Vanishes from face	Present on shoulders
Breast	No palpable tissue	No palpable tissue, areola visible	1 to 2-mm fat nodule in breast, areola raised	5- to 6-mm fat nodule in breast
Ear				
Form	Flat	Flat	Incurving of upper ⅔	Well-defined, incurving
Cartilage	Stays folded	Scant, unfolds slowly	Thin, springs from folding	Firm, erect from head
Genitalia				
Male	Testes at inguinal canal inlet or not palpable	Testes in inguinal canal	Testes in upper scrotum	Testes in lower scrotum
Female	Prominent clitoris	Prominent clitoris; labia majora small	Clitoris nearly covered by labia minora	Labia minora and clitoris covered
Sole of Foot Creases	Smooth, no creases	One or two anterior creases	Creases on anterior ⅔ of sole	Creases on entire sole

Source: From "Assessment of Gestational Age and Development at Birth" by L.O. Lubchenco, 1970, *Pediatric Clinics of North America, 17,* pp. 125–145.

The sole (plantar) creases are entirely absent on the feet of the premature baby of 28 weeks or less. Faint red marks appear over the anterior half of the foot by 30 to 31 weeks, and one or two definite anterior sole creases can be seen by 32 weeks gestation. Generally, by 36 weeks, creases cover the anterior two-thirds of the foot, and the entire sole by full term.

Another well-described physical characteristic that aids in the assessment of gestational age is the sequential regression of vessels in the anterior capsule of the lens of the eye. At 27 to 28 weeks, these vessels cross the entire lens. By 29 to 30 weeks, there is central clearing, which continues until only small remnants can be seen on the periphery at 33 to 34 weeks gestation (Hittner, Hirsch, & Rudolph, 1977).

In general, these physical characteristics should be examined within the first 24 hours. With the predictable loss of extracellular fluid, the characteristics of the skin and the appearance of the sole creases may be altered after that time. Once the infant is cleaned, vernix also is no longer useful for assessment of gestational age.

Neurologic Assessment

While determination of gestational age by physical criteria should be performed immediately after birth, the neurologic evaluation should not be performed until later, when the infant's condition is stable. With the events of transition, this assessment usually cannot be done until the end of the first day or possibly the second or third day. Numerous perinatal factors may affect the neurologic assessment, including asphyxia, maternal anesthesia, maternal medications, and various illnesses and syndromes that may afflict the newborn. Neurologic development of the fetus during the last trimester is characterized, normally, by an increase in muscle mass and tone as well as by changes in reflexes and joint mobility in the extremities. Dutch and French neurologists first provided the details of the neurologic examination by gestational age (Amiel-Tison, 1968; Prechtl & Beintema, 1964). Current neurologic evaluation after birth focuses more specifically on examination of muscle tone (both passive and active), joint mobility, and primitive reflexes.

Infants born at 28 weeks gestation or less have very poor muscle tone and demonstrate a resting posture that is hypotonic, with full extension of the arms and legs. Flexor tone begins to appear at 30 weeks gestation, increasing in the lower extremities before the upper extremities. Characteristically, a 35- to 36-week infant has good muscle tone in the lower extremities but only partial flexion in the arms. By full-term, the resting posture should include full flexion at the joints of both upper and lower extremities. The severely preterm infant does not resist various passive maneuvers, such as movement of the heel to the ear (the scarf sign). Likewise, active tone may be seen as early as 30 weeks when the infant extends the legs in response to stimulation of the soles of the feet. At 32 weeks gestation, the baby straightens the legs when placed in a standing position. By 36 weeks, the neck extensors and flexors begin to function and, by 38 weeks, most infants can hold their heads for a few seconds when pulled to a sitting position.

Trunk tone can be measured by ventral suspension. With the infant prone, chest resting on the examiner's hand, the baby is lifted off the examining surface, and body position is noted. Extremely premature infants of 28 weeks or less have poor trunk tone and will appear to be draped over the hand. By 32 to 34 weeks, the back is straight and, by full-term, the head rises above the straightened back.

Joint mobility or flexibility with respect to gestational age may be examined in the wrist and ankle. With the square window sign, the hand is flexed at the wrist, and the angle between the hand and wrist is measured. In ankle dorsiflexion, the foot is flexed at the ankle with sufficient pressure for maximum change. The angle between the dorsum of the foot and the anterior leg is measured. In the 28-week infant, the wrist does not flex beyond 90 degrees. By 36 weeks, the angle is 45 degrees and, at term, the hand touches the arm. Ankle dorsiflexion reflects a similar pattern of development. In the preterm infant, the angle is generally greater than 45 degrees which progresses to 0 degrees by term. The joints of both wrist and ankle are relatively stiff in early gestation but become more relaxed at term.

Primitive reflexes also have been used to determine gestational age. These reflexes include sucking, rooting, grasping, galant, Moro response, crossed extension, pupillary reflex, glabellar tap, asymmetrical tonic neck reflex, and neck righting. Prior to 32 weeks, virtually all of these reflexes are absent or, at best, are very weak. By term, all are well established. Furthermore, with progressive development of the central nervous system over the first year of life, these reflexes generally disappear. They may persist, however, in infants with central nervous system damage.

Gestational age assessment of newborns now is accomplished most commonly with the use of a combination of both physical and neurologic findings. This current trend was initiated in 1970 by Dubowitz and his colleagues (Dubowitz & Dubowitz, 1977; Dubowitz, Dubowitz, & Goldberg, 1970), who developed a scoring system that used neurologic measures paralleling those of Amiel-Tison as well as the physical characteristics described by Farr and others. Accordingly, 10 neurologic and 11 physical characteristics were weighted, with a higher score assigned for more mature characteristics. A total score then could be obtained, and the gestational age could be determined by means of a graph. Many abbreviations of this assessment have appeared recently (Ballard et al., 1991; Petrucha, 1989). Overall, these are briefer versions that correlate well with the more sophisticated scoring systems. Such examination also allows for less handling and exposure of the acutely ill preterm infant.

As developed by Narayanan et al. (1982), simple measures of gestational age have encompassed examination of the ear, breast tissue, plantar creases, and lens vessels, as described in Table 4–2. An infant of 28 weeks typically scores no more than 1. A full-term infant, on the other hand, achieves 14 points or more. The evaluation is accurate plus or minus11 days, which is within the normal range of the Dubowitz scoring system (Narayanan et al., 1982).

Table 4–2 Rapid Assessment of Gestational Age

Criteria	Score				
	0	1	2	3	4
Ear Firmness (palpate upper pinna and note recoil after folding)	Pinna extremely soft, foldable into bizarre shapes with no recoil	Pinna soft along the edge, easily folded with slow recoil	Pinna with some cartilage, but thin at places, "ready recoil"	Pinna stiffened by cartilage up to periphery, immediate recoil	
Breast Nodule (pick up breast tissue with thumb and forefinger)	No breast tissue palpable	Nodule on one or both sides less than 0.5 centimeter	Nodule on one or both sides 0.5–1.0 centimeter	Nodule on one or both sides more than 1.0 centimeter	
Plantar Creases	No creases	Faint red marks over anterior ½	Reddish marks over anterior ½; definite creases over anterior ⅓	Creases over more than anterior ⅓	Creases all over; deep indentations over anterior ⅓
Lens Vessels (ophthalmoscope set on +12 diopters)	Vessels completely covering lens	Area of central clearing <¼ total lens diameter	Area of central clearing ¼–½ total lens diameter	Small vessel loops at periphery; >½ of lens clear	Lens clear except occasional faint loop or vessel remnant

Source: From "A Simple Method for Assessment of Gestational Age in Newborn Infants" by I. Narayanan et al., 1982, *Pediatrics, 69*, pp. 27–32. Copyright 1982 by American Academy of Pediatrics.

Growth for Gestational Age

Once gestational age of the newborn has been established, growth characteristics of the child can be examined to determine whether intrauterine growth has been appropriate. Unfortunately, there is no uniform definition of *small-for-gestational age* (SGA) infants or *large-for-gestational age* (LGA) infants. Designations of "normal" have been arbitrary. Limits of less than the 3rd percentile, less than the 10th percentile, and less than 2 SD (standard deviations from the mean) all have been used in reference to the SGA infant. For the LGA infant, the limits of "appropriate" variously have been set at greater than the 97th percentile, greater than the 90th percentile, and greater than 2 SD. In addition, the measurements used for these comparisons have differed considerably; they include birthweight, length, head circumference, and length-to-head circumference ratio (Cassady, 1981). As a result of such inconsistencies within the medical literature, comparisons and contrasts of the outcome of premature, low birthweight, SGA, and LGA infants are problematic.

Neonatal Morbidity by Birthweight and Gestational Age

Lubchenco and several colleagues carefully documented the increased mortality risk by birthweight, as matched to gestational age (Lubchenco, Delivoria-Papadopoulos, & Searls, 1972). The group at lowest risk for death in the newborn period (0.1 percent or 1/1,000 live births) not surprisingly are full-term infants with development appropriate for gestational age. On the other hand, neonates born preterm or post-term show an increased incidence of neonatal mortality, which is exaggerated by abnormally small or large fetal growth. For example, LGA term infants may have a neonatal mortality rate as high as 1 percent (or 1/100 live births), a 10-fold increase over that for full-term infants appropriate for gestational age. The mortality risk for the growth-retarded newborn is much greater and may reach 9 percent (or 9/100 live births), a 90-fold increase over that for appropriately grown term newborns. As birthweight and gestational age decrease, infant mortality increases dramatically to virtually 100 percent for infants born at less than 24 weeks gestation and weighing less than 500 grams, barely more than 1 pound. Morbidity statistics parallel figures on neonatal mortality (Lubchenco, 1976).

Despite confusion in the nomenclature and diverse standards of norm, high risk (SGA and LGA) subgroups have been the focus of much attention. The SGA infant, however, has received the greatest amount of study; this group is extremely heterogeneous, with many subpopulations. Numerous causes have been associated with growth retardation of the newborn.

Small-for-Gestational Age Infants

As Exhibit 4–1 shows, many fetal factors may result in decreased growth potential. Just as different populations demonstrate a large variation in birthweight of healthy, full-term infants, familial trends for low birthweight infants have been noted, suggesting a genetic basis (Johnstone & Inglis, 1974). The identification of racial and ethnic differences in expected birthweight has suggested additional inherited influences that may alter growth potential (Barron & Vessey, 1966). Congenital infections that have gained access to the fetus prior to birth may interfere

Exhibit 4–1 Factors Associated with Growth-Retarded (SGA) Newborns

Fetal—Decreased growth potential
- Genetics (population)
- Congenital infection
- Chromosomal syndromes
- Congenital anomalies
- Metabolic errors

Placental
- Decreased placental mass
- Intrinsic placental disease

Maternal
- Reduced uteroplacental blood flow
- Decreased nutrient availability
- Decreased oxygen availability
- Drugs
- Multiple gestation

Sources: Neonatology: Pathophysiology and Management of the Newborn, 2nd ed. (pp. 262–286), by G.B. Avery (Ed.), Philadelphia: J.B. Lippincott Company. Copyright 1981 by J.B. Lippincott Company; and "Intrauterine Growth Retardation" by A.F. DiGaetano and S.G. Gabbe, 1983, *Current Problems in Obstetrics and Gynecology, 6*, 7–30. Copyright 1983 by Year Book Medical Publishers, Inc.

with intrauterine fetal growth (Lubchenco, 1976). Chapter 12 discusses these infections in detail. Among the most common infections are rubella, cytomegalovirus, syphilis, and toxoplasmosis. Infants with these infectious diseases, which impair the development of genetically normal cells, may be born growth retarded, with microcephaly, deafness, cataracts, hepatosplenomegaly, pneumonia, hepatitis, or evidence of multiple-organ infection. Excessive or insufficient chromosomal material may cause a number of chromosomal syndromes (e.g., trisomy 21, trisomy 18, and Turner's syndrome), all of which may be associated with growth retardation. Moreover, even in the absence of specific chromosomal abnormalities, congenital anomalies such as microcephaly result in SGA newborns. Metabolic errors in the handling of nutrients crucial to tissue growth has been identified; yet, in many instances, the precise sequence of events leading to growth deficit still is not well understood.

A second series of factors associated with inadequate health of the placenta can result in poor development of the newborn (Sparks & Catlin, 1992). One such condition is a decreased placental mass that may provide insufficient nutrients for fetal growth and also poor clearance of waste products. These conditions often are seen with placental abruption or infarction, and with the rapidly aging placenta of the mother who has delivered post-term. In addition, growth retardation has been intrinsic to several placental factors including malformations, vascular disease, and poor implantation site (DiGaetano & Gabbe, 1983).

The third large category of factors associated with growth retardation may be classified as maternal variables (Gross & Sokol, 1989). Reduced uteroplacental blood flow, with concomitant decreases in nutrient transfer to the fetus, is the cause of growth retardation in many SGA newborns. Maternal vascular diseases, including advanced diabetes, chronic hypertension, and hypertension associated with toxemia, have been associated with impaired fetal growth (Long, Abell, & Beischer, 1980). Decreased nutrient availability to the fetus may be seen in mothers with poor nutrition or gastrointestinal disease and in women who smoke. Similarly, decreased oxygen availability to the newborn curtails fetal metabolism. The two most common causes of this condition are seen in mothers who live at high altitudes and, again, in those who smoke. More unusual causes are evidenced among mothers with cyanotic heart disease or a hemoglobinopathy such as sickle cell disease.

Drugs have been shown to impair fetal growth through a variety of mechanisms. Thirty years ago, thalidomide produced congenitally abnormal babies with short limbs and reduced body weight. Head growth usually was spared (McBride, 1961). In addition, there is well-documented evidence that alcohol results in fetal growth impairment and mental retardation, along with multiple anomalies of the face, eyes, and the cardiovascular and musculoskeletal systems (Clarren & Smith, 1978). Maternal narcotic addiction, too, has been associated with poor fetal growth and development.

Finally, twin gestation is another important consideration in determining growth (Kochenour, 1992). Over the years, many cases of SGA twins have been cited. In 1966, Gruenwald observed that the growth rate of twins followed that of a singleton fetus until approximately 32 weeks gestation, after which there was a progressive falling off in the development of twins. The incidence of growth retardation in twins was documented to be as high as 17.5 percent (Houlton, Marivate, & Philpott, 1981). Twins, in addition, may be discordant in their weights (Figure 4-1), with one weighing considerably more than the other and placental asymmetry affording insufficient nutrients to the smaller twin.

Typically, the impact of growth retardation on the newborn is varied and pervasive. In general, although weight and length are restricted, head growth tends to be spared (Lubchenco, 1976). More often than not, even at term, these babies have clinical problems similar to those of children born prematurely. For instance, *hypoglycemia* in both groups results from decreased body stores of glycogen, a polymer of glucose normally stored in the liver. Essentially, the stress of adaptation to extrauterine life results in increased glucose utilization with little caloric reserve. Thus, hypoglycemia usually occurs within the first 12 hours after birth and can be treated with intravenous glucose or an early feeding regimen. Both preterm and SGA infants are prone to hypothermia. The ratio of surface area to body mass is decreased, and heat is dissipated more readily. Such newborns have little subcutaneous fat to conserve heat, and, with a poor caloric reserve, heat generation is impaired. Often, growth-retarded infants experience problems arising from increased total numbers of red blood cells (polycythemia). While the etiology of this condition is not known, it has been theorized that intrauterine hypoxia (reduced oxygen content and oxygen tension) results in elevated red blood cell

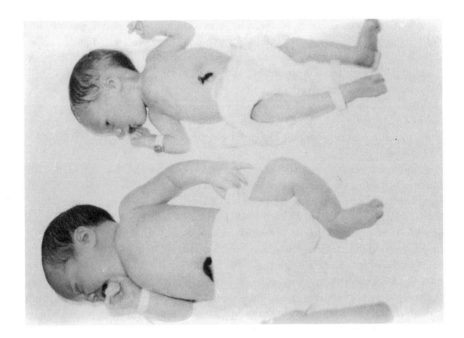

Figure 4–1 Discordant twins

production, probably a form of compensation. These infants with polycythemia usually are asymptomatic, but, if the fraction of red blood cells in the blood exceeds 70 percent, they may show symptoms of respiratory distress, cardiac failure, hypoglycemia, seizures, and/or increased jaundice. The benefits of treatment are controversial, but excess red blood cells can be removed via a partial exchange transfusion, while care is taken to preserve the blood volume by replacement of plasma (Fanaroff, Martin, & Miller, 1989).

In conclusion, we should point out that while maternal and fetal disease may account for abnormalities of growth in many newborns, not every excessively large or small newborn is the result of a pathologic process. Obviously, tall and heavy parents tend to produce large babies, and small, thin parents have small babies.

Large-for-Gestational Age Infants

Our discussion has focused mainly on the SGA baby. Problems of equal seriousness may arise for LGA infants, who generally tend to be more homogeneous than populations of smaller neonates. Commonly, fetal hyperinsulinism is an underlying factor for excessive fetal growth, and this condition most frequently is prompted by maternal diabetes (Coustan, 1992). The maternal pancreas fails to produce quantities of insulin sufficient to prevent the blood glucose of the mother from rising. This maternal hyperglycemia, in turn, results in fetal hyperglycemia. Subsequently, the elevated serum glucose in the newborn provokes excess insulin production and secretion from the fetal pancreas, resulting in overgrowth, especially of fatty tissue, heart, liver, and the adrenal gland. Brain weight is not affected, as evidenced by studies of control subjects matched for gestational age (Naeye, 1965). At birth, LGA infants have hyperinsulinemia. However, when the glucose supply from the mother, which originally stimulated the insulin release is withdrawn, *hypoglycemia* results. Fetal hyperinsulinemia also inhibits lung maturation, causing an increased incidence of respiratory distress in the newborn period.

Congenital anomalies are more frequent among LGA infants born to diabetic mothers. These disorders include cardiac defects, gastrointestinal malformations, spinal anomalies, and the caudal regression syndrome (a malformation of the pelvic region and lower extremities). Pedersen compared infants of diabetic mothers with those of nondiabetic control subjects and discovered a 2-fold increase in congenital anomalies with mild to moderate maternal diabetes and a 4-fold increase in neonatal congenital anomalies with the more severe forms of maternal diabetes (Pedersen, 1977). The large fetal size also predisposes the infants to birth trauma, especially cephalohematomas, brachial plexus injuries, and fractured clavicles, as discussed in Chapter 3.

Other etiologies associated with excessive fetal growth include the *Beckwith syndrome* and *Rh isoimmunization*. The Beckwith syndrome is a clinical disorder consisting of macroglossia (increased size of the tongue), gigantism (abnormal development of the body or parts), large organs, and neonatal hypoglycemia (related to hyperinsulinemia in approximately one-half of the patients). Many newborns have accompanying congenital anomalies, but most evidence normal chromosomes. The neonatal mortality is high, and many babies have residual developmental disabilities (Beckwith, 1969). Rh isoimmunization (see Chapter 8) has been associated with fetal hyperinsulinemia. Commonly, infants with this condition are overgrown and hypoglycemic.

LONG-TERM OUTCOME AS A FUNCTION OF GESTATIONAL AGE

Data on long-term outcome of neonates are difficult to evaluate. Published reports of studies frequently reflect not only the interests, but also the biases of the investigators. Variables included in analyses of children with disabilities often are study specific, making comparisons complex and, not infrequently, ambiguous. Racial, ethnic, social, and economic factors are often ill-defined or hard to interpret. Many follow-up investigations have been conducted retrospectively, with poor matching of case controls. Even in the few prospective studies, it appears that important information may have been missed and that the sample size for follow-up may have been too small for meaningful analysis. Ultimately, prognosis for development of a neonate hinges on gestational age and intrauterine growth and development, as well as on perinatal problems, early childhood illnesses, family dynamics, and other environmental factors much too subtle and complex to quantitate accurately.

Most published studies of long-term outcome in children report only on the first several years of life; rarely are data available beyond 5 years. Intellectual and motor function are virtually always the primary focus, with little attention paid to behavioral and emotional development. To the present time, the mobility of our society and problems in funding have inhibited the duration and completeness of longitudinal follow-up studies.

ROUTINE NEWBORN CARE

Following resuscitation and stabilization of the newborn and an appropriate gestational age assessment, each infant receives specific *prophylactic* health care (Kendig, 1992). This involves proper identification, care of the umbilical cord, eye care, administration of vitamin K, and newborn metabolic screening (Caravella, Clark, & Dweck, 1987). In general, such treatments are designed to prevent infection or other adverse conditions.

Newborn Identification

Before the newborn leaves the delivery room, two identical bands matching the mother's bands with admission number and the sex of the infant are placed on the baby's wrist and ankle. The accuracy of identifiers is checked prior to the baby's leaving the delivery room and again on admission to the nursery. Later, the mother must verify the information on the identification bands both prior to feedings and as a condition of discharge from the hospital (American Academy of Pediatrics and American College of Obstetricians and Gynecologists, 1992).

Although newborns still are being footprinted for identification, this technique has been deemed basically unreliable. Widely available sophisticated blood-typing techniques (human leukocyte antigen [HLA] tissue typing or DNA printing) appear to be more accurate and, concomitantly, more cost-effective (Thompson, Clark, Salisbury, & Cahill, 1981).

Umbilical Cord Care

At delivery, the cord is clamped to prohibit blood loss. It then dries and, in approximately 7 to 10 days, is shed. Much attention has been paid to preventing infection of the cord. Methods include local application of triple dye and various antimicrobial agents such as bacitracin. Although alcohol may hasten drying of the cord, it is not very effective in the healing process (American Academy of Pediatrics and American College of Obstetricians and Gynecologists, 1992). The dried cord is shed by white blood cell enzymatic action in response to normal bacterial colonization. Thus, any antibacterial substance applied to the cord will delay colonization and prolong the time until the cord is shed.

Eye Prophylaxis

Ophthalmia neonatorum (conjunctivitis of the newborn) may be caused by a variety of infectious agents. Approximately 100 years ago, Credé initiated the use of silver nitrate in newborn eye care, and this prophylaxis markedly reduced the incidence of *gonorrheal ophthalmia neonatorum.* The most recent revision of the American Academy of Pediatrics' guidelines directed toward preventing neonatal ophthalmia include (1) installation of a prophylactic agent in the eyes of all newborns and (2) a choice of prophylactic agents including 0.1 percent silver nitrate solution, 0.5 percent erythromycin ophthalmic ointment or drops, or 1.0 percent tetracycline ophthalmic ointment or drops. While all three of these treatments are potent against gonococcal disease, only erythromycin and tetracycline are effective against *chlamydia,* a less serious eye infection with a purulent discharge that limits vision. For those few infants unfortunate enough to develop ophthalmia neonatorum, the specific infectious agent must be identified and treatment must be administered to prevent loss of vision.

Vitamin K

Hemorrhagic disease of the newborn was described first in 1894 as a generalized bleeding that occurred in the first week of life in otherwise healthy infants (Townsend, 1894). It is now known to be caused by a severe depression of *Factors II, VII, IX,* and *X,* which is secondary to a deficiency of vitamin K (Kisker, 1992). These factors are essential to the process of blood clotting. Thus, all newborn infants, as a part of routine care, receive a single dose (0.5 to 1.0 milligrams) of natural vitamin K^1 oxide within 1 hour of birth. Although this prophylaxis generally is given intramuscularly, oral administration also is effective (American Academy of Pediatrics and American College of Obstetricians and Gynecologists, 1992; Hathaway & Bonnar, 1978).

Metabolic Screening

Numerous metabolic diseases can be diagnosed in the early neonatal period. These include *phenylketonuria* (PKU) and *congenital hypothyroidism,* two of many diseases that may result in retarded growth and development. Identification of infants with these conditions and subsequent dietary or therapeutic intervention have been shown to minimize the consequences of these inherited conditions. A blood sample should be obtained from every neonate prior to discharge from the hospital. Small amounts of blood taken by heel-stick are placed on testing cards that then are analyzed in central laboratories in each state. All infants with abnormal results in the screening program must then be tested by more sophisticated methods. Although screening programs are expensive, the long-term cost to the state for infants with developmental delay far exceeds the outlay for screening programs.

Although developmental outcome will be discussed further in Chapter 5, several generalizations are appropriate.

1. Overall, low birthweight infants have a greater likelihood of a poor prognosis (Gunderson, 1990).

2. SGA neonates are more prone to poor neurological and developmental outcomes (Warshaw, 1986).

3. Neonates with severe respiratory distress or intracranial hemorrhage and seizures in the newborn period are at greater risk of neurologic and intellectual deficits (Ross, Lipper, & Auld, 1986; Scott, 1987).

Finally, the long-term developmental prognosis for an individual child only rarely can be predicted with sufficient accuracy to counsel parents with full certainty. However, continuous evaluation of high risk infants and children is helpful, and early intervention should allow high risk infants to reach their fullest potential.

BIBLIOGRAPHY

American Academy of Pediatrics and American College of Obstetricians and Gynecologists (1992). *Guidelines for perinatal care.* Evansville, IN: Author.

Amiel-Tison, C. (1968). Neurological evaluation of the maturity of newborn infants. *Archives of Disease in Childhood, 43,* 89–93.

Ballard, J.L., Khoury, J.C., Wedig, K., Wang, L., Eilers-Walsman, B.L., & Lipp, R. (1991). New Ballard Score, expanded to include extremely premature infants. *Journal of Pediatrics, 119,* 417–423.

Barron, S.L., & Vessey, M.P. (1966). Birthweights of infants born to immigrant women. *British Journal of Preventive and Social Medicine, 20,* 127–134.

Beckwith, J.B. (1969). Macroglossia, omphalocele, adrenal cytomegaly, gigantism, and hyperplastic visceromegaly. In D. Bergsma (Ed.), *The clinical delineation of birth defects* (Vol. 5) (pp. 188–196). New York: National Foundation—March of Dimes.

Caravella, S.J., Clark, D.A., & Dweck, H.S. (1987). Health codes for newborn care. *Pediatrics, 80,* 1–5.

Cassady, G. (1981). The small-for-date infant. In G.B. Avery (Ed.), *Neonatology: Pathophysiology and management of the newborn* (2nd ed.) (pp. 262–286). Philadelphia: J.B. Lippincott.

Clarren, S.K., & Smith, D.W. (1978). The fetal alcohol syndrome. *New England Journal of Medicine, 298,* 1063–1067.

Colman, H., & Rienzo, J. (1962). The small term baby. *Obstetrics and Gynecology, 19,* 87–91.

Coustan, D.R. (1992). Diabetes in pregnancy. In A.A. Fanaroff and R.J. Martin (Eds.), *Neonatal-perinatal medicine: Diseases of the fetus and infant* (5th ed.) (Vol. 1) (pp. 199–204). St. Louis: C.V. Mosby.

DiGaetano, A.F., & Gabbe, S.G. (1983). Intrauterine growth retardation. *Current Problems in Obstetrics and Gynecology, 6,* 7–30.

Dubowitz, L.M.S., & Dubowitz, V. (1977). *Gestational age of the newborn.* Menlo Park, CA: Addison-Wesley.

Dubowitz, L.M.S., Dubowitz, V., & Goldberg, C. (1970). Clinical assessment of gestational age in the newborn infant. *Journal of Pediatrics, 77,* 1–10.

Fanaroff, A.A., Martin, R.J., & Miller, M.J. (1989). Identification and management of high risk problems in the neonate. In R. Creasy & R. Resnick (Eds.), *Maternal-fetal medicine: Principles and practice* (2nd ed.) (pp. 1150–1193). Philadelphia: W.B. Saunders.

Farr, V., Kerridge, D., & Mitchell, R. (1966). The value of some external characteristics in the assessment of gestational age at birth. *Developmental Medicine and Child Neurology, 8,* 657–660.

Farr, V., Mitchell, R., & Neligan, G. (1966). The definition of some external characteristics used in the assessment of gestational age of the newborn infant. *Developmental Medicine and Child Neurology, 8,* 507–511.

Gross, T.L., & Sokol, R. (1989). *Intrauterine growth retardation: A practical approach.* Chicago: Year Book Medical.

Gruenwald, P. (1966). Growth of the human fetus: II. Abnormal growth in twins and infants of mothers with diabetes, hypertension, or isoimmunization. *American Journal of Obstetrics and Gynecology, 94,* 1120–1132.

Gunderson, L. (1990). Infant development. In L.P. Gunderson & C. Kenner (Eds.), *Care of the 24–25 week gestational age infant (small baby protocol)* (pp. 1–22). Petaluma, CA: Neonatal Network.

Hathaway, W.E., & Bonnar, J. (1978). Bleeding disorders in the newborn. In W.E. Hathway & J. Bonnar (Eds.), *Perinatal coagulation* (pp. 115–169). New York: Grune & Stratton.

Hittner, H., Hirsch, N., & Rudolph, A. (1977). Assessment of gestational age by examination of the anterior vascular capsule of the lens. *Journal of Pediatrics, 91,* 455–458.

Houlton, M.C.C., Marivate, M., & Philpott, R.H. (1981). The prediction of fetal growth retardation in twin pregnancy. *British Journal of Obstetrics and Gynaecology, 88,* 264–273.

Johnstone, F., & Inglis, L. (1974). Familial trends in low birth weight. *British Medical Journal, 3,* 659–661.

Kendig, J.W. (1992). Care of the normal newborn. *Pediatrics in Review, 13*(7), 262–268.

Kisker, C.T. (1992). Pathophysiology of bleeding disorders in the newborn. In R.A. Polin & W.W. Fox (Eds.), *Fetal and neonatal physiology* (Vol. 2) (pp. 1381–1394). Philadelphia: W.B. Saunders.

Kochenour, N.K. (1992). Obstetric management of multiple gestation. In A.A. Fanaroff & R.J. Martin (Eds.), *Neonatal-perinatal medicine: Diseases of the fetus and infant* (5th ed.) (Vol. 1) (pp. 225–229). St. Louis: C.V. Mosby.

Long, P.A., Abell, D.A., & Beischer, N.A. (1980). Fetal growth retardation and preeclampsia. *British Journal of Obstetrics and Gynaecology, 87,* 13–16.

Lubchenco, L.O. (1970). Assessment of gestational age and development at birth. *Pediatric Clinics of North America, 17,* 125–145.

Lubchenco, L.O. (1976). *The high risk infant.* Philadelphia: W.B. Saunders.

Lubchenco, L.O., Delivoria-Papadopoulos, M., & Searls, D. (1972). Long-term follow-up studies of prematurely born infants: II. Influence of birth weight and gestational age on sequelae. *Journal of Pediatrics, 80,* 509–512.

McBride, W.G. (1961). Thalidomide and congenital abnormalities. *Lancet, 2,* 1358.

Naeye, R.L. (1965). Infants of diabetic mothers: A quantitative morphologic study. *Pediatrics, 35,* 980–988.

Narayanan, I., Dua, K., Gujral, V., Mehta, D.K., Matthew, M., & Prabhakar, A. (1982). A simple method for assessment of gestational age in newborn infants. *Pediatrics, 69,* 27–32.

Pedersen, J. (1977). *The pregnant diabetic and her newborn.* Baltimore: Williams & Wilkins.

Petrucha, R. (1989). Fetal maturity/gestational age evaluation. *Journal of Perinatology, 9*(1), 100–101.

Prechtl, H.E.R., & Beintema, D. (1964). The neurological examination of the full term newborn infant. *Clinics in Developmental Medicine* (No. 12). Philadelphia: J.B. Lippincott (Spastics International Medicine Publications).

Ross, G., Lipper, E., & Auld, P.E.M. (1986). Early predictors of neurodevelopmental outcome of very-low-birthweight infants at three years. *Developmental Medicine and Child Neurology, 28,* 171–179.

Scott, D.T. (1987). Premature infants in later childhood: Some recent follow-up results. *Seminars in Perinatology, 11,* 191–199.

Sparks, J.W., & Catlin I. (1992). Intrauterine growth and nutrition. In R.A. Polin & W.W. Fox (Eds.), *Fetal and neonatal physiology* (Vol. 1, pp. 179–188). Philadelphia: W.B. Saunders.

Thompson, J.E., Clark, D.A., Salisbury, B., & Cahill, J. (1981). Footprinting in the newborn infant: Not cost effective. *Journal of Pediatrics, 99,* 797–798.

Townsend, C.W. (1894). The haemorrhagic disease of the newborn. *Archives of Pediatrics, 11,* 559–565.

Warkany, J., Monroe, B., & Sutherland, B. (1961). Intrauterine growth retardation. *American Journal of Diseases in Children, 102,* 249–279.

Warshaw, J.B. (1986). Intrauterine growth retardation. *Pediatrics in Review, 8,*107–112.

Chapter 5

Sensory, Motor, and Psychological Development of the High Risk Newborn

With the recent technological advances and environmental changes in neonatal care, survival rates for newborns treated in intensive care nurseries have increased and prognoses have become increasingly optimistic. Some extremely low birthweight infants between 500 and 750 grams, who would have died 5 to 8 years ago, now live; they are treated for multiple insults and hospital stays are prolonged. Longitudinal studies of outcome are underway; in some studies, follow-up has been carried out with children up to 8 years of age.

However, many questions remain concerning the development of seriously ill newborns, as well as that of infants born between 32 and 37 weeks gestation, who continue to surface later in elementary and middle schools as learning disabled. One especially pressing though controversial issue relates to the population of premature and high risk infants. The issue is that, although we may be saving more lives in this group of newborns, the numbers of severely delayed youngsters from certain subgroups of these neonates may be on the rise. One such group are babies suffering chronic lung disease with extended periods of mechanical ventilation.

Another important issue is the interpretation of reports of rapidly expanding research studies in neonatology. First, while the technology of newborn care has changed decidedly for the better, practices still vary from center to center relative to the number of deliveries at Level Three hospitals, the sophistication of transport systems, and the responsiveness of clinical and medical staff to environmental issues within nurseries. Such disparities make it difficult to generalize across facilities. Second, growing numbers of articles on long-term developmental outcome have documented the variability of learning and behavior of infants and young children across time. Children change and evaluation of development in relation to the norm can differ depending on when these children are evaluated in the life span. The findings of these studies highlight the importance of periodic evaluations, as opposed to one-time assessments of developmental progress. A third, related problem that has influenced our knowledge of the developmental status of preterm and high risk infants is the gap between the effectiveness of current treatments and data reported in research journals. Indeed, as a result of dramatic changes in technology, long-term studies often reflect less advanced and sophisticated care. Finally, the effectiveness of contemporary observational and assessment measures to date remain a serious issue. In large part, all of these concerns account for the continuing search for parameters of risk that will best enable us to predict later developmental problems and thus to act preventively to minimize the impact of insults.

In this chapter, we look at the sensory-perceptual, neuromotor, language, cognitive, and psychosocial development of the high risk infant as reflected in research carried out over the past 15 years. In particular, we focus on improvements in neonatal outcome, conditions that consistently tend to be associated with delayed or impaired development, and the educational implications of our knowledge. Since Chapter 13 focuses on developmental difficulties of infants born to substance abusing parents, our discussion here will address prematurity and other conditions that place children at risk.

SENSORY AND PERCEPTUAL SKILLS

Vision

Physiology of the Eye

Any discussion of vision and eye diseases of the newborn needs to be based on a firm grasp of the function of the eye, which resembles the operation of a camera. The outermost layer of the eye is the *conjunctiva*. The most anterior portion of the eye, through which we see, is the *cornea*; and immediately behind this is a layer of fluid, the *aqueous humor,* which separates the cornea from the lens. The *pupil* and *lens* are surrounded by the *iris*, the colored portion of the eye. The lens is attached to a circular muscle that modifies the shape of the lens to allow for the focusing of light on the retina in the back of the eye. Behind the lens is another, more viscous fluid called the *vitreous humor*. The posterior layer of the eye consists of the *retina*, with two major types of sensing cells, the *rods* which distinguish light from dark and are sensitive to the intensity of light, and the *cones*, which are color sensitive. These cells, derived from nerve tissue, send impulses to the posterior portion of the brain, where they are received and interpreted. Thus, the eye functions much like a camera. Light entering the eye is focused by the lens, its intensity is controlled by the size of the aperture (the pupil), and subsequently it strikes the sensitive cells of the retina. Any interference with the transmission of light from the anterior portion of the eye to the retina or with neuron transmission to the brain results in visual impairment.

At birth, the newborn, who has been living in a light-deprived environment, is capable of processing complex visual information. The term infant responds to objects that are bright, with high degrees of contrast, and can fix on and track an object over a limited distance. Although visual acuity is difficult to determine, recent evidence suggests that newborns are able to focus up to approximately 10 inches. They respond to human faces, shiny objects, and preferentially to the color red. To date, studies of vision in neonates have been done nearly exclusively with populations of full-term healthy infants, and virtually no data are available on small premature neonates.

Disorders of the Eye

Despite our lack of research in some areas of newborn capability, vision and hearing losses associated with prematurity have been a long-standing concern of pediatricians and neonatologists. Some historical perspective helps us to comprehend the current problem.

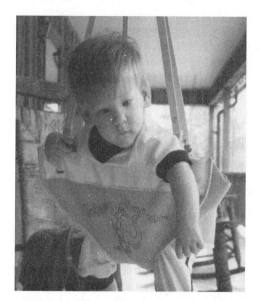

The term *retrolental fibroplasia* (RLF), for example, first was used to describe the clinical appearance of damaged eyes of preterm infants with a vascularized membrane or overgrowth of fibrous tissue behind the lens of the eye. Later, it was discovered that this membrane was, in actuality, the totally detached retina (Friendly, 1987). Terry (1942) was the first ophthalmologist to recognize the condition. So extensive were such insults that by 1945, the condition was identified in 12 percent of all premature infants with birthweights of 1,300 grams or less (Fiedler, Robinson, Shaw, Ng, & Moseley, 1992). By 1950, oxygen had been tentatively identified as an offending agent, and today a new name more commonly is used to refer to the condition—*retinopathy of prematurity* (ROP). At present, both labels are casually used, and it is generally believed that the condition is caused exclusively by the administration of oxygen. In fact, the damage correlates with increased blood oxygen levels beyond the physiologic range, in combination with a number of other factors including elevated blood carbon dioxide levels and nutrition. At present, several trends have been reported, but, unfortunately, predictive patterns are yet to be discovered. Many very immature babies receiving oxygen by mechanical ventilation fail

Figure 5–1 Ben—Born at 25 weeks gestation suffered visual impairment as a result of a Grade 4 hemorrhage

to develop the disease, and other severely premature newborns who never have had supplemental oxygen manifest the problem. Despite conditions requiring intense ventilatory support, ROP (or RLF) rarely is seen in the full-term baby.

Classification systems now have been created in order to describe the abnormal development of the immature retina. While this portion of the eye in babies at full-term is nearly complete, infants born at approximately 28 weeks gestation (12 weeks premature) are still in the formative stages of their growth, with only 50 to 60 percent of the retina fully developed. In such instances, continued appropriate blood vessel growth and nutrients are essential to assure proper maturation. To the experienced ophthalmologist, the retinal lesion (*stage 1*) first appears as a severe constriction of the peripheral vessels, a condition rarely seen before 4 to 6 weeks after birth. In the progression to *stage 2*, there is evidence of dilation and tortuosity, with peripheral new blood vessel ingrowth. This impairment then includes hemorrhage in the retina. By *stage 3*, blood vessels proliferate into the vitreous humor, and there may be localized detachment of the retina. Thus, any light that strikes the detached retinal tissue cannot be converted into an electrical impulse in the brain, and vision is lost. Complete detachment (*stage 4*) obviously results in total blindness. At any early stage of the disease, there may be resolution of the abnormal vascular process, but wherever scarring is present, the retina will be distorted.

In 1981, Phelps projected that approximately 2,100 infants would be affected annually by this troublesome disease. Today, the incidence of ROP continues to be inversely proportional to birthweight and gestational age. Few babies of more than 28 weeks or 1,200 grams develop ROP (Usher, 1987). However, within the population of extremely premature infants delivered at 27 weeks or earlier, the condition continues to be common and occurs often in the most severe stages. One of the leading factors in the growing prevalence of ROP is the increasing number of newborns surviving gestational ages less than 28 weeks, born at 500 to 1,000 grams. Friendly (1987) also observed that ROP is more likely to occur in the event of multiple versus singleton births and, though still not fully understood, remains a function of "multiple causal factors." New techniques in surgical or laser fixation of the retina in most severe stages of ROP hold some promise for treatment. Routinely low birthweight newborns and infants receiving supplemental oxygen for extended periods should receive ophthalmologic examinations prior to discharge or 6 weeks after birth and periodically after leaving the nursery until resolution. In the long term, such children are more prone to myopia (near-sightedness), retinal detachment, and amblyopia (roving eye).

Many other abnormalities of the eyes have been reported in the newborn period. Infants may be born with no eyes or abnormally small eyes. The iris may be missing, have little pigment (albinism), or not be fully formed. The lens may be absent or dislocated. Tumors such as hemangiomas (abnormal growth of blood vessels) may disrupt or distort the developing eye. Retinoblastoma, an aggressive tumor arising in the retina, is found in approximately 1 in 20,000 live births and usually is first recognized after 1 year of age. In cases of retinoblastoma, the mortality rate is 100 percent unless treatment is prompt and includes removal of the affected eye.

Cataracts, opacities affecting the lens of the eye, occur in several forms. About one-third of the newborns with these anomalies have no apparent systemic illness. On the other hand, cataracts may be traumatic or associated with chromosomal disorders such as trisomy 18 and trisomy 13, and approximately 50 percent of the infants with rubella syndrome are thus affected. A number of metabolic diseases, most notably galactosemia, are characterized by cataracts. Neonates with this disorder are able to digest the primary milk sugar lactose for its components, glucose and galactose, but the body then is unable to convert galactose to usable glucose and complexes of the excess carbohydrate are deposited within the lens, impairing vision. Because cataracts interfere with light stimulation of the retina, they should be removed surgically as early as possible in order to promote appropriate development of the retina and, secondarily, the central nervous system.

Unlike *glaucoma* in adults, increased pressure in the anterior chamber of the eye (aqueous humor) is rare in the newborn. Whenever the condition does emerge as a congenital problem, light sensitivity and production of tears are excessive, and the increased pressure in the aqueous humor stretches the cornea and results in blurred vision. Glaucoma is associated with a number of syndromes; it is seen with transplacental infections but also may arise as an isolated defect. Surgery can be performed to re-establish adequate circulation and drainage of the anterior chamber.

Visual Perception

Visual perception, as distinguished from sensory skills, has been studied by evaluating tracking, visual attentiveness, and visual preference during the neonatal period. While this area has been widely investigated with respect to the development of the term baby, less has been done relative to the premature infant. Several types of studies have been conducted. In an evaluation of typical and neurologically impaired preterm and full-term babies, Morante, Dubowitz, Levene, and Dubowitz (1982) found that the visual acuity in low risk preterm infants at 33 to 34 weeks was comparable to that of full-term infants on 60 percent of the tasks, but pattern preference capacities were less well developed. This research was based on the visual discrimination of four different pairs of patterns, and visual perception was assessed by abilities of neonates to distinguish black and white stripes of different widths. The study, in addition, analyzed the performance of neurologically impaired term and preterm infants at 36 and 40 weeks gestation. The researchers found that, as might be expected, abnormal preterm infants showed poorer pattern preference abilities and were not as adept on visual acuity tasks. Further, compared with other preterm babies with known neurological impairment, premature infants with intraventricular hemorrhage revealed even greater problems with visual perception.

In a similar study, Dubowitz, Dubowitz, and Morante (1980) examined the visual performance of the preterm infant by using the tracking techniques of the first edition of the *Neonatal Behavioral Assessment Scale* (Brazelton, 1984) and the pattern preference and fixation strategies of Fantz and Fagan (1975). In a follow-up study of infants of 28 to 37 weeks gestation, Dubowitz and associates demonstrated visual discrimination only after 30 weeks, with maturity equal to that of the full-term infant by 34 weeks. Babies less than 30 weeks gestation, with one exception, showed no fixation or tracking. By 40 weeks gestation, such delays appeared to be resolved, with the few preterm infants included in the sample able to function as well as their full-term counterparts, and in some situations better.

These findings coincide closely with the results of other studies of visual perception. Ruff and colleagues (Ruff, Lawson, Kurtzberg, McCarton-Daum, & Vaughan, 1982) compared the visual following skills of term and preterm infants at 40 weeks postconceptual (chronological) age. In general, the preterm infants did not differ from the term infants. Delays were, however, evident in premature babies who showed other early signs of atypical learning and responsiveness. Likewise, Paine, Pasquali, and Spegiorin (1983) investigated the visually directed prehension of 227 infants in relation to gestational age and intrauterine growth. They also found early developmental delays among preterm and small-for-gestational age infants, compared with full-term infants. Yet, for the majority of premature babies, such problems no longer were apparent by 4 to 5 months of chronological age. Finally, based on their research on the visual response of term and preterm infants, Fantz and Fagan (1975) reported that responsiveness to size and number of pattern details differed markedly for both groups as a function of age during the first 6 months. In addition, the development of the preterm infant varied clearly from that of the term infant by age from birth, but not by age from conception.

Research on the development of sensory and perceptual abilities of high risk infants and young children in relation to later school performance remains an important focus in the current literature. For example, DeGangi and Greenspan (1988) carried out a study of 196 typical infants, 27 babies with developmental delay, and 27 infants with difficult temperament—all 4 to 18 months of age. They used the *Test of Sensory Functions in Infants* (TSFI), a 24-item measure of sensory processing and reactivity in infants. The authors concluded that problems of tactile defensiveness, poor ocular-motor control, and vestibular dysfunction occurred in a "substantial proportion" of the developmentally delayed and temperamentally difficult infants. In addition, problems in visual-tactile integration and adaptive motor responses were evident to a lesser degree. In particular, the study confirmed that ". . . poor performance on the TSFI on the total test was found in 57% to 83% of the developmentally delayed sample and 55% to 86% of the difficult temperament sample for 7- to 18-month-old children" (p. 30). While some caution is needed in drawing conclusions from the data, in view of the very small size and general description of the samples, the preliminary data do point to the importance of identifying early signs of difficulty that later are manifested as learning, emotional, and behavioral disorders in children.

Findings of the DeGangi and Greenspan study, though not stated specifically, parallel results of other studies of low birthweight babies, who similarly evidence problems of developmental delay and temperament difficulties. Although the measures and samples described were different, data of research conducted by Pederson and his colleagues coincide with results of DeGangi and Greenspan's work. The purpose of the Pederson study (Pederson, Evans, Chance, Bento, & Fox, 1988) was "to describe the relationships among various perinatal, environmental, and demographic measures in a sample of low birth weight infants and to relate these measures to 1-year developmental status" (p. 287). Based on the performance and behavior of 160 infants on the *Bayley Scales of Infant Development,* the authors found that the psychomotor scores in the sample were lower than the mental development scores and thus concluded that "low birth weight infants appear to be at particular risk for later learning disabilities" (p. 291). They further noted that the nature of these developmental deficits often does not become clear until the child is older and faces the need for information processing skills necessary for school performance (p. 291). The longitudinal data of a recent study by Saigal and colleagues (Saigal, Szatmari, Rosenbaum, Campbell, & King, 1991) on the intellectual and functional status at school entry of children who weighed 1,000 grams or less at birth also confirms the concerns that such children are at risk for later learning disabilities. These authors wrote:

> The major area of concern identified in our population, even among those with a normal IQ, was in the area of visual-motor integration and motor function. Poor visual-motor performance and problems with spatial relations have been consistently reported in children < 1500 gm BW by previous investigators. We also noted that of the normal group of children at 5 years of age (i.e., neurologically and cognitively intact), approximately half were considered to be at mild to high risk for future learning disabilities. (p. 415)

Rose, Feldman, McCarton, and Wolfson (1988) seemed to confirm the results of Saigal and colleagues when they reported differences between 7-month-old full-term infants and high risk preterm infants (less than 1,500 grams at birth) in regard to problems of visual recognition memory and tasks requiring abilities to recruit, sustain, and shift attention. Specifically, the researchers found that, compared with the full-term infants, preterm infants required longer exposure for familiarization, differed in strategies for examining stimuli, showed no evidence of recognition memory on three types of visual problems, and demonstrated less attentiveness to novelty. In addition, significant perinatal risk factors such as respiratory distress with prolonged mechanical ventilation appeared to be related to poorer performance on measures of visual recognition memory and cross modal transfer, and thus poorer future cognitive outcome.

Finally, Thompson, Fagan, and Fulker (1991) focused on the centrality of visual perception and preference in the scheme of longitudinal prediction of specific cognitive abilities. Maintaining that perceptual tasks require processes involving memory, discrimination, and attention abilities necessary for successful performance on later IQ tests, the authors concluded that infant visual novelty preference correlated significantly with scores on the Bayley scales at 24 months of age and scores on the *Stanford-Binet Intelligence Scale* test at 36 months. The question of the specific nature of the "link" between visual attention measures in infants and tested IQ in later years was left open by the authors, who suggested more detailed assessment of cognitive processing in infancy and early childhood. This recommendation seems to be most appropriate, in light of difficulties of early assessment, the changing nature of perceptual and cognitive abilities throughout the first 5 years of life, and in view of the complexities of understanding the influence of low birthweight and other high risk conditions. Overall, sufficient numbers of studies with long-term follow-up of fragile and high risk children have reported later perceptual, learning, and behavioral problems. They present a convincing case for continued study.

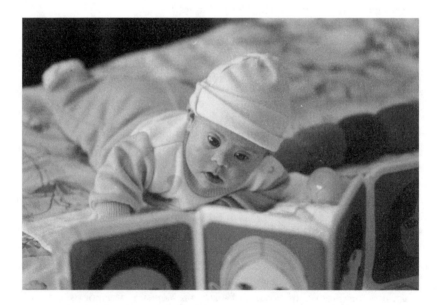

Figure 5–2 Mary Elizabeth at 3 months, weight supporting on arms

Hearing

The Auditory System

Unlike vision, the auditory system is stimulated in its development by sounds reaching the fetus in utero (e.g., maternal heartbeat, bowel sounds, placenta souffle, mother's speech, and external sounds). In normal hearing, sound waves strike the ear drum (tympanic membrane). This energy then is transmitted through three small middle ear bones, the hammer (malleus), anvil (incus), and stirrup (stapes). Vibrations along this bony chain lead to stimulation of a membrane that, in turn, transmits energy to stimulate small hairlike extensions of nerve cells in the inner ear (cochlea). This energy subsequently travels, via electrical nerve impulses (eighth cranial nerve), into the temporal portion of the brain, where sound is differentiated and interpreted. Past research has revealed that full-term newborns are able to discriminate a wide range of frequencies and intensities of auditory stimulation. They also have capacities to habituate to and block out repetitive loud stimuli.

Hearing Disorders

The causes of hearing loss in early childhood are numerous, and the mere fact that an infant has been admitted to a special care nursery increases the likelihood of impairment from 1 chance in 1,000 to 1 chance in 50 (Poland, Wells, & Ferlauto, 1980, p. 31). More particularly, Bergstrom (1980) has reported that "recently developed intensive neonatal detection methods find that 1 in 600 to 800 otherwise normal neonates has a profound congenital hearing loss and that 1 in 60 of the infants in neonatal intensive care units has such a loss" (p. 23). According to Bergstrom, other statistics suggest that approximately 25 percent of the cases of hearing loss are of a genetic etiology, another 42 percent have a nongenetic origin, and about 33 percent have unknown causes. Most nongenetic hearing impairments occur either during the 9 months of pregnancy or within the first 6 months after birth.

In 1972, a Joint Committee on Hearing Screening developed a register for screening high risk infants with potential hearing impairment. The committee cited five indicators: a family history of childhood deafness, maternal rubella during pregnancy, other intrauterine factors such as cytomegalovirus infection, hyperbilirubinemia, maxillofacial anomalies, and birthweight of 1,500 grams or less. To this list of criteria that have documented associations with early hearing loss, some authors (Poland, Wells, & Ferlauto, 1980) have added the problems of anoxia and acidosis. Today, the increased numbers of very low birthweight infants and associated conditions such as intracranial hemorrhage continue to be major determinants of impaired hearing in young children.

Identification of Hearing Problems

Although many special care nurseries still lack early screening procedures, educators and child development specialists are emphasizing the need for systematic identification programs (Cox, Hack, & Metz, 1981; Fitzhardinge, 1987; Salamy, Mendelson, Tooley, & Chaplin, 1980). Every year, pediatricians identify numbers of preschool children with significant disabilities who have gone undetected. If such losses are associated with prematurity, they usually occur in the high frequency range, with total deafness being rare.

In past years, two methods of early identification have been used fairly effectively in intensive care units. The *Crib-O-Gram* records infant reflex responses to narrow-band noise. A motion-sensitive transducer is placed beneath the crib mattress, and the level of arousal of the newborn is scored. This process is repeated several times to obtain a reliable assessment. It is estimated that the possibility for false negative results is about 4 percent and for false positive results, about 15 percent (Poland, Wells, & Ferlauto, 1980). The *brainstem auditory-evoked response* (BAER) is another tool that has been used with the preterm baby (Cox, Hack, & Metz, 1981; Salamy, Mendelson, Tooley, & Chaplin, 1980; Schulman-Galambos & Galambos, 1975). Reportedly, this is one of the most reliable and objective techniques available for assessment of neonatal auditory functioning. Until now, it has been very difficult to obtain evaluations of children younger than 2 to 3 years. BAER technology measures sensory functioning in the subcortical portions of the auditory pathway and allows for objective measurement of peripheral and brainstem auditory function (Cox, Hack, & Metz, 1981, p. 53). Schulman-Galambos and Galambos (1975) have emphasized the important advantages of this method, indicating that responses are not subject to fatigue or habituation with continued stimulation and are not influenced by stages of sleep (p. 462). Thus, it is possible to elicit consistent responses in the newborn, an area of considerable difficulty in the past with the high risk infant. Commenting on the detection of hearing loss in infancy, Poland, Wells, and Ferlauto (1980) have noted:

> It is expensive and does require a person with considerable special training if the technique is to be used reliably. Brainstem-evoked potentials, however, are probably the single most powerful tool that can be used in evaluating the hearing acuity of the hard-to-test child. The method can be used effectively for estimating the learning threshold in babies younger than six months and is also the best method available for determining the symmetry of an already established hearing loss in the child who will not wear earphones. (p. 44)

More recently, Murray (1988) has tempered and refined conclusions with respect to the use of the BAER with children under 9 months of age. Evaluating 93 high and low risk infants with normal and abnormal BAERs, she wrote:

> These findings indicate that the newborn ABR [BAER] has predictive value for developmental outcome over and above predictions that could

be made solely in the child's initial risk status. Newborns with normal and abnormal ABRs differed significantly on seven out of the 20 outcome measures after first adjusting for initial risk status. Thus, the newborn ABR may be useful for identifying which infants requiring neonatal intensive care are most likely to develop deficits and benefit from preventive intervention.

. . . both the individual and group analyses indicate the abnormalities in the newborn ABR are associated with a wider range of impairment than those specific to the auditory system. This finding is consistent with reports from the Vancouver longitudinal study (Clarke et al., 1986) in which sensorineural hearing loss was shown to be a part of a complex of neurological sequelae associated with low birthweight, postnatal illness, and extended ventilation support. (p. 1553)

In the future, new technology (the oto-acoustic response) may replace the BAER to evaluate cochlear function. In conclusion, in view of the fact that the risk of hearing impairment increases substantially with the degree of prematurity and abnormal neurologic patterns, infants who show these very early signs of hearing loss need to have follow-up with initial screening and regular audiometric evaluations.

NEUROMOTOR DEVELOPMENT

Neuromotor patterns of behavior constitute the most widely investigated area of development in the premature and high risk infant. There are obvious reasons for this level of interest. Neuromotor responses comprise the largest repertoire of early observable and well-documented behavior of the newborn. Consequently, scales and other instruments for evaluation of the infant include a fairly extensive collection of items for assessment of this dimension of development. In addition, evaluation of this range of responses generally offers the educator, clinician, and pediatrician an immediate basis for determining the current status of the preterm infant in the special care nursery, as well as the status of the very low birthweight baby and the larger neonate with other medical problems.

As we have indicated in earlier chapters, the increasing survival of smaller infants has generated much research, and this has been particularly focused on short- and long-term neuromotor behavior. It is well recognized that babies born at less than 30 weeks gestational age, weighing less than 1,500 grams, manifest developmental delays. However, given these data, there are four critical questions. How long do these problems persist? Are these babies following slower but typical patterns of development? When should we become concerned? Do certain medical insults seem to predispose babies toward lasting disabilities? These are the issues we will attempt to address relative to the extremely low birthweight infant and the moderately premature baby born between 34 and 37 weeks.

Outcome for Infants Weighing 1,500 Grams or Less

Follow-up of the premature infant has shown that very low birthweight continues to be a critical factor relative to significant neuromotor development and problems (Bennett, Chandler, Robinson, & Sells, 1981; Crowe, Deitz, Bennett, &
Tekolste, 1988; Fitzhardinge, 1987; Gorga, Stern, Ross, & Nagler, 1991; Nickel,
Bennett, & Lamson, 1982; Saigal, Rosenbaum, Stoskopf, & Milner, 1982;
Williamson, Wilson, Lifschitz, & Thurber, 1990). The prevalence of major disabling conditions has declined dramatically within the past 25 years, dropping
from an incidence of 50 to 70 percent in the 1960s to present figures of 8 to 18
percent among extremely low birthweight populations (Doyle et al., 1991; Li,
Sauve, & Creighton, 1990; Saigal, Rosenbaum, Hattersley, & Milner, 1989). Yet,
within this group of the tiniest infants, certain insults tend to be more common and
often are associated with poorer prognoses such as the occurrence of seizures,
cerebral palsy, and mental retardation. Most frequently cited are problems of
perinatal asphyxia, bronchopulmonary dysplasia, and intracranial hemorrhage—
events in which the onset, prevalence, and severity are directly related to extremely low birthweight of 500 to 1,000 grams and gestational ages of 24 to 30
weeks. Most recent studies of infants of 1,000 grams or less consistently bear out
these patterns. For example, reporting on a study conducted at New York Hospital, Cornell Medical Center, Gorga, Stern, Ross, and Nagler (1991) noted that:

> Thirty-six preterm and full-term children were seen during the first year
> of life and at 3 years old. The *Neuromotor Behavioral Inventory*
> (NBI)—Version for 3 Year Olds (a 5-category measure of Gross Motor
> and Fine Motor Development, Reaction to Movement, Neurological
> Reflexes and Reactions, and Neuromotor Outcome) was used with three
> groups: healthy preterm, sick preterm, and healthy full-term. The
> groups differed in gross motor, fine motor, reaction to movement, and
> neuromotor outcome at 3 years of age with the greatest difference be-
> tween the sick preterm group and the other groups. Quality of move-
> ment deteriorated between 12 months and 3 years. . . . Prematurity,
> perinatal illness, and frequency of unfavorable outcome during the first
> year were found to have an adverse impact on neuromotor behavior. (p.
> 102)

Similarly, Yip and Tan (1991) carried out a study of 110 very low birthweight
infants admitted to the National University of Singapore neonatal intesive care
unit (NICU) between October 1985 and January 1989 to determine the incidence
of bronchopulmonary dysplasia (BPD) within this selected population. Of the 110
infants, 32 died; the survival rate was 70.9 percent. Sixty (54.5 percent) of the 110
newborns required mechanical ventilation during the first week of life; 24 of the
60 died. Of the surviving 36 infants, 23 (64 percent) continued to require oxygen

28 days after birth and met the criteria for BPD. Two factors appeared to influence heavily the occurrence of BPD: birthweight and gestational age. All of the survivors in the group weighing 500 to 750 grams developed long-term respiratory problems, compared with 6.25 percent of the infants born at 1,240 grams or more. None of the infants delivered at more than 30 weeks gestation had BPD.

As with many of these studies, the very small numbers are not an adequate basis for firm conclusions about development, and it is nearly impossible to predict, at the outset, the particular course that any given baby will take. Parents, educators, and physicians must "wait and see" in most situations.

In addition to these findings regarding the correlation of neuromotor development with gestational age and birthweight, poor head growth appears to be another characteristic closely related to less advantageous developmental outcome (Eckerman, Sturm, & Gross, 1985; Gross, Kosmetatos, Grimes, & Williams, 1976; Lipper, Lee, Gartner, & Grellong, 1981). In particular, some researchers now make a distinction between very low birthweight babies who are merely small-for-gestational age and infants who also show small head circumference and, later, delayed neurodevelopmental outcome. Lipper and colleagues (1981) have pointed out that "small birthweight in relation to gestational age" has often been associated with a poor prognosis (p. 505). The authors suggest, however, that perhaps the key predictor is head growth retardation. These findings relative to small head size again were confirmed in a more recent study conducted by Hack and her associates (Hack, Breslau et al., 1991). An 8-year follow-up of 249 very low birthweight infants admitted to the neonatal intensive care unit at Rainbow Babies and Children's Hospital in Cleveland revealed that the 33 children with "subnormal head sizes at the age of eight months had significantly lower mean birth weights (1.1 vs. 1.2 kg) and higher neonatal risk scores (71 vs. 53) and at the age of eight years had a higher incidence of neurologic impairment (21 percent vs. 8 percent) and lower IQ scores (mean verbal, 84 vs. 98)" (p. 231).

Based on considerable data from studies of preterm and high risk newborns, it would be reasonable to assume that the astute clinician should be able to identify those babies who will have long-term and/or severe neuromotor problems. Often, such is not the case initially, with the exception of the most extreme impairments. For this reason, babies falling within the realm of severe prematurity (1,500 grams or less) and having documented high risk medical complications need to have follow-up on a periodic schedule for evaluation of neuromuscular development. In line with this strategy, experts in the field have attempted to describe typical patterns of behavior of the preterm infant and significant ways in which these patterns differ from those for the full-term baby (Carter & Campbell, 1975; Fox & Lewis, 1982; Illingsworth, 1983; Kurtzberg, Vaughan, & Daum, 1979; Palmer, Dubowitz, Verghote, & Dubowitz, 1982; Prechtl, Fargel, Weinmann, & Bakker, 1979; Saint-Anne Dargassies, 1966, 1979). Palmer, Dubowitz, Verghote, and Dubowitz (1982) have pointed out the difficulties associated with attempting to arrive at such generalizations.

> The variability of response of preterm infants was apparent in this study and has been commented on by several authors. . . . Many studies comparing preterm and full-term infants have attempted to characterize the neurological development of the preterm infant as accelerated or retarded. . . . Because of the specific problems of preterm birth and the large number of variables affecting the preterm infant we consider it impossible to characterize the preterm infant as more or less neurologically mature than the full-term but rather as different in several important respects. (p. 188)

Further addressing the issue of variability of developmental outcome, two recent studies highlight the importance of setting and individualized behavioral and environmental care in the very low birthweight premature infant. In the first piece of research, a retrospective study of all infants weighing 701 to 1,500 grams, born at 11 neonatal intensive care centers during 1983 and 1984, was carried out to determine 28-day outcomes in terms of survival and treatment without the need for supplemental oxygen (Horbar et al., 1988). Over the 2-year period, 1,776 live infants were delivered. Of the total, 85 percent (1,512 newborns) survived for a period of at least 28 days, with a range of 80 to 90 percent at individual centers (p. 554). Differences across participating units were even more significant in terms of survival without supplemental oxygen. A total of 60 percent (1,056 infants) did not require treatment by day 28, with a range of 51 to 70 percent at individual centers. The authors further indicated that "predicted survival rates varied by as much as 15% and the predicted rates for survival without supplemental oxygen varied by nearly 17% between centers with the highest and lowest rates" (p. 554). Undetected population differences and variability in techniques of obstetrical and neonatal care were cited as potential factors accounting for these irregularities.

Paralleling findings of the research by Horbar et al., Als and her colleagues examined individualized behavioral and environmental care for very low birthweight infants at risk for bronchopulmonary dysplasia (Als et al., 1986). Based on a controlled study of two groups of eight consecutively born infants randomly assigned to control and treatment groups, the authors concluded that:

> . . . in the very low birthweight, initially critically ill and premature experimental group, the individualized behavioral developmental approach to care, emphasizing from early on stress reduction and increase of self-regulating competence, may improve outcome not only medically, as shown in reduced respirator and oxygen dependency and improved feedings, but also behaviorally and developmentally, as shown in significantly better mental and motor performance as well as overall better differentiation and modulation of functioning in the first 9 months post-term. These results acknowledge the complexity and sensitivity of the early born preterm infant who is, in essence, a displaced fetus and, as such, appears keenly sensitive to all environmental impingements. The

sensitivity of the young nervous system engenders a unique opportunity for the caregiver to provide a developmentally supportive environment, rather than hazardous, stressful surroundings. We hypothesize that stress avoidance may improve developmental outcome by preventing active inhibition of CNS pathways due to inappropriate impact during a highly sensitive period of brain development. (p. 113)

Given the difficulties of prediction and well-documented variation in medical and developmental outcome as a result of complex influences, many extremely low birthweight infants (see Figure 5-3) of 28 weeks or less initially exhibit several patterns of neuromotor development that are important to monitor into at least the 3rd and 4th months after birth. For example, asymmetries of the trunk, shoulders, arms, and legs often are seen with the head turned to the right or left side.

Usually, there is a high incidence of random movement, characterized by a jerky and arrhythmic quality. Similarly, these babies startle frequently in response to any change in position or external stimulation such as the ringing of a bell or twirling of a red ring within visual range. The asymmetrical tonic neck reflex predominates, with the head turned toward the extended arm and leg, the opposite arm and leg observed in flexed positions. Often, an exaggerated Moro response is present, with extension and abduction of the arms to 180 degrees.

Neonates born prior to 32 weeks gestation are characteristi-

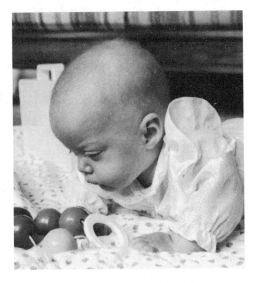

Figure 5-3 Jennifer—Born at 28 weeks gestation

cally hypotonic. but, later, one frequently sees the infant, supine or prone, in a position of full flexion of the arms and extension of the legs so that two or more extremities are off the floor. When arms and legs are moved through the passive range of motion, there often is a maximal resistance of both extremities, with only limited mobility possible. A recoil response consisting of immediate and full flexion of the arms and legs generally is present. In a prone position, infants are able to lift their heads only to a 5 to 10 degree angle, so as to clear the nose in turning from one side to the other. As might be expected, there is no evidence of weightbearing or weightshifting, as is seen within the first month or two in a full-term baby. In response to ventral suspension (the Landau reaction), these babies remain in a draped position, with the head, arms, and legs well below the horizontal plane. In either the prone or supine position, the hands are held fisted most of the time, with thumbs flexed inside the palm. When pulled to a sitting position, infants are unable to maintain the range and their heads passively hang backward. Moreover, in sitting with support, these babies make no attempt to bring their heads to an upright position, even momentarily, but passively hang forward. In addition, especially in the earliest weeks after birth, nurses and clinicians frequently observe behavioral indicators of overstimulation, such as an arching of the extremities, gaze aversion, hiccoughs, yawning (see Figure 5–4), and a furrowing of the brow, all indicating the need for decreasing or terminating interaction (Barb & Lemons, 1989; Catlett & Holditch-Davis, 1990).

By the 4th month of chronological age, most of these immature behaviors are being integrated into more typical and directed activity, and the majority of the newborn responses are seen less than 50 percent of the time or not at all. Yet, other significant milestones may remain delayed. For instance, purposeful reaching, hands-to-midline, and hand regard, which ordinarily appear in the 4th or 5th month, may not be readily evident until the 6th or 7th month of chronological age, and the skill of independent sitting may be acquired only as the baby approaches the 9th or 10th month of chronological age.

Within the full-term population, the typical range for the development of reciprocal crawling lies between 6 and 9 months of age. The severely premature baby may not reach this milestone until 10 to 12 months of age. Transitions from and into sitting usually are beginning to emerge for the full-term baby between 7 and 10 months. The preterm youngster still may have difficulty with falling at 12 months of age, and backward protective responses may not be available to these babies until a still later age of 13 to 14 months. There is much variability among full-term babies in the development of walking, some starting at an early 9 months, with others taking their first steps at 13 to 14 months. For the extremely premature baby, it is not uncommon for independent walking to be delayed until about 16 to 17 months. Once the skill is developed, on the other hand, many babies are as coordinated as their full-term counterparts.

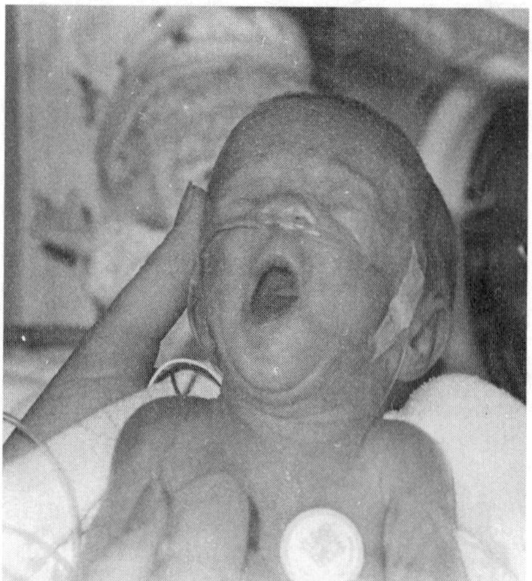

Figure 5–4 Very low birthweight infant born at 26 weeks gestation, showing signs of overstimulation (yawning)

Being able to determine problems that are surfacing requires an experienced and sensitive educator or child development specialist. For still unknown reasons, many severely premature babies between 6 and 8 months of age seem to manifest higher muscle tone than is normally found in full-term youngsters. Such symptoms naturally bear careful watching. Yet, if other skills appear to be evolving regularly within the time frame of adjusted age and without obviously atypical development, these children often perform well within the typical range of development by the time they reach their second birthday. Furthermore, whether this group of children will show signs of more subtle difficulties once they are in school is a subject of keen interest in a number of current follow-up programs (Baroni, 1991; Crowe, Deitz, Bennett, & Tekolste, 1988; Doyle et al., 1991; Forslund & Bjerre, 1990; Gardner, Karmel, Magnano, Norton, & Brown, 1990; Grögaard, Lindstrom, Parker, Culley, & Stahlman, 1990; Hoffman & Bennett, 1990; Slater, Naqvi, Andrew, & Haynes, 1987; Williamson, Wilson, Lifschitz, & Thurber, 1990). As reflected in the research described here, neurobehavioral outcome of the very low birthweight infant depends on a number of variables including the characteristics of the population studied, the site and geographic location of the neonatal intensive care unit, and the nature of medical and psychoeducational interventions used at a given nursery.

Developmental Outcome for Borderline to Moderately Premature Infants (Born at 34 to 37 Weeks of Gestation)

The infant weighing more than 1,500 grams and/or delivered at 34 weeks or more gestational age (see Figure 5–5) responds very differently from the smaller and shorter-term newborn and, in general, carries a far better prognosis for a healthy developmental outcome (Bennett, Chandler, Robinson, & Sells, 1981; Drillien, 1972; Palmer, Dubowitz, Verghote, & Dubowitz, 1982; Saint-Anne Dargassies, 1966, 1979). The "evolutionary patterns to normalization" (Saint-Anne Dargassies, 1979) are more immediate, more direct, and less guarded. Usher (1981) has commented:

> The many physiologic handicaps of the infant born 1 to 2 months prematurely can be dealt with effectively using modern therapeutic techniques. Rare prematurity-related deaths are the result of specific disease entities, either respiratory distress syndrome or severe infection. (p. 230)

Developmental outcome for the moderately preterm infant, like that for the extremely low birthweight infant, is influenced by many medical/biologic and environmental considerations. In addition, more and more child development specialists, educators, and psychologists are recognizing the fact that high risk infants who appear to be free of developmental problems at one point in their infant and preschool years may show learning disabilities later when they are in school.

Moreover, research on the predictions of developmental status of the moderately premature baby, overall, has been less consistent than follow-up of the extremely low birthweight infant. Study findings are complicated by inadequate descriptions of subject populations, in which outcome varies markedly as a result of whether or not infants are appropriate-for-gestational age or small-for-gestational age (Cassady & Strange, 1987; Fitzhardinge, 1987). While the "light-for-dates" baby has been found to be at risk for neurologic and behavioral problems, the severity of these difficulties depends on the specific cause and degree of impaired growth (Cassady & Strange, 1987). Generally, however, the prognosis is good in terms of the absence of major disabilities.

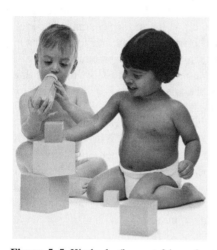

Figure 5–5 Kimberly (born at 34 weeks gestation) and Dale

Infants appropriate-for-gestational age who are born at 34 weeks or later may manifest some variations in neuromotor development such as problems with feeding as a result of poor sucking ability, but usually they do not suffer the severe complications and delays seen in the extremely premature baby. Typically, both the quality and rate of development within the first 18 months is much less adversely affected than that of the extremely low birthweight neonate. Notably, the baby delivered between 34 and 37 weeks gestation is not troubled with the excessive random and tremulous movement and extremes in flexion and extension tone that are markedly apparent with the severely premature baby. Major milestones such as reaching, transferring objects (see Figure 5–6), rolling, sitting, crawling, and standing may be delayed, but, often if there are no other significant complications, these milestones lag by periods of only 4 to 6 weeks. Obviously, the earlier the gestational age and the lower the birthweight, the greater the gap between the observed and the normal. In addition, typical newborn behaviors such as the Moro response, asymmetrical tonic neck reflex, fisted hands, and the placing foot response may be a bit more exaggerated in the initial stages and persist by 2 to 4 weeks longer than these behaviors in a typical population of full-term babies. However, in our experience, by 6 to 8 months of chronological age, premature youngsters delivered at 34 to 37 weeks gestation reveal no greater variation than do infants born at 38 to 41 weeks. Saint-Anne Dargassies (1979) has suggested:

The pediatrician who is responsible for the developmental follow-up of children born prematurely must know that normalization is seldom rapid (only 16%), or belated (i.e., at the age of 3 years). Normalization occurs between age one and age two in 64% of cases. But the preliminary signs should be known; the child must begin to emerge from its pathological condition at about 6 months in some cases, more often at about 9 months. (p. 243)

Moreover, clinicians should be alert to warning signs when reflexes or variations in muscle tone persist beyond expected periods, given the degree of prematurity. In such cases, babies need to have appropriate follow-up and receive services as necessary.

MENTAL DEVELOPMENT

Data on the long-term effects of prematurity on mental development do not lead to clear-cut conclusions. Furthermore, accurate predictions about future development in the areas of language and cognition are difficult

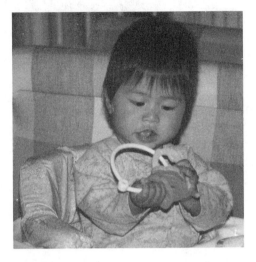

Figure 5–6 Olivia transferring a rattle from hand to hand

to make because they are a function of many factors. Today, despite the overwhelming medical problems of preterm and high risk infants, professionals who work with and follow the development of such groups often agree that the influence of home experiences after discharge, in most situations, far outweighs the impact of hospitalization and initial impairment. One needs only to spend time with families and young children to understand why this is the case. Some parents constantly talk to their babies, encouraging them to pay attention, to survey their environment, to vocalize, to explore, and to problem solve. Within the first year to 18 months, these mothers, fathers, and siblings are well involved in looking at books (see Figure 5–7), reading, and sampling the rich experiences of words and the symbolic world with the newest family member. Other parents are more subdued in their approach—sometimes stifling the young inquiring mind or not knowing how to help it grow toward fulfillment. In a lifetime, these differences make a difference, and the data on language and cognitive development exemplify this observation.

Language of the High Risk Infant

In the normal course of events, infants develop very early a diverse repertoire of behavior for communicating with their immediate environment. They cry to make

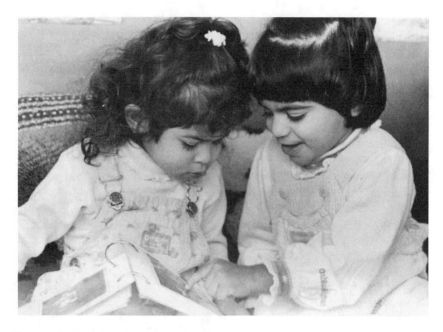

Figure 5–7 Ali and Lindsey reading together

their needs known. Usually within the first month, they smile in response to soft voices and familiar faces, particularly those of the primary caregiver. They can be soothed and quieted by being held, walked, and patted or by the voice of a significant family member, frequently the mother. Their vocalizations may increase or decrease in response to external stimulation such as a schematic or doll face or in response to soft talking of a familiar person. While the infant pays attention to an object or person, sucking patterns may be interrupted for brief periods of high interest and visual scanning. Typically, infants react by eye blinking, eye widening, or startle to the ringing of a bell, and by the 5th or 6th month they are able to determine the direction of a sound. The infant begins to coo and to make differentiated short vowel sounds within the first 2 months. These sounds are followed later by initial consonant sounds such as "g," "b," "d," "p," "m," and "n." Vocal play with repetitive sounds, yells, laughs, and squeals increases through the first 6 months, although there is much variability in the amount and type of vocalization among babies. Some are spontaneously verbal when alone, while others respond more directly to personal interaction. By 7 months, babies are beginning to make two-syllable repetitions such as "da-da" and "ma-ma," and as they reach 12 to 14 months, they should be using one or two of these words in appropriate context. Often at this age, babies also want to sit with a book to look at pictures, jabbering, and pointing as they turn the pages.

Between 15 and 24 months, typical development of speech and language accelerates. Toddlers begin to involve themselves in a great deal of symbolic play with dishes, dolls, and other favorite toys. They can follow one direction by 19 months, and often say "bye-bye" when putting on a hat and coat. Some children even have a gross sense of time at this age and begin to look for Mommy and Daddy at a certain hour of the day in day-care or baby-sitting situations. By 19 months, too, they should have an expanding vocabulary of 20 to 35 words. They point to body parts on themselves and on a doll and can name pictures of familiar people in a photograph. By 19 to 20 months, babies typically are beginning to put together two- or three-word sentences such as "more juice" or "juice all gone." As he or she approaches the second birthday, the child should be able to select two or three objects correctly from a familiar series such as a ball, shoe, spoon, or cup.

Research on the development of speech and language in the very low birthweight baby seems to bear out evidence of consistent delays in language development (Casiro, Moddemann, Stanwick, & Cheang, 1991; Field, Dempsey, & Shumar, 1981; Fitzhardinge & Pape, 1981; Janowsky & Nass, 1987; Knobeloch & Kanoy, 1982; Landry, Schmidt, & Richardson, 1989; Vohr, Garcia-Coll, & Oh, 1989). Without question, problems stem from different factors at varying stages. Initially, the rate of development is more directly related to the predominant effects of prematurity and other medically related variables, such as the duration of intubation, evidence of Grades 3 or 4 intraventricular hemorrhage, or occurrence of apnea and asphyxia. Later, experience and the environment appear to play a major role in language developmental outcome (Parker, Greer, & Zuckerman, 1988).

The interface between biological and psychosocial factors is clearly reflected in the frequent observation that infants with severe medical complications in the early months after birth, given a facilitating environment, may manifest fewer problems than children with lesser initial insults who suffer adverse family situations.

In our experience, specific patterns of development among extremely premature babies may take the following course. For example, it is common for the very low birthweight infant to make few sounds other than high-pitched crying up to the 4th or 5th month and to experience frequent periods of irritability, so that it is difficult to assess differentiation of the infant's needs. Furthermore, the social smile in response to the familiar voice of the mother and father may not appear until the 4th month, which is a source of great frustration to parents.

In the absence of obvious neurologic insults, the appearance of vocal play, reduplicated and variegated babbling, and first words usually follow a typical pattern of development, but both the onset and frequency of behavior often are depressed. This situation appears to be especially prevalent among boys. Although some studies have not revealed such differences in middle and upper income families (Aram, Hack, Hawkins, Weissman, & Borawski-Clark, 1991), without the direct attention and intervention of the parents or primary caregivers in facilitating these skills and abilities, babies may continue to manifest significant delays up to 25 months of age. Perhaps this is one of the reasons that, over the first 3 years, in our experience, neuromotor lags typically seem less persistent in comparison with the emergence of delayed communicative skills.

The point at which an early intervention program should be initiated is a difficult clinical judgment. Professionals should not overreact, and certainly if a toddler is beginning to use even a few familiar words appropriately at about 20 months, there is justification for cautious expectations that the child will achieve a normal range of performance by 3 years. Such hopes probably are warranted if delays are uncomplicated by symptoms of excessive drooling, feeding difficulties, tongue thrusting, hearing impairment, or other obvious abnormalities. On the other hand, if a child appears frustrated in not being able to communicate, does not appear to understand what is said, and lacks a minimal level of intelligible expressive language of a few words, assistance before age 3 is indicated. There are, of course, differing points of view on these issues, some professionals taking a conservative approach, and merely waiting. We differ with this position because language is so crucial to later learning and school performance. If the cooperation of parents can be enlisted in the face of early developmental lags, problems frequently can be ameliorated or at least greatly minimized. We have seen dramatic changes in young children born at risk, given the benefit of formal programing and family support.

To make reasonable judgments about early intervention, we suggest the following guidelines:

- Evaluate the quality and level of home interaction with the child and offer directed guidance to the parents.
- If gains in patterns of communication begin to surface, perhaps further intervention is not necessary.
- If such gains are not observed, however, families should usually seek additional assistance.

The optimistic side of this discussion is that, although many very low birthweight children, at 24 months, reveal serious speech and language delays, research indicates that for a "good portion of children, the speech defect is temporary and is not apparent by school age" (Fitzhardinge, 1987, p. 410), in the absence of more global mental retardation or other complications. This statement is reinforced by the findings of Aram and her colleagues (1991), who compared the speech and language development of 249 very low birthweight and 363 normal birthweight 8-year-olds, randomly sampled in a geographic area. The authors concluded that:

> . . . the present study suggests that at 8 years of age, specific language impairment, as defined and measured here, is no more frequent among VLBW children. The major qualification to this finding is, however, the

acknowledgment by these authors that within the population of very low birthweight children, there still remains a higher incidence of language deficits and delays that are "accompanied" by more generalized developmental problems including reduced IQ, hearing loss, and/or major neurological abnormalities. (p. 1179)

Cognitive Skills of the Preterm Infant

By far, the overwhelming numbers of studies on the cognitive or mental development of preterm populations have been based on general standardized measures such as the *Denver Developmental Screening Test*, the *Gesell Scales*, the *Bayley Scales of Infant Development*, or at latter stages, the *Stanford-Binet Intelligence Scale*, the *Wechsler Preschool and Primary Scale of Intelligence*, and the *Wechsler Intelligence Scale for Children* (Fitzhardinge, 1987; Gibbs, 1990). In recent years, efforts to analyze specific components of cognitive competence have changed (Odom & Karnes, 1988), and these investigations are sorely needed in order to gain a better understanding of the wide range of abilities that constitute infant cognition, the significance of diversity among high risk populations, and the long-term implications. With the intense interest in growing populations of extremely low birthweight infants, follow-up studies have escalated over the past decade. Nevertheless, as Kopp (1987) has pointed out:

Despite numerous new studies, the overall gain in recent knowledge has been modest. It is absolutely clear, for example, that virtually any group of infants who are at risk and who are studied with virtually any paradigm will show some variation in behavior (sometimes a lot, sometimes just a bit) when compared with normally developing, non-risk infants. *But it is not at all clear when and how these differences are developmentally meaningful for the short and for the long term.* (p. 882)

In the areas of language, motor, and sensory skill development, we have discussed the fact that the preterm infant initially and sometimes thereafter may differ significantly from the full-term baby. Our experience has led us to similar conclusions with respect to cognitive functioning. During the first 12 months of life, infants ordinarily make remarkable progress toward knowledge of the world about them. This process starts with the objects and the people closest at hand and takes place through mutual and regular daily interaction. Babies by 4 months of age (Olson, 1981) learn to distinguish their parents and siblings from other individuals. They tend to smile more in response to the familiar face of their mother and can be soothed by her comforting when all other attempts prove unsuccessful. Within the first 2 to 3 months, infants are especially attracted to bright contrasting colors such as yellow and red, and gaze for sustained periods of 2 minutes or more at novel patterns and schematic faces. By 4 months, babies are beginning to reach for rattles and other attractive objects held at midline and may make gross attempts to grasp them. However, the skill of following objects held and dropped or looking for partially covered playthings will not be acquired until the 5th or 6th month. Typically, babies become more socially interactive at this stage—laughing and gaining enjoyment from games such as "Peek-A-Boo." Increasingly, they become aware that objects can be manipulated, transferred, and banged, and they do so with spoons, blocks, rattles, and other materials small enough to hold. Also at this age, they begin to search for objects that are partially covered and understand that toys can be pulled toward them with an attached string.

The period from 6 to 12 months is a stage of rapid physical growth, active exploration, and the appearance of several critical milestones. By 7 to 8 months, babies are capable of responding to hand clapping with imitation or, on verbal command, to "Patty-Cake." They can be taught to throw a ball reciprocally and are interested in more independent hand-to-mouth activities, such as self-feeding with Cheerios and other table foods. Two months later, the skill of object permanence is well established. Babies search for toys dropped or completely hidden. They play with containers, taking objects out of canisters or dishes and putting them back. Some children at 9 to 10 months are beginning to develop a basic cause-and-effect relationship with pop-up and musical toys. Finally, the child near his or her first birthday begins to evidence simple problem-solving skills. For example, if Cheerios are hidden behind a plexiglass screen, the 12-month-old child is able to figure out how to retrieve these attractive bits successfully. Likewise, if raisins are placed in toy milk cartons, the child typically attempts several strategies by probing, dumping, or pouring. Basic round block recognition, too, is seen at this age, although for some youngsters this skill is not evident consistently until 13 to 14 months.

From 15 months to the end of the second year, the development of language and cognition are closely intertwined. These abilities, coupled with an emerging social autonomy, dramatically change the ways in which the now skillful toddler relates to the immediate environment (see Figures 5–8, 5–9, and 5–10). The child makes his or her needs known by telling someone. Most youngsters at this age have a desire to feed and dress themselves and like to play dress-up. They know their own names well and those of friends with whom they associate daily. They can demonstrate the utility of many common objects, such as a toothbrush, comb, tissues, or play dishes. They have a basic comprehension of how puzzles fit together and can place two or three pieces successfully. Light switches and other gadgets are a great fascination and a wonderful source of amusement. With amazing dexterity, 20- to 24-month-old children understand how to get to what they want, whether or not an object is within apparent grasp. In part, this capacity is a result of new opportunities open to the toddler, as he or she develops a firmer grasp of cause-and-effect relationships. The world has now become a place where the child can act more independently in the environment without repeated demonstration.

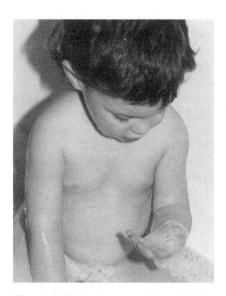

Figure 5–8 Matthew examining bubbles of his bath

The preterm infant and toddler present a very different pattern of behavior, especially if the child has sustained an insult of prematurity of less than 28 to 30 weeks gestation. Wide variations from the norm are seen in the initial capacity of the severely low birthweight baby to respond to any stimuli, which frequently prove disruptive. The simple task of focusing on a directed object or face for a period of 1 to 5 seconds may elude the infant within the first 2 to 3 months of life. As a result, it is not surprising that such a child does not actively survey the immediate surroundings, as the full-term baby does at 6 to 8 weeks. Likewise, attempts to search for partially or fully covered objects or efforts to play appropriately with pull toys are delayed by several weeks. Some of this disparity may be a function of physical limitations, but even among babies of 34 to 35 weeks gestation who are able to sit at 6 months, a lack of awareness of objects that are out of sight is not uncommon.

How young children manipulate objects tells us a great deal about their cognitive level of understanding. Instead of interest in playing with two or more toys, banging, or attention to detail—milestones usually evident between 5 and 6 months—the preterm baby may be content even beyond the 8th or 9th month only to hold a toy and mouth it. Play with cars, books, and problem-solving toys such as pop-up and musical boxes similarly may be reduced to mouthing or to play that lacks purposeful behavior. These observations often accompany delays in symbolic language development. Finally, the constructive placing and stacking of nesting or

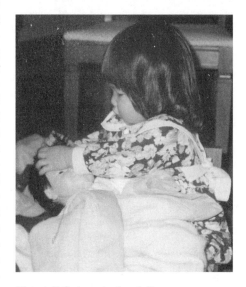

Figure 5–9 Ana playing dolls

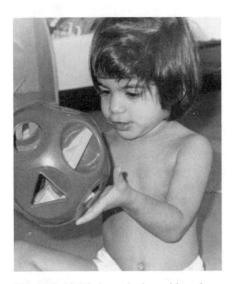

Figure 5–10 Lindsey playing with a shape sorter at 18 months

concentric cups, discrimination of round block shapes, and scribbling with crayons which are expected in the 11- to 12-month-old child, typically appear 4 to 6 months later in the severely premature toddler. Taking the place of more refined skills, banging is the primary source of play and satisfaction.

The cognitive development of the premature baby raises a number of critical issues and remains, to date, a fertile area for study. In the total pattern of growth and later school performance, delays of 6 to 8 weeks may not be significant enough to upset the timetable of acquisition and organization on a permanent basis. Within the normal population, full-term children without insult at or before birth vary widely in skill development, and we should expect no less among babies at risk. On the other hand, we know that the severely preterm infant is unable to focus on persons and surroundings and interact in a sustained and coherent way, often for extended periods of several weeks or months. As long as this condition persists, milestones such as recognition of object permanence and cause-and-effect relationships, as well as problem solving and other dimensions of cognition may continue to be delayed.

Much research now is being done in medical centers across the country to determine the effect and appropriateness of early stimulation in intensive care nurseries. Such studies should shed light on the development of cognition in the premature baby in relation to gestational age at birth, birthweight, and varying medical conditions. Thus far, the results are sparse and inconclusive. Presently in question are such issues as the substance of effective intervention, optimal gestational ages and duration for stimulation, the impact on various aspects of infant behavior, and effective ways of intervening with parents of high risk babies in home settings. As we begin to answer a few of these questions prospectively, some of the concerns and enigmas about cognitive development in the high risk infant—in terms of why some children do better than others—can be examined more closely. Certainly, we know from the substantial body of research on "disadvantaged" youngsters that a large part of the puzzle involves families, the nature of their interactions, and the ways in which they offer appropriate stimulation for their babies.

To date, the question of whether the incidence of cognitive delays has increased, decreased, or remained the same in the face of improved mortality rates is an extremely controversial and unresolved issue of high interest in the fields of neonatology, child development, and education (Escobar, Littenberg, & Petitti, 1991; Hack, Horbar et al., 1991; Lowe & Papile, 1990; Luchi, Bennett, & Jackson, 1991; Resnick et al., 1992; Saigal, Szatmari, Rosenbaum, Campbell, & King, 1991; Schmidt & Wedig, 1990; The Victorian Infant Collaborative Study Group, 1991). Numerous factors have influenced widely variant findings. These factors include the following:

- sample size
- characteristics of neonates in the particular sample(s)
- sites of NICUs involved in the research
- timing of evaluations in the life span of the children
- duration of follow-up
- methods and measures for determining developmental outcome
- definitions of delay used in the research and degrees of correction for prematurity
- rapidly changing technologies in medical treatment of the infant at risk.

Illustrating these points, Escobar, Littenberg, and Petitti (1991) have published the conclusions of a meta-analysis of outcome studies of very low birthweight infants (less than 1,500 grams). After a search of 1,136 published English language references, 161 outcome studies that met the authors' criteria for inclusion were grouped into 111 article clusters. This meta-analysis revealed several interesting results (pp. 209–210):

1. The data base was very small. Studies reported data for only 26,000 babies over a 30-year period. (Each year 4 million infants are born in the United States alone.)
2. The data bases of vital statistics across studies were not comparable.
3. Most studies presented outcome data on follow-up of less than 3 years. This point is especially important in view of another finding that the reported incidence of disability was higher among those studies with longer follow-up programs.
4. The authors' best estimate for the incidence of disability among very low birthweight infants was approximately 25 percent.
5. Most striking was the finding that the incidence of disability reported in studies from the United States was substantially higher (by about 50 percent) than the incidence reported in studies conducted in other countries. The authors discussed this conclusion in light of such differences being a reflection of variations in health care technology or delivery around the world, differences in definitions of disability across countries, or differences in the physiology or mortality of very low birthweight neonates in various centers.

6. Finally, the authors emphasized that, since the 1960s, there has been surprisingly little improvement in the ways in which research has been conducted.

In conclusion, despite dramatic changes in saving infants with complicated medical histories, it is still very difficult to know how survivors of NICU experiences are "faring."

PSYCHOSOCIAL DEVELOPMENT

Within the first few hours of life, babies begin to interact with persons of their immediate environment in ways that are mutually satisfying to infant and caregiver. The subsequent unfolding of these relationships thus becomes the building block of infant social cognition and later personality development (see Figures 5–11 and 5–12). The crying newborn can be brought to a quiet state by one or both parents almost instantly. In response to a familiar voice, the infant typically reacts with a noticeable change in activity level, some babies becoming very still and others showing a dramatic increase in their rate of movement. By 3 to 6 months, the alert and socially attentive baby plays and skillfully anticipates parental interaction by smiling, cooing, and expressing obvious excitement. Sometime between the 6th and 9th month, babies clearly become distressed by the presence of a nonfamily member or by separation of any kind from mother or father. The degree to which such stranger anxiety persists is variable in duration and intensity and frequently is difficult to cope with; yet, it is a healthy sign in the overall schema of psychosocial development and usually diminishes by the beginning of the 10th month.

The period extending from the first to the second year is marked by a growing awareness of the child's affective world and social autonomy. Youngsters, for instance, may cry in reaction to verbal reprimands or expressions of anger directed toward others or themselves. Playful teasing with games of "Hide and Seek" is common. Sometime after the end of the first year, the child learns well the meaning and use of the word "No." Usually, toddlers look to their mothers and fathers for reinforcement and censoring of their behavior. Indeed, before "the act," many children seem fully aware that their behavior may draw a negative response and appear *intent* on testing the limits of their freedom. In a similarly positive fashion, the 21-month-old child may reveal innermost desires of acquisition by responding "*Thank you*," before claiming an attractive object. Finally, the 24-month-old child understands and uses, at will, the giving and withholding of affection with people, as well as with toy dolls and favorite animals. The toddler is able to delay immediate wants, if only for a few seconds, and, with some verbal reassurance, comprehends the fact that the parent will return before long. The child now is prepared to interact more fully with peers and adults and to meet the world with an unbridled curiosity and quest for learning that brings new knowledge and insight day by day.

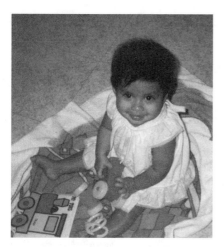

Figure 5–11 Helen at 9 months, smiling at her mother

As a whole, the development of motor abilities, language, cognition, and psychosocial skills has superbly equipped the young child to accomplish this task.

For the high risk infant, the course of psychosocial development is as variable as in full-term populations, but, as we have discussed, distinguishing trends repeatedly are cited in the literature. Our discussions have centered primarily around the earliest patterns of social awareness and interaction of the preterm and high risk infant after hospital discharge. In this context, irritability and inattentiveness commonly have characterized behaviors of the premature newborn. Moreover, certain medical centers have carried out follow-up programs and have reported that the incidence of child abuse is high. Researchers have speculated that events may be closely linked to problems of bonding and the extraordinary demands of caring for preterm and high risk infants in the early weeks and months of life (Field, 1987; Landry, Chapieski, Richardson, Palmer, & Hall, 1990; Riese, 1988).

As we have visited and worked with families, we too have observed stress and sometimes discord between caregiver and child. It is not uncommon for these difficulties to persist throughout the first 5 months. On the other hand, our evaluations of a comparison group of full-term babies has rendered us a firm basis for a second judgment; that group is by no means free from problems of frequent irritability, which may occur from six to a dozen times a day or continuously from the afternoon into the evening hours. More importantly, for both high risk and full-term babies, these troublesome events usually have passed by 6 months of age. Continuation of such behavior beyond this age may suggest other underlying medical or environmental contributors that require closer scrutiny.

The preterm baby experiences delays in social and emotional develop-

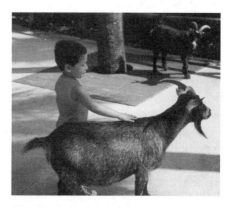

Figure 5–12 Stephen at a game farm socially interacting with his environment

ment that parallel the milestones in other areas of development. Thus, for example, we have frequently observed strong anxiety reactions in babies of less than 32 weeks gestation, which begin to be manifested at about the 9th or 10th month or later and last until the first birthday. Again, in our 2-year follow-up program with selected babies, we did not see persistent negative effects. What *is* certain are the pervasive hazards of some environments and the acceleration of these difficulties throughout the preschool years. Furthermore, as our research has taken us into homes over the past 15 years, we have been truly impressed with the consistency of psychosocial patterns within families among siblings who were not even the target of our study. Our work has led us to believe that the progress of social and emotional growth is much more inherent in the child's home setting than contingent on the early prematurity or the nature of the particular medical insult. The togetherness of families, the affection expressed toward children, the consistency of behavioral management, the use of positive rather than negative discipline, and the appropriateness of parental expectations are a few of the factors—irrespective of income or educational level—that influence psychosocial development in negative or positive directions.

In combination with characteristics of arrhythmicity, low adaptability and low persistence during the toddler and preschool years (Schraeder & Tobey, 1989), and delays in stability of temperament during the first 24 months in very low birthweight children (Riese, 1988), persistent dysfunctional relationships specific to this high risk population are not surprising. Much research still remains to be done before some basic questions about the development of infant affective disturbances can be answered. Circumstances carry varying degrees of impact on individual children at different stages. For instance, is discord or asynchrony of behavior between parent and child more devastating at particular periods of development than at others? Are such disturbances long term? What are the resolving or mediating factors or events for families and children? The introduction of substance abuse of parents and behavioral disorganization of infants adds another layer of complexity to the task of sorting out issues and understanding how best to intervene in cycles of disturbance. Studies examining infant attentiveness and positive affect modulated by mother and father behavior in interactive coaching studies (Field, 1987) hold considerable promise for learning about ways in which to help parents in reading the cues of their children, to respond appropriately, to offer nurturing feedback, and to foster in their young children a growing sense of social and emotional competence. The concept of the Individual Family Service Plan of PL 99-457 (Part H) and emerging infant-toddler assessment measures focused on family-child interaction clearly distinguish the priority of continued study of healthy psychosocial development.

In summary, there is a wealth of information available on the sensory, motor, and psychological development of the preterm and high risk infant. At present, the data suggest a higher incidence of developmental problems among infants weigh-

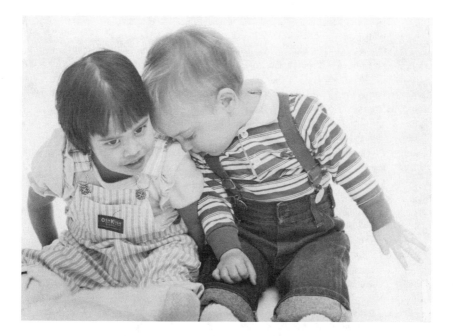

Figure 5–13 Kimberly and Dale at 18 months

ing less than 1,500 grams or born at less than 28 to 30 weeks gestation. However, noteworthy among these studies are prevalent exceptions and the candid acknowledgment of researchers that it is very difficult at the earliest stages of treatment and recovery to make unqualified predictions. There are few medical conditions for which the type and severity of developmental difficulty can be specified unquestionably. In the process of growing, environment and experience make the critical difference, especially for the young child born early. Parents share a lasting frustration because they want guarantees. There are none! On the other hand, families consistently are revealing great hope for the tiniest and most critically ill newborns. Should impairments surface with some of these children, we have the secure knowledge that such variations are not as limiting as they might have been, given a loving home with parents who care and know how to spend quality time with their babies and young children.

BIBLIOGRAPHY

Als, H., Lawhon, G., Brown, E., Gibes, R., Duffy, F.H., McAnulty, G., & Blickman, J.G. (1986). Individualized behavioral and environmental care for the very low birth weight preterm infant at high risk for bronchopulmonary dysplasia: Neonatal intensive care unit and developmental outcome. *Pediatrics*, *78*(6), 1123–1132.

Aram, D.M., Hack, M., Hawkins, S., Weissman, B.M., & Borawski-Clark, E. (1991). Very-low-birthweight children and speech and language development. *Journal of Speech and Hearing Research, 34,* 1169–1179.

Barb, S.A., & Lemons, P.K. (1989). The premature infant: Toward improving neurodevelopmental outcome. *Neonatal Network, 7*(6), 7–15.

Baroni, M.A. (1991). Apparent life-threatening events during infancy: A follow-up study of subsequent growth and development. *Developmental and Behavioral Pediatrics, 12*(3), 154–161.

Bennett, F.C., Chandler, L.S., Robinson, N.M., & Sells, C.J. (1981). Spastic diplegia in premature infants. *American Journal of Diseases in Children, 135,* 732–737.

Bergstrom, L. (1980). Causes of severe hearing loss in early childhood. *Pediatric Annals, 9,* 23–30.

Brazelton, T.B. (1984). *Neonatal behavioral assessment scale*, 2nd ed. Spastics International Medical Publications Clinics in Developmental Medicine Monograph, no. *88.* Cambridge, MA: Blackwell Scientific Publications.

Carter, R.E., & Campbell, S.K. (1975). Early neuromuscular development of the premature infant. *Physical Therapy, 55,* 1332–1341.

Casiro, O.G., Moddemann, D.M., Stanwick, R.S., & Cheang, M.S. (1991). A natural history and predictive value of early language delays in very low birthweight infants. *Early Human Development, 26,* 45–50.

Cassady, G., & Strange, M. (1987). The small-for-gestational age (SGA) infant. In G.B. Avery (Ed.), *Neonatology: Pathophysiology and management of the newborn* (3rd ed.) (pp. 299–331). Philadelphia: J.B. Lippincott.

Catlett, A.J., & Holditch-Davis, D. (1990). Environmental stimulation of the acutely ill premature infant: Physiological effects and nursing implications. *Neonatal Network, 8*(6), 19–26.

Cox, C., Hack, M., & Metz, D. (1981). Brainstem-evoked audiometry: Normative data from the preterm infant. *Audiology, 20,* 53–64.

Crowe, T.K., Deitz, J.C., Bennett, F.C., & Tekolste, K. (1988). Preschool motor skills of children born prematurely and not diagnosed as having cerebral palsy. *Developmental and Behavioral Pediatrics, 9*(4), 189–193.

DeGangi, G.A., & Greenspan, S.I. (1988). The development of sensory functions in infants. *Physical and Occupational Therapy in Pediatrics, 8*(4), 21–33.

Doyle, L.W., Kitchen, W.H., Ford, G.W., Rickards, A.L., Kelly, E.A., Callanan, C., Raven, J., & Olinsky, A. (1991). Outcome to eight years of infants less than 1,000-g birthweight: Relationship with neonatal ventilator and oxygen therapy. *Journal of Pediatrics and Child Health, 27,* 184–188.

Drillien, C.M. (1972). Etiology and outcome in low birthweight infants. *Developmental Medicine and Child Neurology, 14,* 563–574.

Dubowitz, L.M.S., Dubowitz, V., & Morante, A. (1980). Visual function in the newborn: A study of preterm and full-term infants. *Brain and Development, 2,* 15–27.

Eckerman, C.O., Sturm, L.A., & Gross, S.J. (1985). Developmental courses for very-low-birthweight infants differing in early head growth. *Developmental Psychology, 21,* 813–827.

Escobar, G.J., Littenberg, B., & Petitti, D.B. (1991). Outcome among surviving very low birthweight infants: A meta-analysis. *Archives of Disease in Childhood, 66,* 204–211.

Fantz, R.L., & Fagan, J.F., III. (1975). Visual attention to size and number of pattern details by term and preterm infants during the first six months. *Child Development, 46,* 3–18.

Fiedler, A.R., Robinson, J., Shaw, D.E., Ng, Y.K., & Moseley, M.J. (1992). Light and retinopathy of prematurity. Does retinal location offer a clue? *Pediatrics, 89*(4), 648–653.

Field, T. (1987). Affective and interactive disturbances in infants. In J.D. Osofsky (Ed.), *Handbook of infant development* (2nd ed.) (pp. 972–1005). New York: John Wiley & Sons.

Field, T., Dempsey, J., & Shumar, H. (1981). Developmental follow-up of pre-term and post-term infants. In S. Friedman & M. Sigman (Eds.), *Preterm birth and psychological development* (pp. 299–312). New York: Academic Press.

Fitzhardinge, P.M. (1987). Follow-up studies of the high-risk newborn. In G.B. Avery (Ed.), *Neonatology: Pathophysiology and management of the newborn.* (3rd ed.) (pp. 400–417). Philadelphia: J.B. Lippincott.

Fitzhardinge, P.M., & Pape, K.E. (1981). Follow-up studies of the high risk newborn. In G.B. Avery (Ed.), *Neonatology: Pathophysiology and management of the newborn* (2nd ed.) (pp. 350–367). Philadelphia: J.B. Lippincott.

Forslund, M., & Bjerre, I. (1990). Follow-up of preterm children: II. Growth and development at four years of age. *Early Human Development, 24,* 107–118.

Fox, N., & Lewis, M. (1982). Motor asymmetrics in preterm infants: Effects of prematurity and illness. *Developmental Psychobiology, 15,* 19–23.

Friendly, D.S. (1987). Eye disorders in the neonate. In G.B. Avery (Ed.), *Neonatology: Pathophysiology and management of the newborn.* (3rd. ed.) (pp. 1298–1316). Philadelphia: J.B. Lippincott.

Gardner, J.M., Karmel, B.Z., Magnano, C.L., Norton, K.I., & Brown, E.G. (1990). Neurobehavioral indicators of early brain insult in high risk neonates. *Developmental Psychology, 26*(4), 565–575.

Gibbs, E.D. (1990). Assessment of infant mental ability: Conventional tests and issues of prediction. In E.D. Gibbs & D.M. Teti (Eds.), *Interdisciplinary assessment of infants: A guide for early intervention professionals* (pp. 77–89). Baltimore: Paul H. Brookes.

Gorga, D., Stern, F.M., Ross, G., & Nagler, W. (1991). The neuromotor behavior of preterm and full-term children by three years of age: Quality of movement and viability. *Developmental and Behavioral Pediatrics, 12*(2), 102–107.

Grögaard, J.B., Lindstrom, D.P., Parker, R.A., Culley, B., & Stahlman, M.T. (1990). Increased survival rate in very low birth weight infants (1500 grams or less): No association with increased incidence of handicaps. *Journal of Pediatrics, 117*(1, Pt. 1), 139–146.

Gross, S.J., Kosmetatos, N., Grimes, C.T., & Williams, M.L. (1976). Newborn head size and neurological status: Predictor of growth and development of low birthweight infants. *American Journal of Diseases of Children, 132,* 753–756.

Hack, M.B., Breslau, N., Weissman, B., Aram, D., Klein, N., & Borawski, E. (1991). Effect of very low birth weight and subnormal head size on cognitive abilities at school age. *The New England Journal of Medicine, 325*(4), 231–236.

Hack, M., Horbar, J.D., Malloy, M.H., Tyson, J.E., Wright, E., & Wright, L. (1991). Very low birth weight outcomes of the National Institute of Child Health and Human Development Neonatal Network. *Pediatrics, 87*(5), 587–597.

Hoffman, E.L., & Bennett, F.C. (1990). Birthweight less than 800 grams: Changing outcomes and influences of gender and gestation number. *Pediatrics, 86*(1), 27–34.

Horbar, J.D., McAuliffe, T.L., Adler, S.M., Albersheim, S., Cassady, G., Edwards, W., Jones, R., Kattwinkel, J., Kraybill, E.N., Krishnan, V., Raschko, P., & Wilkinson, A.R. (1988). Variability in 28-day outcomes for very low birth weight infants: An analysis of 11 neonatal intensive care units. *Pediatrics, 82*(5), 554–559.

Illingsworth, R.S. (1983). *The development of the infant and young child: Normal and abnormal* (8th ed.). New York: Churchill Livingstone.

Janowsky, J.S., & Nass, R. (1987). Early language development in infants with cortical and subcortical perinatal brain injury. *Developmental and Behavioral Pediatrics, 8*(1), 3–7.

Knobeloch, C., & Kanoy, R.C. (1982). Hearing and language development in high risk and normal infants. *Applied Research in Mental Retardation, 3,* 293–301.

Kopp, C.B. (1987). Developmental risk: Historical reflections. In J.D. Osofsky (Ed.), *Handbook of infant development* (2nd ed.) (pp. 881–912). New York: John Wiley & Sons.

Kurtzberg, D., Vaughan, H.G., Jr., & Daum, C. (1979). Neurobehavioral performance of low birthweight infants at 40 weeks conceptual age: Comparison with normal full-term infants. *Developmental Medicine and Child Neurology, 21,* 590–607.

Landry, S.H., Chapieski, M.L., Richardson, M.A., Palmer, J., & Hall, S. (1990). The social competence of children born prematurely: Effects of medical complications and parent behaviors. *Child Development, 61,* 1605–1616.

Landry, S.H. Schmidt, M., & Richardson, M.A. (1989). The effects of intraventricular hemorrhage on functional communication skills in preterm toddlers. *Developmental and Behavioral Pediatrics, 10*(6), 299–306.

Li, A.K., Sauve, R.S., & Creighton, D.E. (1990). Early indicators of learning problems in high-risk children. *Developmental and Behavioral Pediatrics, 11*(1), 1–6.

Lipper, E., Lee, K., Gartner, L.M., & Grellong, B. (1981). Determinants of neurobehavioral outcome in low birthweight infants. *Pediatrics, 67,* 502–505.

Lowe, J., & Papile, L. (1990). Neurodevelopmental performance of very-low-birth-weight infants with mild periventricular, intraventricular hemorrhage. *American Journal of Diseases of Children, 144,* 1242–1245.

Luchi, J.M., Bennett, F.C., & Jackson, J.C. (1991). Predictors of neurodevelopmental outcome following bronchopulmonary dysplasia. *American Journal of Diseases of Children, 145,* 813–817.

Morante, A., Dubowitz, L.M.S., Levene, M., & Dubowitz, V. (1982). The development of visual function in normal and neurologically abnormal preterm and full-term infants. *Developmental Medicine and Child Neurology, 24,* 771–784.

Murray, A.D. (1988). Newborn auditory brainstem evoked responses (ABRs): Longitudinal correlates in the first year. *Child Development, 59,* 1542–1554.

Nickel, R.E., Bennett, F.C., & Lamson, F.N. (1982). School performance of children with birth weights of 1,000 grams or less. *American Journal of Diseases of Children, 136,* 105–110.

Odom, S.L., & Karnes, M.B. (Eds.). (1988). *Early intervention for infants and children with handicaps: An empirical base.* Baltimore: Paul H. Brookes.

Olson, G.M. (1981). The recognition of specific persons. In M.E. Lamb & L.R. Sherrod (Eds.), *Infant social cognition: Empirical and theoretical considerations* (pp. 37–59). Hillsdale, NJ: Lawrence Erlbaum.

Paine, P.A., Pasquali, L., & Spegiorin, C. (1983). Appearance of visually directed prehension related to gestational age and intrauterine growth. *The Journal of Genetic Psychology, 142,* 53–60.

Palmer, P.G., Dubowitz, L.M.S., Verghote, M., & Dubowitz, V. (1982). Neurological and behavioral differences between preterm infants at term and full-term newborn infants. *Neuropediatrics, 13,* 183–189.

Parker, S., Greer, S., & Zuckerman, B. (1988). Double jeopardy: The impact of poverty on early child development. *Pediatric Clinics of North America, 35*(6), 1227–1238.

Pederson, D.R., Evans, B., Chance, G.W., Bento, S., & Fox, A.M. (1988). Predictors of one-year developmental status in low birth weight infants. *Developmental and Behavioral Pediatrics, 9*(5), 287–292.

Phelps, D.L. (1981). Retinopathy of prematurity: An estimate of vision loss in the United States— 1979. *Pediatrics, 67,* 924–925.

Poland, R.M., Wells, D.H., & Ferlauto, J.J. (1980). Methods for detecting hearing impairments in infancy. *Pediatric Annals, 9,* 31–44.

Prechtl, H.F.R., Fargel, J.W., Weinmann, H.M., & Bakker, H.H. (1979). *Developmental Medicine and Child Neurology, 21,* 3–27.

Resnick, M.B., Roth, J., Ariet, M., Carter, R.L., Emerson, J.C., Hendrickson, J.M., Packer, A.B., Larsen, J.J., Wolking, W.B., Lucas, M., Schenck, B.J., Fearnside, B., & Bucciarelli, R.L. (1992). Educational outcome of neonatal intensive care graduates. *Pediatrics, 89*(3), 373–378.

Riese, M.L. (1988). Temperament of full-term and preterm infants: Stability over ages 6 to 24 months. *Developmental and Behavioral Pediatrics, 9*(1), 6–11.

Rose, S.A., Feldman, J.F., McCarton, C.M., & Wolfson, J. (1988). Information processing in seven-month-old infants as a function of risk status. *Child Development, 59,* 589–605.

Ruff, H.A., Lawson, K.R., Kurtzberg, D., McCarton-Daum, C., & Vaughan, H.G., Jr. (1982). Visual following of moving objects by full-term and preterm infants. *Journal of Pediatric Psychology, 7,* 375–386.

Saigal, S., Rosenbaum, P., Hattersley, B., & Milner, R. (1989). Decreased disability rate among 3 year old survivors weighing 501 to 1,000 grams at birth and born to residents of a geographically defined region from 1981 to 1984 compared with 1977 to 1980. *Journal of Pediatrics, 114,* 839–846.

Saigal, S., Rosenbaum, P., Stoskopf, B., & Milner, R. (1982). Follow-up of infants 501 to 1,500 gm. birth weight delivered to residents of a geographically defined region with perinatal intensive care facilities. *Journal of Pediatrics, 100,* 606–613.

Saigal, S., Szatmari, P., Rosenbaum, P., Campbell, D., & King, S. (1991). Cognitive abilities and school performance of extremely low birth weight children and matched term control children at age 8 years: A regional study. *Journal of Pediatrics, 118*(5), 751–760.

Saint-Anne Dargassies, S. (1966). Neurological maturation of the premature infant of 28 to 41 weeks gestational age. In F. Falkner (Ed.), *Human development* (pp. 306–325). Philadelphia: W.B. Saunders.

Saint-Anne Dargassies, S. (1979). Normality and normalization as seen in a long-term neurological follow-up of 286 truly premature infants. *Neuropediatrics, 10,* 227–244.

Salamy, A., Mendelson, T., Tooley, W.H., & Chaplin, E.R. (1980). Differential development of brainstem potential in healthy and high risk infants. *Science, 210,* 553–555.

Schmidt, R.E., & Wedig, K.E. (1990). Very low birth weight infants—Educational outcome at school age from parental questionnaire. *Clinical Pediatrics, 29*(11), 649–651.

Schraeder, B.D., & Tobey, G.Y. (1989). Preschool temperament of very-low-weight infants. *Journal of Pediatric Nursing, 4*(2), 119–126.

Schulman-Galambos, C., & Galambos, R. (1975). Brainstem auditory-evoked responses in premature infants. *Journal of Speech and Hearing Research, 18,* 456–465.

Slater, M.A., Naqvi, M., Andrew, L., & Haynes, K. (1987). Neurodevelopment of monitored versus nonmonitored very low birthweight infants: The importance of family influences. *Developmental and Behavioral Pediatrics, 8*(5), 278–285.

Terry, T.L. (1942). Extreme prematurity and fibroblastic overgrowth of persistent vascular sheath behind each crystalline lens. I. Preliminary Report. *American Journal of Ophthalmology, 25,* 203.

Thompson, L.A., Fagan, J.F., & Fulker, D.W. (1991). Longitudinal prediction of specific cognitive abilities from infant novelty preference. *Child Development, 62,* 530–538.

Usher, R.H. (1981). The special problems of the premature infant. In G.B. Avery (Ed.), *Neonatology: Pathophysiology and management of the newborn* (2nd ed.) (pp. 230–261). Philadelphia: J.B. Lippincott.

Usher, R.H. (1987). Extreme prematurity. In G.B. Avery (Ed.), *Neonatology: Pathophysiology and management of the newborn* (3rd ed.) (pp. 264–298). Philadelphia: J.B. Lippincott.

The Victorian Infant Collaborative Study Group. (1991). Improvement of outcome for infants of birth weight under 1,000 g. *Archives of Diseases in Childhood, 66,* 765–769.

Vohr, B.R., Garcia-Coll, C., & Oh, W. (1989). Language and neurodevelopmental outcome of low-birthweight infants at three years. *Developmental Medicine and Child Neurology, 31,* 582–590.

Williamson, W.D., Wilson, G.S., Lifschitz, M.H., & Thurber, S.A. (1990). Nonhandicapped very-low-birth weight infants at one year of age: Developmental profile. *Pediatrics, 85,* 405–410.

Yip, Y.Y., & Tan, K.L. (1991). Bronchopulmonary dysplasia in very low birthweight infants. *Journal of Paediatric Child Health, 27,* 34–38.

Chapter 6

Neonatal Care on the International Scene

Although physicians from France, the Netherlands, Sweden, and England have made important contributions to the care of newborns, the majority of the scientific advances in neonatology and the leadership in research have come from the United States. The purpose of this chapter is to present an overview of the care of newborns as it is practiced around the world, especially in underdeveloped countries.

To date, the unwritten contract for neonatal care in the United States has been: If technology is available, it should be applied, even if the chance for survival and a normal neurologic outcome is small. This approach has led to technological advances that are routinely saving the lives of babies who were considered hopeless as little as 10 years ago. This level of care depends on many factors:

1. commitment by both private and public sectors to fund these services adequately
2. availability of advanced technology
3. access to care by skilled health professionals
4. regionalization of care
5. existence of national standards of quality of care.

Many of the countries in the developing world are deficient in one or more of these areas.

AUSTRALIA

Australia is an advanced country, but it is somewhat isolated geographically from its western heritage. The large population centers of Sidney, Melbourne, Brisbane, Adelaide, and Perth all have a well-established infrastructure with advanced university facilities. The majority of mothers deliver babies in a hospital, and maternal and neonatal problems can be identified readily and addressed. There is a firm financial commitment to the critically ill neonate, as well as to the availability of excellent technology.

Personnel issues are the greatest single concern. There are no training programs in Australia for pediatricians to become neonatologists. Pediatricians seeking advanced training usually travel, either to the United States or to England, to further their education. While many physicians have become skilled using this approach, the training of other health care professionals still lags somewhat behind that in the United States. There are too few well-trained critical care nurses and few respiratory therapists. Young women from countries in Southeast Asia often come to Australia for nursing education and many work in intensive care nurseries (see Figure 6–1).

The population of the country is heterogeneous, with many descendants of European stock, especially from England, Italy, and Greece. The native population, the aborigines, have a higher infant mortality rate than the general population; this results partly from alcohol abuse, cigarette smoking, little prenatal care, and habitation of settlements far from medical care.

In Australia, there are few social, legal, or financial impediments to provision of a quality of care similar to that available in neonatal intensive care units in the United States.

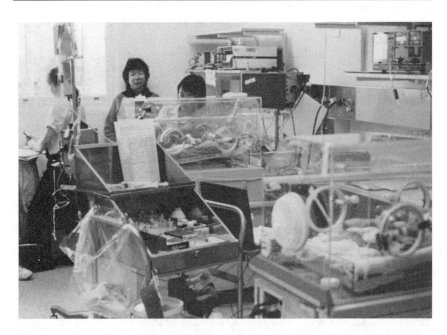

Figure 6–1 Australia—Modern, well-equipped nursery in Sidney (King's Hospital)

INDIA

India is the prototype of the crowded, overpopulated developing nation. There is a wide variety of impediments to adequate critical care. While advanced technology may be available, it often is reserved only for those who can afford to pay. The cost per day in an intensive care nursery is 25 to 75 rupees ($1 to $3). This cost is borne directly by the family. Insurance is uncommon, and if a family has no resources, the baby may be discharged to be taken home (see Figure 6–2). The vast majority of babies are born at home or in a neighboring house, and the mothers are attended by local midwives. Babies with anomalies or of very low birthweight routinely are not even brought to the few critical care facilities that do exist. The mother must remain hospitalized for the duration of her premature baby's course because she is the baby's food supply (Figure 6–3). Preterm infant formulas are not available and the mother must be able to provide sufficient breast milk for a child to thrive. Rather than feeding by tube, as would be customary in the West, the infants are fed their mother's breast milk via special feeding devices that pour small quantities of milk into the baby's mouth.

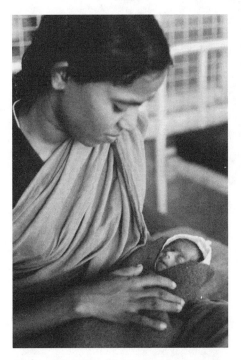

Figure 6–2 India—Three-pound baby being sent home with his mother after she has learned to keep him warm and fed (Madras)

Most intensive care nurseries have very limited technology, and it is uncommon to see more than one baby receiving ventilator care. Often, several babies share a heating unit (Figure 6–4) or even one bed (Figure 6–5). Surfactant replacement therapy, costing $500 to $1,000 a treatment, is not widely available and is far too costly. Virtually no transport systems for critically ill neonates are available. The most common "transport" to the hospital is the 1-day-old, full-term neonate who has suffered severe perinatal asphyxia, frequently from a traumatic delivery. Since the mother has just delivered the baby, such a baby usually is brought to the hospital by a grandmother on public transportation, usually by bus. Typically, the baby is unable to suck and swallow, is lethargic and hypotonic, and may have seizures. Little can be done for such a child, and the family usually takes the baby home to die.

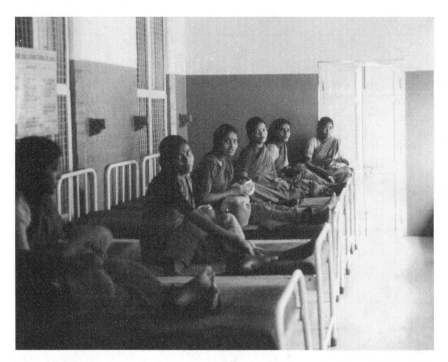

Figure 6–3 India—Mothers of premature babies required to remain in hospital to provide breast milk (Madras)

Bhargava and colleagues have reported on the delivery of prenatal care in India (Bhargava, Ramji, Sachev, & Iyer, 1986). They indicated that, in India, the prenatal mortality rate varied from as low as 12.5/1,000 live births to as high as 147/1,000. Most study sites reported rates of 70/1,000 to 90/1,000 live births, which is approximately 6 to 7 times the rate in the United States. According to these authors, the primary reported causes of mortality were perinatal asphyxia, pulmonary conditions, birth trauma, and neonatal infections. Bhargava and colleagues (1986) concluded that many perinatal deaths are preventable. They also suggested that high fetal and childhood mortality interfered with the acceptance of family planning programs.

There are many well-trained physicians in India who are capable of caring for the critically ill newborn, but resources are limited. There are few well-trained nurses and respiratory therapists, and funding is limited. In addition, all of those who practice neonatology spend most of their time providing for the vast needs of more healthy children in ambulatory clinics.

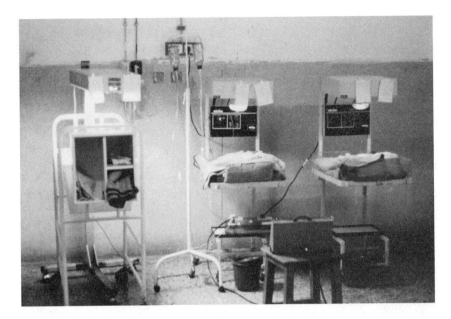

Figure 6–4 India—Only pieces of equipment in Bombay intensive care nursery were heating units that had to be shared

---

CHINA

The situation in China is similar to that in India. However, a study by Peabody, Hesketh, and Kattwinkel (1992) reported on Project Hope efforts to develop a neonatal intensive care in the Children's Hospital in Hangzhou, China. The approach was comprehensive, including renovation of facilities and purchase of modern equipment and supplies. Several experienced neonatologists worked as short-term consultants in the unit to demonstrate the use and effectiveness of the equipment, and selected physicians were brought to the United States for training. At 18 months after initiation of the project, an evaluation revealed poor leadership and organization, inconsistent clinical care, and unacceptable maintenance of equipment and facilities. A more intense approach, using long-term physician and nursing consultants in combination with formal education programs, was undertaken. After 4 years, this effort resulted in a functioning, independent, intensive care nursery with budding effective leadership, continuing education activities, and well-coordinated maintenance programs. Relatively little progress was made with laboratory capabilities, however, and an adequate transport system is yet to be developed. These experiences demonstrate that, in a developing nation, an intense effort must be maintained to ensure progress toward high quality health care.

SOVIET UNION

Although the Union of Soviet Socialist Republics (USSR) no longer exists, there has been little change in the care of critically ill neonates. In this former socialist state, in which the government exercised tight control, rubles were carefully allotted to health care. Given the advanced age of the members of the former Politburo, it is not surprising that the government selectively promoted health care services that would meet the needs of government officials. The Soviet Institutes of Cardiology and Oncology are well funded and well staffed, rivaling similar facilities in the Western world. Thus, up-to-date care for heart disease and cancer, the primary diseases of the elderly, is readily available. At the opposite extreme, however, only the healthy full-term newborn is considered valuable. In many intensive care facilities in Leningrad, Moscow, Tashkent, and Samarkand, obstetrical and neonatal care is virtually the same. Deliveries of babies are scattered in small facilities and attended by nurse midwives. Babies born at or near term with mild infections or readily correctable surgical problems receive care. Infants with more complex malformations and very low birthweight routinely are allowed to die. The infant mortality rate is estimated to be between 35/1,000 and 50/1,000 live births. Since the society has chosen not to fund intensive neonatal care, there

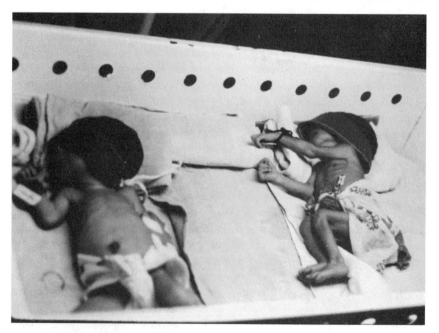

Figure 6–5 India—Two infants sharing nursery bed in Bombay

are few medical and nursing personnel well trained in this field, technology is limited, and there are no standards or expectations at the national level. However, the Soviet citizens value their healthy children and invest vast amounts of time and money in education, preventive health care, and sports training.

COLOMBIA

As in many developing countries, there is a wide disparity of wealth in Colombia, South America. Its close proximity to the United States allows the wealthy to bring their complex health care problems for state-of-the-art care in any one of a number of facilities in California, Texas, Louisiana, and Florida. In addition, many South American physicians have received advanced training in the United States (Figure 6–6). In the private sector, funding is good, although the source of funding may be questionable (e.g., money from the sale of drugs). Funding is more limited in the public sector. The equipment available is modern, and there is much technical expertise. There are no national standards of care, however, and the expectations of the population regarding outcome are relatively low.

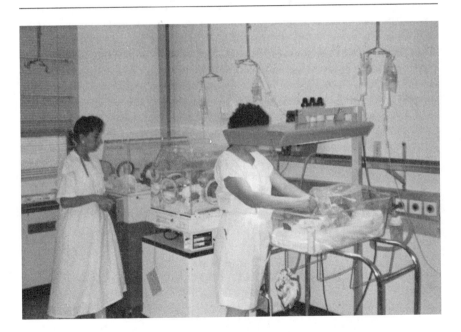

Figure 6–6 Colombia—Excellent warming units, phototherapy, oxygen therapy, limited ventilator therapy, quality intravenous solutions, and excellent nursing care—all available in the largest neonatal intensive care unit in Cali, with 12 beds

INTERNATIONAL CONSIDERATIONS

Beyond the variations of care already discussed, there may be cultural and societal pressures that differ by specific populations. Since the male newborn is more valued than the female in China and in much of the Middle East, the existing technology may be utilized selectively, discriminating against the female. The common practice of placing animal dung on the umbilical cord stump of the newborns in native populations in Africa leads to neonatal tetanus with a high mortality. Both mothers and children in poor countries and countries at war suffer greatly from poor nutrition and widespread infections. Advanced neonatal care cannot compensate for malnutrition, poor prenatal care, and other endemic societal problems.

CONCLUSION

Neonatal care is advanced in Western Europe, Canada, and the United States because of a 25-year commitment to the well-being of mothers and children. In underdeveloped countries, it is far more cost-effective to spend limited funds on nutrition and immunizations rather than on the intensive care of newborns with complex medical problems. In many of these countries, limited critical care facilities will be developed as the technical expertise becomes available, but, in general, only upper class families with adequate funds will have access to these facilities. Even for such families, however, there are few resources to turn to for continued intervention to maximize the potential of disabled infants and young children.

BIBLIOGRAPHY

Bhargava, S.K., Ramji, S., Sachev, H.P., & Iyer, P.U. (1986). Delivery of perinatal care in India: Priorities and policies. *Annals of Tropical Paediatrics, 6,* 225–231.

Peabody, J.W., Hesketh, T., & Kattwinkel, J. (1992). Creation of a neonatology facility in a developing country: Experience from a 5-year project in China. *American Journal of Perinatology, 9,* 401–408.

Part II

Clinical Issues: Problems, Identification, Assessment, and Prognosis

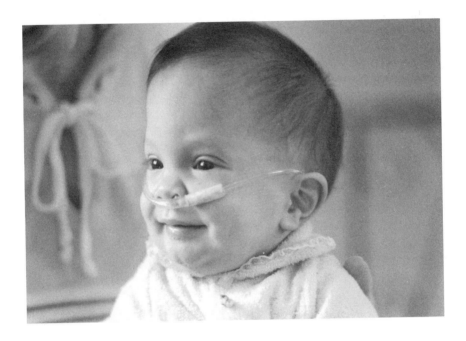

Modern techniques for identifying and monitoring medical conditions of high risk and disabled infants have played a major role in reducing the severity of developmental problems. Today, there is an increasingly healthy awareness among physicians, educators, therapists, and other professionals that, while many neonates experience significant complications that place them at risk for central nervous system damage, such events do not inevitably lead to negative outcome. New and innovative strategies for developmental and behavioral screening and assessment, as well as long-term follow-up of graduates of the neonatal intensive care unit (NICU) into the adolescent years, are positive steps that have begun to address some important questions about prognosis and vulnerable populations.

Chapter 7

Neurology of the Newborn

Potential damage to the developing central nervous system is a substantial concern with the ever-increasing survival of the very low birthweight (less than 1,500 grams) infant. The overwhelming numbers of articles and chapters now appearing in the literature make it clear that many investigators are exploring the subtleties of the neurological examination with the hope of predicting the neonate's developmental outcome. Since Chapter 5 has covered the sensory and psychological development of the high risk infant, this discussion will concentrate primarily on the medical neurological examination and on insults to the central nervous system.

NEUROLOGICAL EXAMINATION OF NORMAL NEWBORN

The neurological examination is limited in the newborn. The neonate obviously can offer no verbal input as to the subjective function of the central nervous system. Also, the integration of sensory processes such as vision and hearing is incomplete (Pomeroy & Volpe, 1992). Consequently, the evaluation must be restricted to the general neurological condition or level of alertness and responsiveness of the child and an examination of the specific cranial nerves, neuromotor development, and primary neonatal reflexes (Dubowitz, 1988). As previously mentioned, portions of the neurological examination of the newborn are included in the assessment of gestational age.

Behavior

Responsiveness or level of alertness varies considerably with gestational age and with recent life experiences. Infants beyond 30 weeks gestation have distinct periods of wakefulness and can be stimulated to open their eyes and be alert. Beyond 30 weeks, responsiveness and periods of wakefulness increase and occur without external stimulation. By 36 weeks, the infant is attentive to both visual and auditory stimuli. In general, the extent of alertness is crucial to evaluating the quality of the newborn's responses, especially the reflex reactions (Saint-Anne Dargassies, 1974).

More specific dimensions of the newborn neurological examination entail an assessment of behavior governed by the 12 cranial nerves that are connected directly to the brain, without involvement of the spinal cord. The *first cranial nerve*, the olfactory neuron, is responsible for the sense of smell. Because relatively little work has been done on olfactory perception in the newborn, this sense is usually not tested as part of the routine examination (Sarnat, 1978). The *second cranial nerve* is the primary neuron of visual function. It connects with the retina of the eye and transmits electrical impulses to the posterior portion of the brain. Appropriate function is evidenced by the fact that full-term newborns typically have a preference for the color red, patterns with heavy contrast, and facial features (Isenberg, 1989; Peeples & Teller, 1975). The *third, fourth,* and *sixth cranial nerves* govern muscle movements of the eyes. Since most newborns do not fix on and track an object, changes in the baby's head position must suffice for adequate evaluation of movement. The *fifth cranial nerve* controls sensation to the face and also provides motor input for the facial muscles. The *seventh cranial nerve* directs the muscles of the face and is important to symmetry and expression that can be best estimated by facial movement in a crying state. The *eighth cranial nerve* connects the inner ear to the brain and directs the sense of hearing. Sophisticated auditory testing has demonstrated that most healthy newborns can discriminate sounds by intensity and pitch. Sucking, swallowing, palate, and tongue functions are integrated through the *fifth, seventh, ninth, tenth,* and *twelfth cranial nerves.* The sucking, rooting, and gag reflexes most often are tested to ensure that the functions of these neurons are appropriate. The *eleventh cranial nerve* provides motor tone to the major muscles of flexion in the neck, primarily the sternocleidomastoid muscle. However, these responses are difficult to test in the newborn with any degree of reliability (England, 1988).

Muscle Tone and Reflexes

The motor system can be examined by observing the resting posture of the infant and various spontaneous movements, along with several newborn reflexes that can be elicited specifically (Hill, 1992). General observation alone reveals that there is a progression of development of muscle tone by gestational age. Although lower extremity flexor tone is well established by 32 weeks, it is not until approximately 36 weeks that upper extremity flexor tone is apparent (Harris & Brady, 1986). When the baby is handled, muscle tone can be assessed subjectively by the resistance of the extremities, trunk, and head with changes in position. Recoil of the extremities, foot and head flexion, head lag, back extension, and ventral suspension—elements of the Dubowitz examination—are all useful in estimating muscle tone (Dubowitz, Dubowitz, & Goldberg, 1970).

In addition to more generalized observations, several reflexes, including the Moro, tonic neck, walking, and grasp responses, have been found helpful in the neurological evaluation. Perhaps most familiar among these is the Moro reflex, which should be integrated and disappear by 4 months of age. Typically in the newborn, several reactions initially are present. In sequence, these consist of arms and legs abducting (drawing away) from the body, followed by an adduction of the arms, as if the new baby were hugging. Once the arms return to the body, the infant usually cries. Characteristically, asymmetric responses are seen in children with birth injuries or in those with fractures of the clavicle or upper arm bones (Parmalee, 1964).

The asymmetrical tonic neck reflex (ATNR), a second commonly observed response in the newborn, often is referred to as the reflex of the fencing position. As the infant's head is turned to one side, on the nonface side the arm and leg are flexed. If the baby's head then is passively turned in the opposite direction, a reversal of position of the extremities usually occurs. The reflex tends to disappear in the first 3 to 4 months, although some of the responses may persist for several years. Tonic neck reflex that continues and is easy to elicit is usually a sign of serious central nervous system pathology (Bly, 1981). The placing response can be elicited if the infant is held so that the sole of one foot touches a smooth surface. Reciprocal flexion and extension occurs, simulating walking (i.e., the walking or stepping response). This reflex usually dissipates by approximately 4 weeks. The palmar and plantar reflexes are prompted readily by placing a finger in the palm or on the sole of the baby's foot. In response, the fingers or toes curl around the finger. This reflex occurs naturally in the infant, indicates normal neurological development, and generally disappears at approximately 3 months (Hogan & Milligan, 1971). Numerous other neonatal reflexes have been described, but most of these seem to have limited value in the evaluation of the newborn.

MAJOR NEUROLOGICAL INSULTS

Birth Asphyxia

As we have discussed previously, birth asphyxia causes a major insult to the brain (Goldstein, Johnston, Donn, & Custer, 1989). The result may be insufficient oxygen and elevated tissue acid concentrations, along with poor blood flow. Any portion of the brain may be affected with birth asphyxia, and the causes vary (Levene, 1988). Infants born prematurely, however, are more prone to have intraventricular hemorrhage than are full-term neonates. The staging of damage to the brain can be estimated fairly accurately. Obviously, the more prolonged the asphyxia, the more severe the manifestations. In such instances, loss of consciousness may be progressive, proceeding to coma. Muscle tone may span a range from normal through hypotonic to flaccid. The primitive reflexes, as well as the complex reflexes, may be absent. In the more severe states, respiratory effort may be diminished or absent and the heart rate may slow.

Management of the asphyxiated infant includes adequate correction of blood pressure, blood oxygen and carbon dioxide levels, and acidosis (Novotny, 1989). The baby should receive temperature support, and blood glucose should be maintained. Infants who develop seizures obviously should be treated with an anticonvulsant, usually phenobarbital.

Surprisingly, the developmental outcome of newborns with birth asphyxia is not as grim as might be expected. Neonates are particularly resistant to the effects of acidosis and hypoxia (Fawer & Calame, 1988). In absolute numbers, there have been more children with moderate to severe cerebral palsy who were full-term babies than who were low birthweight or premature babies. It is therefore critical that all infants experiencing birth asphyxia be evaluated carefully and serially for developmental disability (Volpe, 1981).

Intracranial Hemorrhage

Intracranial hemorrhage refers to bleeding in or around the brain tissue. Although intracranial hemorrhage may rarely occur in utero, the trauma of the delivery process is the greatest risk factor for central nervous system bleeding. Until the mid-1970s, when new technology became available, such insult was difficult to confirm. Now, as a result of cranial ultrasonography, computerized axial tomography (CAT) scanning, and magnetic resonance imaging (MRI), new information has come to light. Findings indicate that as many as 30 percent of infants smaller than 1,500 grams have some variety of intracranial hemorrhage (Volpe, 1989). The ultimate prognosis, of course, depends on the type and severity of the bleeding (Brann & Schwartz, 1987).

Basically, there are two major subgroups within this primary category of insult: (1) hemorrhage in and around the membranes that cover the surface of the brain and (2) bleeding into the brain tissue. *Subdural hemorrhage* is a collection of blood that results from tearing of the vessels between the brain and the dura (the outermost thick membrane covering the surface of the brain). This is a traumatic lesion found predominantly in the full-term baby. Subsequently, the collection of blood results in compression of the brain, which may progress to a compromise of the controlling centers of respiration in the brainstem. Once this condition is properly identified, the only available therapy is surgical decompression and removal of the blood clot.

In comparison, *subarachnoid hemorrhage* is bleeding beneath the arachnoid membrane, which is the layer immediately covering the brain. This condition is most commonly seen with asphyxia, and minor degrees may be completely asymptomatic. On the other hand, blood on the surface of the brain may result in local irritation and seizures. At an extreme, damage may be massive and acute, resulting in death. Unfortunately, since the blood generally extends over the surface of the brain without a localization that would be amenable to surgical removal, no specific therapy is presently available.

The second major type of hemorrhage is bleeding into the brain tissue (*parenchymal hemorrhage*), which also includes the ventricular system deep inside the brain. By way of explanation, the brain ventricles comprise an interconnected system of reservoirs that contain spinal fluid. The two lateral cavities, one on each side of the brain, are slitlike and extend from the anterior to the posterior portion of the brain. Cerebrospinal fluid is produced from collections of blood vessels (choroid plexus) found within the lateral ventricles and then circulates to a midline third cavity. From this point, the fluid flows to the fourth ventricle through the aqueduct of Sylvius, which is a very small canal (less than the size of a pencil lead, even in an adult). Subsequently, the cerebral spinal fluid passes from deep inside the brain tissue (fourth ventricle) through three connections to the subarachnoid space over the surface of the spinal cord and brain, and finally is reabsorbed by another blood vessel complex located between the two halves of the brain. This continuous process of circulation results in an exchange of spinal fluid approximately four or five times a day.

Some specific variations in severity of hemorrhage within the brain are shown in Table 7–1. A periventricular insult refers to bleeding adjacent to the lateral ventricles inside the brain where spinal fluid is produced (grade 1 hemorrhage). Such bleeding then may break into the ventricular system, developing into a grade 2 hemorrhage. If enlargement of the ventricular system occurs following this damage, the condition is designated as a grade 3 hemorrhage. Blood increases the viscosity of the spinal fluid from its normal watery consistency, which may result in an obstruction of the aqueduct of Sylvius, either mechanically or from secondary inflammation induced by the blood in the cerebral spinal fluid. If this blockage

Table 7–1 Neonatal Intraventricular Hemorrhage (IVH)

Grade of Severity	Incidence in Infants at less than 1,500 grams (%)	Mortality (%)	Progressive Ventricular Dilation (% survivors)	Major Neurological Sequelae (%) (by 3 years)
1	35	15	5	15
2	40	20	25	30
3	25	40	55	40
4	15	60	80	90

Sources: From "Major Problems in Clinical Pediatrics" in *Neurology of the Newborn* by J.J. Volpe, pp. 1–46. Copyright 1987 by W.B. Saunders Company, and "Neonatal Neurology" by J.J. Volpe, *Clinics in Perinatology, 16*, pp. 2–8. Copyright 1989 by W.B. Saunders Company.

is not relieved, *hydrocephalus*, an enlargement of the ventricular system, then occurs. Most serious is bleeding into the brain tissue itself, which is considered to be a grade 4 hemorrhage (Hambleton & Wigglesworth, 1976).

Clinical Signs and Symptoms

The clinical presentations or manifestations of these hemorrhagic insults vary considerably with the amount and location of the bleeding (Papile, Burstein, Burstein, & Koffler, 1978; Goldstein & Donn, 1984). Recent studies have reported evidence of periventricular hemorrhage to be as high as 50 percent among infants with birthweights of 1,500 grams or less, but grade 1 hemorrhage is frequently "silent" (Volpe, 1989). However, as the severity of hemorrhage increases, the presentation tends to be more catastrophic and may involve rapid deterioration, progressing to coma, hypoventilation, and respiratory arrest within a short time. Occasionally, in conjunction with intraventricular or periventricular bleeding, newborns have *intracerebellar* hemorrhage, which is thought to result primarily from asphyxia. Often, these insults are fatal or, among the survivors, are manifested in uniformly poor developmental prognoses.

In summary, it is important to emphasize that bleeding alone is not the primary issue, because the blood is broken down and reabsorbed into the body within a week after the hemorrhage. Local changes in blood flow to the brain and the initial pressure effects in the brain are much more critical. Since brain tissue has a high metabolic rate that must be maintained by adequate provision of nutrients through appropriate blood flow, those portions of the organ that are deprived may be irreversibly damaged.

The techniques available to document intracranial hemorrhage have improved rapidly over the past several years. Unfortunately, we are unable to document hemorrhage that may have no prognostic significance. Studies that compare infants who have periventricular-intraventricular hemorrhage with control groups of the same birthweight and gestational age reveal that neonates with grade 1 or 2 hemorrhage have the same risk for major neurodevelopmental disability by 2 years, with an incidence in both groups of approximately 10 to 15 percent. In infants with grade 3 or 4 hemorrhage, the risk for major disabilities increases 3- to 10-fold. Although hydrocephalus that develops from the obstruction of cerebrospinal fluid flow does not by itself seem to increase the risk for developmental disability, the lesion and its surgical intervention tend to increase the risk of neuromotor and cognitive disabilities. The ventricular dilation resulting from diffuse cerebral atrophy (hydrocephalus ex vacuo) has been linked with severe developmental disability. Limited longtitudinal studies suggest that surgical intervention does not change the rate of major disability and that approximately 50 percent of these children will require special education.

Pharmacological Intervention

The best means of eliminating intracranial hemorrhage is the prevention of premature birth. Because the incidence of premature birth has decreased only minimally in the last several decades, other approaches, using medications, are under investigation in an attempt to reduce the incidence and severity of intracranial hemorrhage. Available studies do not support routine clinical use of any drug to prevent intracranial hemorrhage. However, medications that are being investigated include phenobarbital, which may decrease the incidence but perhaps not the severity of hemorrhage when given postnatally. When phenobarbital is given prophylactically to the mother in active labor or with premature rupture of the membranes, there is a lowering of both the incidence and the severity of intracranial hemorrhage. Unfortunately, studies to date are few and the results cannot yet be applied widely.

Indomethacin, an inhibitor of prostaglandin metabolism in animal models, has decreased the incidence and severity of hemorrhage. There are, however, conflicting data in prospective, randomized, controlled clinical studies (Hanigan et al., 1988; Ment et al., 1988).

In infants receiving mechanical ventilation, changes in intracranial blood flow may be responsible for loss of vascular integrity or overdistention of cerebral capillaries and veins. Agents that paralyze the baby and allow for greater control of ventilation may improve intracranial blood flow, but they may have so many adverse effects on other organ systems, including renal failure and hypotension, that routine use cannot be advocated.

Ethamsylate, a medication that reduces capillary bleeding, is widely available in Europe (Benson et al., 1986). It increases platelet activity and strengthens the capillary wall. In one study, frequency of hemorrhage was reduced in infants treated within 2 hours of birth. At present, there are insufficient data to determine the effectiveness of this agent.

Vitamin E, an antioxidant, has been promoted for the prevention of chronic lung disease and retinopathy of prematurity. Vitamin E supplementation after birth may decrease the incidence of the less significant forms of hemorrhage but does not appear to affect the frequency of severe hemorrhage.

In summary, the use of any medication to prevent hemorrhage, especially in premature infants, needs to be evaluated by careful, well-designed research protocols before it can be applied on a broader basis.

Seizures

Seizures resulting from abnormal transmission of electrical impulses in the brain are a fairly frequent occurrence in the neonatal period (Clancy, 1989; Craig, 1960). Similarly, tremors may result from minor metabolic disturbances or from a catastrophic central nervous system insult. In essence, abnormal electrical activity that may emerge from any portion of the brain is communicated much more rapidly in the neonatal period than in later life. In part, this condition arises because of incomplete myelinization. (Myelin is the fatty material that surrounds the mature nerves and functions as an insulator to electrical impulses.) Abnormal motor movements or seizures are the manifestations of this condition (Brown & Minns, 1988).

In general, neonatal seizures have been described according to four varieties of clinical presentation. The categories of neonatal seizure are subtle, tonic, multifocal clonic, and myoclonic. *Subtle seizures* occur most frequently, and often are overlooked. They may include staring, lip smacking, sucking, a swimming/rowing motion of the arms and legs, apnea, rapid heart rate, or a change in blood pressure. Although such seizures may last only a few seconds, they may be harmful to the infant. Their relationship to long-term disability has not been clearly established. The generalized *tonic seizure* includes extension of the trunk, neck, and extremities and has been likened to the decerebrate posturing of older individuals. This condition is found primarily in the premature infant who has experienced periventricular or intraventricular hemorrhage. In such cases, it is difficult to distinguish whether the seizures are merely a manifestation of the insult or whether they themselves add to the poor developmental outcome of babies with the most serious impairment (Scher & Painter, 1989; Volpe, 1981, 1987).

In contrast with the subtle and generalized tonic varieties, the *multifocal clonic seizure* is found more commonly in full-term infants and is usually characterized as repetitive jerking movements of one or two limbs; the seizure then may migrate to other portions of the body. The etiology is thought to be primarily birth asphyxia, and the electroencephalogram (EEG) in these infants commonly shows abnormal repetitive spikes. Finally, *myoclonic seizures* are seen in both the premature and full-term infant and are symptomatic single or repeated synchronous jerks of the entire body or limbs, with an EEG pattern that often is abnormal. Although numerous causes of seizure disorders have been identified, no specific etiology has been determined for myoclonic seizures.

Virtually any insult to the brain may precipitate seizures. The single and most frequent origin is an asphyxial event, in which brain tissue is compromised as a result of inadequate oxygen, excess acid, and changes in blood flow—with or without overt evidence of hemorrhage. In the first week of life, metabolic disturbances such as hypoglycemia, hypocalcemia (low blood calcium), hypomagnesemia (low blood magnesium), and elevated blood phosphate commonly have been cited as responsible agents. Usually, these problems are very amenable to therapy that corrects the metabolic disorder, and it is rare that long-term developmental disabilities ensue. However, other metabolic disturbances may have a much more serious and lasting prognosis. For example, seizures associated with a deposition of abnormal compounds in the brain tissue seldom have a favorable outcome. Included in this group are genetic defects resulting in inborn errors such as amino acid disorders (e.g., phenylketonuria) and lipid metabolism disturbances (e.g., Tay-Sachs disease) (Volpe, 1981).

Another large group of problems well known for altering or disrupting brain development are perinatal infections such as toxoplasmosis, herpes, and rubella. Whether or not seizures are a prominent part of the presentation, developmental outcome is poor. Likewise, malformations of the central nervous system that include seizures rarely are associated with typical patterns of growth and maturation.

One very old problem, witnessed with increased frequency, is the delivery of infants born to mothers taking drugs (Zelson, Rubio, & Wasserman, 1971) (see Chapter 13). Babies addicted to narcotics or barbiturates frequently have withdrawal symptoms including a high-pitched cry, high muscle tone, increased activity, vomiting, respiratory distress, and loose stools. Overt seizures may be seen in approximately 3 percent of these newborns. The judicious use of medication can control the symptoms and thus allow for gradual drug withdrawal. The little information that is available on the long-term development of these infants, including social and environmental factors, unfortunately precludes any firm prognosis (Wilson, McCleary, Kean, & Baxter, 1979).

The diagnosis of seizure disorders is accomplished by careful observation in conjunction with an EEG. While an abnormal EEG in the full-term infant more likely increases the risk of future developmental difficulties, serious sequelae may be seen in newborns with seizures who have a normal EEG. Consequently, it is no surprise that studies generally have failed to demonstrate the prognostic value of the EEG in premature infants (Volpe, 1981). In any event, the treatment of seizures must be tailored to the specific etiology. In most cases, for example, correction of a metabolic disturbance leads to prompt resolution of the pathology. Today, the primary medication for neonatal seizures is phenobarbital, which is not only safe and effective but relatively inexpensive (Goldbarg & Yeh, 1991). Less frequently, additional medications such as diphenylhydantoin (Dilantin) or diazepam (Valium) may be necessary. Although most infants are treated for a minimum of 6 months, the duration of therapy again is dependent on the severity of seizures, their recurrence, and periodic re-evaluation (Ellison, 1984).

Apnea

As many as 50 percent of all premature newborns experience irregular respiratory patterns, often characterized by 10- to 15-second pauses in the breathing cycle (periodic breathing). If these hesitations last more than 20 seconds or are accompanied by a slowing of the heart rate or cyanosis (low blood oxygen), they are termed *apnea* (Miller & Martin, 1992).

Two centers in the brainstem exercise control over the respiratory cycle. These centers receive cues from inspiration and expiration not only from a constant monitoring of the blood oxygen and carbon dioxide levels, but also from stretch and pressure receptors within the lungs and chest wall. In the immature central nervous system, the peripheral signals may not be of sufficient magnitude or the central receptor may not be adequately sensitive to coordinate the respiratory cycle. Hemorrhagic, metabolic, or infectious damage to the central nervous system also may affect the centers for control of respiration.

The treatment of apnea is relatively straightforward. If a specific metabolic basis can be determined, the problem may be resolved easily with its correction. On the other hand, if no specific etiology can be ascertained, tactile stimulation may be effective. In the event that these therapies alone are inadequate, several medications including theophylline and caffeine may be helpful in reducing the frequency of apnea. With a few infants, none of these treatments is sufficient; such children may require intense intervention with intubation and mechanical ventilation.

In retrospect, apnea per se has not been responsible for poor developmental outcome and, with time and maturation of the central nervous system, the frequency of apnea generally decreases. Those infants who do not seem to respond to therapy or who fail to reach mature respiratory development require continuous monitoring, even after discharge to the home.

Developmental Abnormalities

The mature central nervous system is a highly complex and organized network. At approximately 3 to 4 weeks gestation, the neural tube is formed. On the back portion of the embryo, crests of nerve tissues on each side of an open groove of tissue meet and then progressively close, by fusion, in both the cephalic direction (toward the head) and the rostral direction. Failure of the tissue around this tube to join is referred to as a *neural tube defect*. These problems are the most common developmental abnormalities of the central nervous system and include anomalies such as *anencephaly*, *meningomyelocele* (see Figure 7-1), and *spina bifida occulta* (Lyon & Beaugerie, 1988). Anencephaly occurs where the anterior neural tube fails to grow closed, and any or all of the brain may have failed to develop. Most babies with this type of defect die within the first several weeks of life.

Failure of the *posterior* neural tube to join may be manifested as a myeloschisis (open

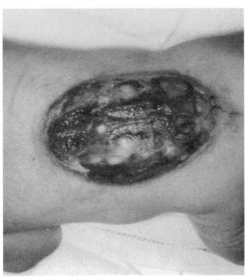

Figure 7–1 Infant with meningoschisis

nerve tissue) or as a meningomyelocele, which usually is a sac composed of the meninges (the outer membranes of the brain), with nerve tissues (myelo-) in the lower portion of the back. This impairment frequently is associated with a developmental defect of the lower portion of the brain, where there is an obstruction to the flow of cerebrospinal fluid through the aqueduct of Sylvius or a blockage to its path from the lower portion of the brain. In over 90 percent of the children with meningomyelocele, hydrocephalus (see Figure 7–2) is present (Punt, 1988). Although intellect often is spared, profound motor effects can be seen, depending on the level of the spinal malformation. Most lesions of the lower back have accompanying loss of nerve function to the legs, resulting in paralysis and a lack of innervation to the sphincters for bladder and bowel control. Early repair of the meningomyelocele minimizes the risk of the infection in the central nervous system. However, progressive hydrocephalus (enlarge-

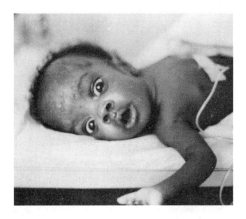

Figure 7–2 Newborn with early hydrocephalus, manifesting setting sun sign

ment of the ventricles in the central nervous system) does lead to abnormal head growth and nearly always requires a shunting procedure to drain the fluid through a catheter from the head, underneath the skin, and into the abdominal cavity in order to relieve the intracranial pressure (Silver, Marzocchi, Farrell, & McLone, 1989).

Spina bifida occulta differs from meningomyelocele in that the lesion consists of a defective bony formation of the lower back, without exposed nerve or meningeal tissue. The condition is common and may be seen in as much as 25 percent of the population. Although the majority of individuals have no associated disability, deficits such as gait disturbance, muscle weakness, or problems with bowel and bladder sphincter control may occur in early childhood (Volpe, 1981).

Many other developmental abnormalities of the central nervous system have been described in the literature. These include disordered growth of brain tissue, either the nerve cells or the nerve cells and the supportive tissue, the glial cells. Abnormal growth of blood vessels, too, may occur. Depending on the portion of brain affected, children with such conditions may have persistence of the primitive reflexes (e.g., rooting and Moro). As might be expected, the developmental outcome usually is poor.

In summary, the brain is a marvelously complex organ that integrates all of our body functions. Unfortunately, relatively little can be done once serious damage has taken place. The magnitude of the insult, its duration, and the location within the brain all determine the severity of residual dysfunction. In these instances, careful sequential evaluation is necessary to determine the degree of developmental disability and to design intervention strategies to minimize the impact of such impairments.

BIBLIOGRAPHY

Benson, J.W.T., Hayword, C., Osborne, J.P., Schulte, J.F., Drayton, M.R., Murphy, J.F., Rennie, J.M., Speidel, B.D., & Cooke, R.W.I. (1986). Multicentre trial of ethamsylate for prevention of periventricular hemorrhage in very low birth-weight infants. *Lancet, 2,* 1297–1302.

Bly, L. (1981). The components of normal and abnormal movements during the first year of life. In D.E. Slaton (Ed.), *Development of movement in infancy* (pp. 8–17). Chapel Hill, NC: University of North Carolina.

Brann, A.W., & Schwartz, J. F. (1987). Central nervous system disturbances. In A.A. Fanaroff & R.J. Martin (Eds.), *Neonatal-perinatal medicine: Diseases of the fetus and infant* (4th ed.) (pp. 495–553). St. Louis: C.V. Mosby.

Brown, J.K., & Minns, R.A. (1988). Seizure disorders. In M.I. Levene, M.J. Bennett, & J. Punt (Eds.), *Fetal and neonatal neurology and neurosurgery* (pp. 487–514). Edinburgh: Churchill Livingstone.

Clancy, R.R. (1989). Neonatal seizures. In D.K. Stevenson & P. Sunshine (Eds.), *Fetal and neonatal brain injury* (pp. 123–140). Toronto: B.C. Decker.

Craig, W.S. (1960). Convulsive movements occurring during the first 10 days of life. *Archives of Diseases in Childhood, 35,* 336–344.

Dubowitz, L.M.S. (1988). Neurological assessment of the full term and preterm newborn infant. In X. Harel & N.Y. Anastolsion (Eds.), *The at-risk infant: Psycho/social/medical aspects* (pp. 185–196). Baltimore: Paul H. Brookes.

Dubowitz, L.M.S., Dubowitz, V., & Goldberg, C. (1970). Clinical assessment of gestational age in the newborn infant. *Journal of Pediatrics, 77,* 1–10.

Ellison, P.H. (1984). Management of seizures in the high risk infant. *Clinics in Perinatology, 11,* 175–188.

England, M.A. (1988). Normal development of the central nervous system. In M.I. Levene, M.J. Bennett, & J. Punt (Eds.), *Fetal and neonatal neurology and neurosurgery* (pp. 3–27). Edinburgh: Churchill Livingstone.

Fawer, C.L., & Calame, A. (1988). Assessment of neurodevelopmental outcome. In M.I. Levene, M.J. Bennett, & J. Punt (Eds.), *Fetal and neonatal neurology and neurosurgery* (pp. 71–88). Edinburgh: Churchill Livingstone.

Goldbarg, H., & Yeh, T.F. (1991). Seizures. In T.F. Yeh (Ed.), *Neonatal therapeutics* (pp. 313–325). St. Louis: Mosby-Year Book.

Goldstein, G.W., & Donn, S.M. (1984). Periventricular and intraventricular hemorrhages. In H.B. Sarnat (Ed.), *Topics in neonatal neurology* (pp. 83–108). New York: Grune & Stratton.

Goldstein, G.W., Johnston, M.V., Donn, S.M., & Custer, J.R. (1989). Birth asphyxia: Issues in neurologic management. In J.S. Wigglesworth & K. Pape (Eds.), *Perinatal brain lesions* (pp. 99–113). Boston: Blackwell Scientific.

Hambleton, G., & Wigglesworth, J.S. (1976). Origin of intraventricular hemorrhage in the preterm infant. *Archives of Diseases in Childhood, 51,* 651–659.

Hanigan, W.C., Kennedy, G., Roemisch, F., Anderson, R., Cusak, T., & Power, W. (1988). Administration of indomethacin for the prevention of periventricular-intraventricular hemorrhage in high risk neonates. *Journal of Pediatrics, 112*, 941–946.

Harris, S.R., & Brady, D.K. (1986). Infant neuromotor assessment instruments: A review. *Physical and Occupational Therapy in Pediatrics, 6*, 121–124.

Hill, A. (1992). Development of tone and reflexes in the fetus and newborn. In R.A. Polin, & W.W. Fox (Eds.), *Fetal and neonatal physiology* (Vol. 2, pp. 1578–1586) Philadelphia: W.B. Saunders.

Hogan, G.R., & Milligan, J.E. (1971). The plantar reflex of the newborn. *New England Journal of Medicine, 285*, 502–503.

Isenberg, S.J. (1989). How to examine the eyes of the neonate. *Clinical Modules for Ophthalmologists, 7*, 1–6.

Levene, M.I. (1988). The asphyxiated newborn infant. In M.I. Levene, M.J. Bennett & J. Punt (Eds.), *Fetal and neonatal neurology and neurosurgery* (pp. 371–382). Edinburgh: Churchill Livingstone.

Lyon, G., & Beaugerie, A. (1988). Congenital developmental malformations. In M.I. Levene, M.J. Bennett, & J. Punt (Eds.), *Fetal and neonatal neurology and neurosurgery* (pp. 231–247). Edinburgh: Churchill Livingstone.

Ment, L.R., Duncan, C.C., Ehrenkranz, R.A., Kleinman, C.S., Taylor, K.J.W., Scott, D.T., Gettner, P., Sherwonit, E., & Williams, J. (1988). Randomized low dose indomethacin trial for the prevention of intraventricular hemorrhage in very low birth weight infants. *Journal of Pediatrics, 112*, 948–953.

Miller, M.J., & Martin, R.J. (1992). Pathophysiology of apnea of prematurity. In R.A. Polin & W.W. Fox (Eds.), *Fetal and neonatal physiology* (Vol. 1, pp. 872–884). Philadelphia: W.B. Saunders.

Novotny, E.J. (1989). Hypoxic-ischemic encephalopathy. In D.K. Stevenson & P. Sunshine (Eds.), *Fetal and neonatal brain injury* (pp. 141–145). Toronto: B.C. Decker.

Papile, L., Burstein, J., Burstein, R., & Koffler, H. (1978). Incidence and evolution of subependymal and intraventricular hemorrhage: A study of infants with birth weights less than 1,500 g. *Journal of Pediatrics, 92*, 529–533.

Parmalee, A.H., Jr. (1964). A critical evaluation of the Moro reflex. *Pediatrics, 33*, 773–788.

Peeples, D.R., & Teller, D.Y. (1975). Color vision and brightness discrimination in two-month-old human infants. *Science, 189*, 1103–1105.

Pomeroy, S.L., & Volpe, J.J. (1992). Development of the nervous system. In R.A. Polin & W.W. Fox (Eds.), *Fetal and neonatal physiology* (Vol. 1, pp. 1490–1509). Philadelphia: W.B. Saunders.

Punt, J. (1988). Hydrocephalus. In M.I. Levene, M.J. Bennett, & J. Punt (Eds.), *Fetal and neonatal neurology and neurosurgery* (pp. 586–591). Edinburgh: Churchill Livingstone.

Saint-Anne Dargassies, S. (1974). Confrontation neurologique des concepts: Maturation et development, chez le jeune. *Revue Neuropsychiate Infant, 22*, 227–235.

Sarnat, H.B. (1978). Olfactory reflexes in the newborn infant. *Journal of Pediatrics, 92* (4), 624–626.

Scher, M., & Painter, M. (1989). Controversies concerning neonatal seizures. *Pediatric Clinics of North America, 36*, 281–288.

Silver, R.K., Marzocchi, M., Farrell, E.E., & McLone, D.G. (1989). The perinatal management of central nervous system anomalies. *Clinics in Perinatology, 16*, 939–944.

Volpe, J.J. (1981). *Neurology of the newborn*. Philadelphia: W.B. Saunders.

Volpe, J.J. (1987). Major problems in clinical pediatrics, *Neurology of the Newborn, 22*, 1–46.

Volpe, J.J. (1989). Neonatal neurology. *Clinics in Perinatology, 16*, 2–8.

Wilson, G.S., McCleary, R., Kean, J., & Baxter, J.C. (1979). The development of preschool children of heroin-addicted mothers: A controlled study. *Pediatrics, 63*, 135–141.

Zelson, C., Rubio, E., & Wasserman, E. (1971). Neonatal narcotic addiction: 10 year observation. *Pediatrics, 48*, 178–189.

Chapter 8

Jaundice

Jaundice is the most prevalent problem that pediatricians confront in dealing with newborns, full-term as well as premature infants. The yellowish skin hue results from the deposition of bilirubin in the skin when the blood level of this chemical becomes elevated. Although it is not common knowledge, *all* newborns have an elevated blood level of bilirubin, and the condition is more difficult to detect in dark-skinned infants. Children with mild elevation of serum bilirubin may not be considered jaundiced because the perception of yellow varies among observers. The major concern in the neonatal period, however, is not the discolored skin but the elevated serum bilirubin, which at high levels has been associated with developmental disability in infants. Since jaundice is a treatable potential insult to all high risk babies, it is important that educators and clinicians have a basic understanding of this condition.

UNDERSTANDING JAUNDICE

Production of Bilirubin

Bilirubin is a chemical that results from breakdown of the hemoglobin pigment of red blood cells. (Hemoglobin in the red blood cells is responsible for oxygen transport from the lungs to body tissue.) As an aged red blood cell is destroyed, *hemoglobin* is released and catabolized (see Figure 8–1). The *globin* portion of hemoglobin is a protein that can be metabolized to its constituent amino acids, which are recycled in the body. The iron within the heme ring also can be recycled as new red blood cells are produced. When the *heme* ring is broken, the enzyme *heme oxygenase* converts the heme to a harmless green pigment called *biliverdin*. This compound, in turn, is altered by another enzyme, *biliverdin reductase,* to form bilirubin. Each of these enzymatic steps occurs within the *reticuloendothelial system*, which includes the liver and the spleen. Approximately 75 percent of

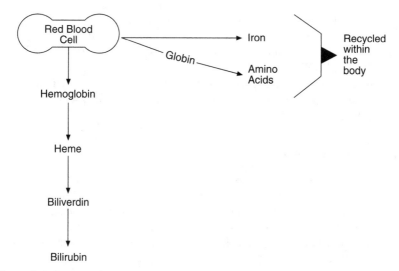

Figure 8–1 Schema of bilirubin production within the newborn

the total amount of bilirubin is formed by the destruction of old red blood cells, with as much as 15 percent resulting from ineffective red blood cell formation within the bone marrow. Several other heme-containing compounds within the body are degraded in the same fashion (Gartner & Arias, 1969).

Prior to birth, bilirubin is produced from the degradation of heme, but it is cleared rapidly by one of two mechanisms (Billing, 1987). Copious bilirubin is found in meconium, the sterile intestinal contents of the newborn, indicating that the fetal liver excretes a large amount of bilirubin. In conditions such as premature birth or hypothyroidism, with decreased intestinal motility, a substantial amount of bilirubin may be reabsorbed from the intestinal tract. The second major mechanism for clearance of fetal bilirubin involves the placenta; bilirubin is transported through the placenta to the mother's liver and cleared in small amounts in comparison to the amount her own body produces. Thus, it is obvious that, if the mother is jaundiced as a result of conditions such as hepatitis, the clearance of bilirubin from the fetus to the mother likewise is reduced and the baby consequently may be born with jaundice.

Transport of Bilirubin

Leaving the reticuloendothelial system, bilirubin is transported in the blood plasma, where it is bound to albumin, the primary circulating protein (Rosenthal, 1992). Because the solubility of unbound bilirubin is very low, the link to albumin is essential and may relate to the potential toxicity of bilirubin. There are two potential binding sites on albumin, but only one of these is a tight linking site (Brodersen, 1979). Moreover, the second site is more easily influenced by environmental conditions such as acidosis, which may allow the bilirubin to be displaced. When the bilirubin-albumin complex reaches the liver cell (hepatocyte), the bilirubin is transferred to the cell, presumably by a receptor protein on the cell surface. The albumin then is free to circulate and perhaps bind with bilirubin or some other substance such as a fatty acid or medication.

Conjugation of Bilirubin

Within the cytoplasm of the liver cell, the bilirubin is transformed, by *conjugation*, into a compound that can be excreted into the intestinal tract. Through an enzymatic process, two glucose molecules are attached to the *unconjugated* bilirubin molecule to form *conjugated* bilirubin. After conjugation, the bilirubin is rapidly discharged into bile by the hepatocytes (liver cells) (Wolkoff, Ketley, Waggoner, Berk, & Jakoby, 1978).

Elimination of Bilirubin

Once it reaches the small intestine, the conjugated bilirubin is not normally reabsorbed. In the adult, the intestinal bacteria convert the conjugated bilirubin to stercobilin (a brown pigment derived from bile), which is excreted in the stool, and urobilinogen (a colorless derivative), which is absorbed from the intestine and excreted in the urine. In the newborn, however, an enzyme in the intestinal tract may strip the glucose molecule from the bilirubin, allowing reabsorption of the unconjugated bilirubin. Less commonly, bilirubin can be excreted in stools without alteration by the bacteria (Maisels, 1987).

Physiologic versus Pathologic Jaundice

Earlier, we noted that virtually all newborns have elevated levels of serum bilirubin. Two conditions account for this finding. First, a much higher percentage of the total blood volume of the fetus is composed of red blood cells. In utero, this state allows for the fetus to extract oxygen from the mother's blood in sufficient amounts to meet the demands of growth and development. Second, following birth, there is an increased breakdown of red blood cells (shorter red blood cell survival), yielding a large quantity of hemoglobin that is converted to bilirubin. Each gram of hemoglobin is converted to approximately 34 milligrams of bilirubin. Rarely is the fetus jaundiced because the placenta clears bilirubin.

There is a gradual rise in serum bilirubin in the healthy full-term baby until approximately 3 or 4 days after birth, with resolution usually by 7 to 10 days (Maisels & Gifford, 1986). In babies that are small-for-gestational age, the mean peak levels of bilirubin are approximately 7 milligrams per deciliter, appearing 4 to 5 days after birth. In preterm babies, the mean peak level is approximately 9 milligrams per deciliter, on the 4th or 5th day with gradual resolution over the next 7 to 10 days. These findings were determined during the course of a National Collaborative Perinatal Project, which examined the clinical progress of over 35,000 newborns (Hardy, Drage, & Jackson, 1979). This study also demonstrated that Caucasian infants are more likely to have higher levels of serum bilirubin than African-American infants.

Because jaundice is common in newborns, researchers have sought to distinguish normal physiologic conditions from pathologic conditions. For this reason, the following criteria have been developed to establish the diagnosis of pathologic jaundice:

1. clinical jaundice within the first 24 hours of life
2. total serum bilirubin concentration (unconjugated plus conjugated) that increases by more than 5 milligrams per deciliter per day
3. total serum bilirubin concentration exceeding 12.9 milligrams per deciliter in a full-term infant or 15 milligrams per deciliter in a preterm infant
4. conjugated serum bilirubin concentration exceeding 1.5 milligrams per deciliter
5. clinical jaundice persisting for more than 1 week in a full-term infant or more than 2 weeks in a preterm infant.

It is important to recognize that the absence of pathologic criteria does not necessarily guarantee that the jaundice is physiologic (Maisels, 1987).

Numerous theories have been postulated to explain the progression and resolution of jaundice in infants, especially those who have been breast-fed. It has been long believed that breast-fed infants have higher bilirubin levels than formula-fed infants in the first week of life. To the contrary, over one-half of the studies addressing these questions have been unable to verify this association. The majority of infants with prolonged jaundice have not been breast-fed. Instead, prolonged jaundice most likely arises from an excess bilirubin load on the newborn liver, which results from increased red blood cell destruction; increased fatty acids in the serum, which bind to albumin and displace bilirubin; and the relative deficiency of hepatic enzymes such as glucuronyl transferase.

CAUSES OF JAUNDICE

Increased Bilirubin Production

The most common reason for neonatal jaundice or *hyperbilirubinemia*, an elevated blood level of bilirubin with or without clinical jaundice, is accelerated destruction of red blood cells (hemolysis) (Cashore, 1992). The most common serious problem of accelerated hemolysis is Rh isoimmunization, a condition resulting from blood group incompatibility between the mother and the baby. The fetus possesses an antigen (protein) on the red blood cell surface that is not present in the mother. If the mother is exposed to these red blood cells as they cross the placenta in a small quantity, her immune system produces antibodies (immunoglobulins) that will attempt to neutralize and eliminate the foreign fetal red blood cell protein. In repeated pregnancies, the antibody response may be enhanced. As a consequence, the antibodies cross the placenta, attach to the red blood cells of the newborn, and subsequently cause them either to be destroyed in circulation or to become misshapen and removed from the bloodstream by the spleen. This condition results in increased bilirubin production.

In some pregnancies, the problem may be severe; the fetus may be so compromised by such rapid destruction of red blood cells that extreme anemia ensues and the blood has insufficient capacity to carry oxygen to the tissues. This problem may result in fetal death or birth of an infant with hydrops fetalis, with severe respiratory distress (Oski & Naiman, 1982).

Within the Rh system, there are at least five major antigens that may result in Rh isoimmunization. The most common of these is the D antigen Rh factor. Whether or not someone is "Rh positive" or "Rh negative" relates specifically to the presence or absence of the D antigen, a cell surface protein. Other Rh factors (antigens) may cause similar disease.

The severe fetal disease caused by the D antigen has become less frequent in infants from subsequent pregnancies, now that mothers can be given RhoGAM following delivery or abortion of an Rh positive (D antigen) infant. RhoGAM is a gamma globulin, virtually identical to the protein that the mother produces in response to the red blood cell D antigen. The fetal D antigen is bound by the RhoGAM antibody, and the mother does not respond and produce antibodies. As a result, in subsequent pregnancies, she does not become sensitized to the fetal red blood cell protein and, therefore, no antibody crosses to the fetus. The administration of RhoGAM does not guarantee lack of a maternal antibody response. There are situations in which the mother has been sensitized during pregnancy by early transfer of fetal red blood cells, so that RhoGAM given at delivery does not prevent the subsequent immune response. There also may be a large fetal-to-maternal transfusion at the time of delivery, and the typical RhoGAM dosage may be insufficient to neutralize the antigen exposure the mother has received (Queenan, 1977).

There are other blood group incompatibilities in which the fetal antigen may trigger a maternal antibody response (Oski & Naiman, 1982). The most common of these is the ABO blood type incompatibility. The mother's blood type may be O, A, or B. The baby may be blood type A, B, or AB. The mother does not possess the fetal red blood cell antigen A or B, and produces antibodies that cross the placenta to the baby. This difficulty may occur in the first pregnancy, since the A and B antigens are universal proteins occurring in plants and animals, and the mother will have already produced antibodies to neutralize natural antigens absorbed from the intestine. These naturally occurring antibodies subsequently may cross in sufficient amounts, even during the first pregnancy, to produce neonatal disease.

There are many other etiologies of hemolysis in a newborn (Oski & Taeusch, 1991), including biochemical defects in red blood cells (erythrocytes). The most common disease is leukocyte G6PD deficiency, in which the red blood cell's ability to maintain its shape is dependent on an internal energy source. If this source is stressed, especially by a sulfur-containing antibiotic, the red blood cells may be destroyed rapidly. Biochemical defects in the red blood cells include pyruvate kinase deficiency, hexokinase deficiency, and congenital erythopoietic porphyria. These are defects within the biochemical apparatus of the red blood cells that cause them to become susceptible to rapid destruction.

An anatomic malformation or sequestered blood in a newborn may lead to trapping and accelerated destruction of red blood cells. One example of an anatomic malformation is a hemangioma, especially the cavernous hemangioma—a vascular tumor with many large spaces. The hemangioma traps and destroys red blood cells. A malformation within the cardiovascular system (e.g., severe coarctation, a narrowing of the aorta) or an abnormality of a heart valve may result in turbulent blood flow and shorten red blood cell survival. Blood trapped in a bruise or hematoma results in excess production of bilirubin. In addition, certain hereditary structural abnormalities of the red blood cells allow excessive clearance of red blood cells by the reticuloendothelial system. In hereditary diseases, the red blood cell may take the shape of a sphere (hereditary spherocytosis) or an ellipse (hereditary elliptocytosis) rather than the normal shape of a biconcave disk.

Finally, the production of red blood cells and their life span may be adversely affected by infections, especially transplacental infections. These include: syphilis, rubella, cytomegalovirus, and toxoplasmosis. After birth, bacterial infection similarly may lead to accelerated red blood cell destruction.

Decreased Bilirubin Clearance

Once bilirubin is formed in the reticuloendothelial system, its clearance may be delayed by several factors. The first factor is decreased transport via the blood to the liver. If albumin is diminished, as is common with premature infants, less bilirubin can be carried efficiently to the liver cells. Second, as we have mentioned, many compounds may compete with bilirubin for various binding sides on albumin. These agents include salicylates (aspirin or any salt of salicylic acid), sulfa drugs, vitamin K, fatty acids, and the heme pigment itself from the red blood cell. Third, once bilirubin has been conjugated and excreted into bile, a fraction of it may be reabsorbed from the intestinal tract. This process is known as *enterohepatic circulation*, which implies a necessary reprocessing of bilirubin through the liver. Any condition that delays intestinal motility (e.g., hypothyroidism or delayed feeding) may result in elevated serum bilirubin levels (Johnson, 1975).

Several types of hereditary disease are responsible for inducing a congenital hyperbilirubinemia that is related to an excess of unconjugated bilirubin in the blood. The most common of these diseases is a mild disorder known as Gilbert syndrome, an autosomal dominant disorder that may affect as much as 3 to 5 percent of the population. Bilirubin clearance is decreased to approximately 30 percent of normal process. The syndrome never has been associated with neurological disability. In comparison, the most severe form of hereditary jaundice is the Crigler-Najjar syndrome, in which bilirubin clearance is markedly impaired as a result of the absence of an enzyme necessary for conjugation. Bilirubin blood levels rise rapidly, and bilirubin encephalopathy (brain damage) is often present.

Bilirubin Toxicity

A direct association has been established between hyperbilirubinemia, with elevated unconjugated bilirubin, and neurological damage (Cashore, 1990). This relationship was first described in 1875, and the link has been well documented in work in the 1950s, when correlations were made between the yellow staining of brain tissue and hyperbilirubinemia (Hsia, Allen, Gellis, & Diamond, 1952). While it is well established, both epidemiologically and experimentally, that unconjugated bilirubin is toxic to the central nervous system, the exact mechanism of this toxicity is not well known. The term *kernicterus* refers specifically to bilirubin staining of the brain, particularly of basal ganglia and cranial nerve nuclei, found at autopsy. The term more appropriately used for neurological disease resulting, presumably, from elevated serum bilirubin is *bilirubin encephalopathy* (Connolly & Volpe, 1990). This clinical syndrome includes a high-pitched cry, lethargy, poor feeding, and hypotonia. In the later stages, irritability, seizures, and opisthotonos (arching of the body) may occur. Long-term sequelae include athetosis (writhing movements), spasticity, sensorineural hearing loss, and dental dysplasia (deVries, Lary, & Dubowitz, 1985).

Many clinical circumstances may increase the risk of elevated serum bilirubin and subsequent toxic effects in the brain (Bratlid, 1990). Injury to the blood-brain barrier, occurring more commonly in premature infants, may result from rapid change of serum osmolarity, acidosis, infection, or intracranial hemorrhage (Levine, Fredericks, & Rapoport, 1982). A high unconjugated bilirubin concentration may exceed the bilirubin-binding capacity of the plasma proteins. This situation is seen more commonly in the preterm infant with low serum albumin concentration. Bilirubin rapidly may be displaced from the bilirubin-albumin complex by medications commonly used in the neonatal period.

Bilirubin has an affinity for the lipids in the cell membrane and may also be bound to proteins within the neuron. The specific toxicity of bilirubin in the neuron most likely results from its ability to disrupt cellular processes. Bilirubin appears to inhibit water and salt transport across the cell membrane. It also binds to and inhibits selected intracellular enzymes, which are responsible for energy production and waste elimination.

Based on research of the 1950s, it was determined that kernicterus was more likely to occur in infants in whom serum bilirubin levels were higher than 30 milligrams per deciliter and unlikely to occur in newborns with levels lower than 20 milligrams per deciliter (Mollison & Cutbush, 1954). However, as with many diseases of the newborn, there have been numerous case reports of infants with elevated levels of bilirubin who have not developed bilirubin encephalopathy and also many instances of low birthweight, high risk neonates with levels much below 20 milligrams per deciliter who developed neurological symptoms (most likely secondary to bilirubin toxicity to the central nervous system) (Gartner, Snyder, Chabon, & Bernstein, 1970; Turkel, Guttenberg, Moynes, & Hodgman, 1980).

There are new approaches to assessing the risks of neonatal hyperbilirubinemia (Vohr, 1990). The brainstem auditory-evoked response (BAER) measures the response of the acoustic nerve (eighth cranial nerve) to a specific aural stimulus. The conduction of nerve impulses is delayed in babies whose serum bilirubin levels exceed 15 milligrams per deciliter and normalizes as the jaundice resolves. A computerized analysis of the cry of a jaundiced newborn reveals changes in pitch and phonation from the baseline (Golub & Corwin, 1982). Jaundiced infants evaluated by the *Brazelton Neonatal Behavioral Assessment Scale* (BNBAS) have scored lower than control subjects in orientation, habituation, and autonomic stability (Leijon & Finnstrom, 1981).

TREATMENT

The treatment of jaundice is directed toward reduction of the serum bilirubin level. In 1958, Cremer and others observed that the exposure of infants to light produced a decline in blood bilirubin levels (Cremer, Perryman, & Richards, 1958). This finding led to widespread use of phototherapy as an adjunct to exchange blood transfusion, a procedure that is performed when serum bilirubin reaches levels considered potentially toxic (Tan, 1976).

Several processes need to be understood in order to comprehend the effectiveness of phototherapy in resolving jaundice (National Institute of Child Health and Human Development, 1985). First, bilirubin is a photoactive molecule that absorbs light at 440 to 460 nanometers. Blue or green lights provide the greatest energy in the wavelengths that modify bilirubin and are more effective than phototherapy with white light (Ennever, 1990). A high energy light source is positioned 16 to 20 inches from the unclothed baby (Figure 8–2). A plexiglass shield is placed between the light source and the infant to absorb potentially harmful ultraviolet light and to prevent injury in case the lamp explodes. With phototherapy, bilirubin is cleared from the body by two mechanisms. In the photoconversion pathway, light energy changes the unconjugated bilirubin molecule into a photoisomer, which reaches a stable concentration in 2 to 4 hours in the blood, which is a high protein solution. This compound can be discharged into the bile by the liver cell without conjugation (McDonagh & Lightner, 1988). Once the bilirubin is in the bile, which is a low protein solution, it reverts to its native form. Photo-

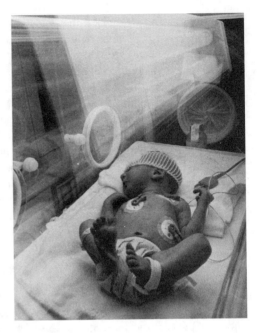

Figure 8–2 Preterm infant under phototherapy lights

oxidation is a minor pathway in which the energy of phototherapy converts bilirubin to water soluble compounds that can be excreted in urine and bile. Once phototherapy is stopped, the liver alone is responsible for bilirubin clearance.

Exhibit 8–1 lists the adverse effects of phototherapy. It routinely increases insensible water loss through the skin, making infants more prone to dehydration. Phototherapy increases bile secretion, and stools become loose and are more frequent. Since phototherapy is commonly administered to babies in incubators, a "green house" effect may occur, causing the infants to overheat. The skin of dark-skinned babies pigments more rapidly. In addition, animal research demonstrates

---

Exhibit 8–1 Complications of Phototherapy

• Increased insensible water loss	• Hypocalcemia—white light
• Loose stools, lactose intolerance	• Decreased riboflavin (vitamin B_6)—blue light
• Accelerated skin pigmentation	• Possible retinal degeneration
• Overheating	

degeneration of the retina with exposure to bright lights, although this condition may be averted by the use of eye patches. White-light phototherapy affects the pineal gland, causing a mild reduction in blood calcium. Phototherapy with blue light lowers blood riboflavin (vitamin B_6). However, since observation of cyanosis is more difficult under blue or green light, phototherapy with white light is more commonly used. Long-term effects of neonatal phototherapy are not well documented. Investigators have expressed concerns about possible endocrine effects, especially the potential for precocious sexual maturation.

Exchange Blood Transfusion

When phototherapy does not blunt a rapid rise of serum bilirubin, an unacceptable level may be reduced by an exchange blood transfusion (Allen & Diamond, 1958). A catheter is inserted into an umbilical artery and/or vein and, over the course of several hours, small aliquots of blood are removed from the baby and replaced with anticoagulated blood from an adult donor, to a total blood volume of approximately twice that of the baby (e.g., a 1,000-gram baby with a blood volume of 100 cubic centimeters would require an exchange transfusion of 200 cubic centimeters). In general, there is a 50 percent reduction in the serum bilirubin level following an exchange transfusion. The serum level then will gradually rise, as bilirubin equilibrates from the tissues to the blood, and a subsequent exchange transfusion may be necessary. Rare complications of the procedure include infection, vascular accidents, and metabolic disturbances.

Medications

Many medications are capable of stimulating hepatic conjugation and excretion of bilirubin (Vales & Harvey-Wilkes, 1990). Although phenobarbital has been used in the United States, medications are seldom given to enhance bilirubin clearance. The primary exception is the jaundice resulting from type II Crigler-Najjar syndrome, which can be ameliorated effectively with barbiturates.

Within the last several years, a novel approach has emerged (Rodgers & Stevenson, 1990). Tin or zinc protoporphyrin is used to block the enzyme heme oxygenase. Consequently, nontoxic heme is not degraded to biliverdin and bilirubin but is excreted directly by the liver. There is no jaundice to treat!

In summary, there is much yet to be learned about the subtle and long-range physical and developmental influences of jaundice (Kemper, Forsyth, & McCarthy, 1990). Similar to many other newborn conditions, hyperbilirubinemia affects each child on an individual basis. Although most neonates fully recover, educators and clinicians responsible for infant intervention programs must be cognizant of the potential adverse impact of neonatal jaundice.

BIBLIOGRAPHY

Allen, F.H., & Diamond, L.K. (1958). *Erythroblastosis fetalis including exchange transfusion technique.* Boston: Little, Brown.

Billing, B. (1987). Bilirubin metabolism. In L. Schiff & E.R. Schiff (Eds.), *Diseases of the liver* (6th ed.) (pp. 103–127). Philadelphia: J.B. Lippincott.

Bratlid, D. (1990). How bilirubin gets into the brain. *Clinics in Perinatology, 17,* 449–466.

Brodersen, R. (1979). Bilirubin, solubility, and interaction with albumin and phospholipid. *Journal of Biological Chemistry, 254,* 2364–2369.

Cashore, W.J. (1990). The neurotoxicity of bilirubin. *Clinics in Perinatology, 17,* 437–448.

Cashore, W.J. (1992). Bilirubin metabolism and toxicity in the newborn. In R.A. Polin & W.W. Fox (Eds.), *Fetal and neonatal physiology* (pp. 1160–1164). Philadelphia: W.B. Saunders.

Connolly, A.M., & Volpe, J.J. (1990). Clinical features of bilirubin encephalopathy. *Clinics in Perinatology, 17,* 371–380.

Cremer, R.J., Perryman, P.W., & Richards, D.H. (1958). Influence of light on the hyperbilirubinemia of infants. *Lancet, 1,* 1094–1097.

deVries, L.S., Lary, S., & Dubowitz, L.M.S. (1985). Relationship of serum bilirubin levels to ototoxicity and deafness in high risk low birth weight infants. *Pediatrics, 76,* 351–354.

Ennever, J.F. (1990). Blue light, green light, white light, more light: Treatment of neonatal jaundice. *Clinics in Perinatology, 17,* 467–482.

Gartner, L.M., & Arias, I.M. (1969). Formation, transport, metabolism, and excretion of bilirubin. *New England Journal of Medicine, 280,* 1339–1345.

Gartner, L.M., Snyder, R.M., Chabon, R.S., & Bernstein, J. (1970). Kernicterus: High incidence in premature infants with low serum bilirubin concentrations. *Pediatrics, 45,* 906–917.

Golub, H.L., & Corwin, M.J. (1982). Infant cry: A clue to diagnoses. *Pediatrics, 69,* 197–201.

Hardy, J.B., Drage, J.S., & Jackson, E.C. (1979). *The first year of life: The collaborative perinatal project of the National Institutes of Neurological and Communicative Disorders and Stroke.* Baltimore: Johns Hopkins University Press.

Hsia, D.Y., Allen, F.H., Gellis, S.S., & Diamond, L.K. (1952). Erythroblastosis fetalis: VIII. Studies of serum bilirubin in relation to kernicterus. *New England Journal of Medicine, 247,* 668–671.

Johnson, J.D. (1975). Neonatal nonhemolytic jaundice. *New England Journal of Medicine, 292,* 194–197.

Kemper, K.J., Forsyth, B.W., & McCarthy, P.L. (1990). Persistent perceptions of vulnerability following neonatal jaundice. *American Journal of Diseases of Children, 144,* 238–241.

Leijon, I., & Finnstrom, O. (1981). Studies on the Brazelton neonatal behavioural assessment scale. *Neuropediatrics, 12,* 242–252.

Levine, R.L., Fredericks, W.R., & Rapoport, S.I. (1982). Entry of bilirubin into the brain due to opening of the blood-brain barrier. *Pediatrics, 69,* 255–259.

Maisels, M.J. (1987). Neonatal jaundice. In G.B. Avery (Ed.), *Neonatology: Pathophysiology and management of the newborn* (3rd ed.) (pp. 534–629). Philadelphia: J.B. Lippincott.

Maisels, M.J., & Gifford, K. (1986). Normal serum bilirubin levels in the newborn and the effect of breast feeding. *Pediatrics, 78,* 837–843.

McDonagh, A.F., & Lightner, D.A. (1988). Phototherapy and the photobiology of bilirubin. *Seminars in Liver Disease, 8,* 272–277.

Mollison, P.L., & Cutbush, M. (1954). Haemolytic disease of the newborn. In D. Gairdner (Ed.), *Recent advances in Pediatrics* (pp. 110–118). New York: Blakiston.

National Institute of Child Health and Human Development (1985). National Institute of Child Health and Human Development: Randomized, controlled trial of phototherapy for neonatal hyperbilirubinemia. *Pediatrics, 72*(Suppl. 1), 384–441.

Oski, F.A., & Naiman, J.L. (1982). *Hematologic problems in the newborn* (3rd ed.) (pp. 83–132, 176–235). Philadelphia: W.B. Saunders.

Oski, F.A., & Taeusch, H.W. (1991). Disorders of bilirubin metabolism. In H.W. Taeusch, R.A. Ballard, & M.E. Avery (Eds.), *Diseases of the newborn* (6th ed.) (pp. 749–776). Philadelphia: W.B. Saunders.

Queenan, J.T. (1977). *Modern management of the Rh problem* (2nd ed.). Hagerstown, MD: Harper & Row.

Rodgers, P.A., & Stevenson, D.K. (1990). Developmental biology of heme oxygenase. *Clinics in Perinatology, 17*, 275–292.

Rosenthal, P. (1992). Bilirubin metabolism in the fetus and neonate. In R.A. Polin & W.W. Fox (Eds.), *Fetal and neonatal physiology* (Vol. 2, pp. 1154–1159). Philadelphia: W.B. Saunders.

Tan, K.L. (1976). Phototherapy for neonatal hyperbilirubinemia in healthy and ill infants. *Pediatrics, 57*, 836–838.

Turkel, S.B., Guttenberg, M.E., Moynes, D.R., & Hodgman, D.E. (1980). Lack of identifiable risk factors for kernicterus. *Pediatrics, 66*, 502–506.

Vales, T.N., & Harvey-Wilkes, K. (1990). Pharmacologic approaches to the prevention and treatment of neonatal hyperbilirubinemia. *Clinics in Perinatology, 17*, 245–274.

Vohr, B.R. (1990). New approaches to assessing the risks of hyperbilirubinemia. *Clinics in Perinatology, 17*, 293–306.

Wolkoff, A.W., Ketley, J.N., Waggoner, J.G., Berk, P.D., & Jakoby, W.B. (1978). Hepatic accumulation and intracellular binding of conjugated bilirubin. *Journal of Clinical Investigation, 61*, 142–149.

Chapter 9

Respiratory Distress

Respiratory distress is one of the most familiar and critical problems of the newborn period, for both preterm and full-term babies. Without appropriate intervention, poor oxygenation of the blood (hypoxia) and retention of carbon dioxide (hypercarbia), which lead to acidosis, almost inevitably occur. The result is multiple-organ dysfunction, especially dysfunction of the central nervous system. In recent years, as medical technology has continued to increase survival of smaller premature infants, there has been high interest in various forms of respiratory distress, along with the concern that the incidence of developmental disabilities may be high in the extremely low birthweight infant (less than 1,000 grams). In this chapter, we review normal lung development, acute respiratory distress, and chronic lung disease, and discuss current medical treatment and information regarding outcome.

NORMAL LUNG DEVELOPMENT

Typical lung development proceeds as follows. At approximately day 24 of embryonic life, a lung bud appears from the rudimentary intestinal tract (Hodson, 1992; Reid, 1967). This pouch elongates and begins to branch to form what eventually becomes the airways leading to the alveoli (air sacs), where oxygen and carbon dioxide are exchanged (Hislop, 1986). The process is complete by about 16 to 18 weeks gestation. Subsequently, primitive air sacs evolve; the first functional alveoli appear at about 24 weeks gestation. Their activity is limited by the ingrowth of blood vessels, which, for adequate exchange of gas, must closely parallel the development of air sacs. The *arterial system* supplies the lung from the right side of the heart and emerges from a primitive arch artery in the embryonic neck. In turn, the *venous system* grows backward from the left side of the heart.

124

These two networks must join to form capillaries (the smallest blood vessels), which are adjacent to alveoli for optimum gas transfer. Prior to 26 weeks gestation, this process is not sufficiently advanced for blood to acquire oxygen or to rid the body of carbon monoxide, a waste product of metabolism. From 26 to 32 weeks gestation, the small terminal air sacs give way to larger alveolar spaces with a complex branching pattern. Between 32 and 36 weeks, further budding occurs, followed by development of the type of alveoli that are present in the adult lung.

Lung growth continues even after birth, and the adult lung volume is finally attained in the midteens. The lungs of a full-term newborn have approximately one-tenth of the alveolar surface area available to an adult. Accordingly, an infant born at 28 weeks gestation has about one-eighth of the alveolar surface area of a full-term baby. Thus, a neonate delivered 12 weeks prematurely, although approximately one-third the size of a full-term baby, has disproportionately less lung tissue according to body weight.

Just as the anatomy of the lung is ever changing prior to birth, there are rapidly evolving simultaneous biochemical changes (Jobe, 1992). Specifically, the adult alveoli are lined with a complex fat, containing small amounts of protein called *surfactant* (Harwood, 1987). This substance reduces the surface tension within the alveoli. The presence of this chemical is essential in preventing the air sacs from collapsing during expiration of air in the breathing cycle. Surfactant is virtually absent before 26 weeks gestation; the primary pathway for its production is not very active until 34 to 36 weeks gestation in most fetuses. Furthermore, recent studies have demonstrated that females mature biochemically approximately 2 weeks before males, which may help to explain the disproportionate numbers of premature boy infants who have respiratory distress. There also is some evidence that the early surfactant of African-American babies is more physiologically effective than that of Caucasian babies at less than 36 weeks gestation.

ACUTE RESPIRATORY DISTRESS

Various types of respiratory distress occur in the newborn; not all respiratory failure in the neonate is caused by intrinsic lung disease. Medications given to the mother may cross the placenta and depress the respiratory effort of the newborn. Neurological disease or a malformation of the chest may restrict expansion of normal lungs, and massive abdominal distention with fluid or tumors may limit movement of the diaphragm and, therefore, restrict respiratory function. Malformations or tumors of the upper airway also may inhibit airflow into and out of the lungs. However, these impairments are all relatively uncommon causes of respiratory failure in the newborn (Avery, Fletcher, & Williams, 1981).

The signs and symptoms of respiratory distress in the neonate do not necessarily help to differentiate specific etiologies. Most infants with respiratory distress have an increased respiratory rate (tachypnea) and may be cyanotic (blue in color) because of decreased blood oxygenation. Because the chest wall musculature and rib strength (mineralization) are not yet well developed, the chest wall is less capable of resisting the strong negative pressure exerted by the diaphragm against diseased lungs. Hence, retractions (collapsing chest, especially between ribs) are frequently seen, resulting from downward movement of the diaphragm and creating a negative pressure within the chest. Under these conditions, the lungs are unable to expand adequately to fill the potential space and thus the more compliant chest wall collapses. The more immature infant with poor total body caloric reserve is not able to maintain such labored respiratory effort without serious metabolic compromise.

Retained Lung Fluid and Transient Tachypnea

Prior to birth, the lungs are filled with fluid. This substance is not amniotic fluid but is produced within the lung and contributes to amniotic fluid, especially in the 3rd trimester of pregnancy. At birth, this liquid must be cleared rapidly to allow for appropriate respiratory function. It has been shown that the biochemical processes initiating labor begin to shift fluid from the air spaces of the baby's lungs into the bloodstream 3 to 5 days prior to labor, in preparation for birth (Bland, 1992). Much of the remaining fluid then is expelled as the chest is squeezed in the process of delivery. Subsequently, the residual fluid in the lungs is absorbed into the circulatory system and excreted through the kidneys.

Transient tachypnea refers to a mild form of respiratory distress that requires brief oxygen supplementation (Rawlings & Smith, 1984). Essentially, this condition results from increased retention of lung fluid. It is more commonly seen in babies born prematurely and in those delivered by cesarean section, especially in infants whose mothers have had no labor. By chest X-ray, it may be noted that the lungs have a normal volume and often have fluid in the fissures between the lung lobes. In the typical course of the illness, respiratory symptoms disappear in the first 24 to 48 hours after birth, as the lung fluid is absorbed and excreted (Halliday, McClure, & McCreid, 1981).

Surfactant-Deficiency Syndrome

Surfactant-deficiency syndrome (Exhibit 9–1) is the current name for respiratory distress syndrome (hyaline membrane disease), which is seen in premature infants who lack surfactant in the alveoli (Avery, 1984; Hansen & Corbet, 1991a and 1991b). As the result of this condition, the alveoli collapse and the total area for absorption of oxygen into the body and elimination of carbon dioxide is markedly reduced. This is a progressive illness, which becomes worse over 3 to 4 days, as the small amount of surfactant remaining in the lungs is degraded faster than it can be replaced. Proteins leak from the capillaries into partially or completely

Exhibit 9–1 Relative Risk of Surfactant Deficiency

Factors for Decreased Risk	*Factors for Increased Risk*
• Fetal growth retardation • Narcotic addiction • Prenatal corticosteroids • Ruptured membranes >24 hours after birth • Toxemia of pregnancy	• Maternal diabetes • Maternal hemorrhage • Multiple gestation

collapsed air sacs, and this material forms a *hyaline membrane*, which further limits the exchange of gases from the alveoli back and forth to the capillaries. The disease begins to resolve as the lungs begin to synthesize the adult form of surfactant, which provides for stability of the alveoli. Reabsorption of the proteinaceous hyaline membrane then follows over the next several weeks.

Most newborns with surfactant deficiency require supplemental oxygen and many need mechanical ventilatory support. Although the pathophysiology was described over two decades ago in the early 1960s, surfactant-replacement therapy first became available in the United States in August 1990 (Shapiro, 1992). In the United States, two products are available for this therapy: *Exosurf Neonatal*, which is a synthetic product, and *Survanta,* which is derived from an extract of calf lung. Babies who have severe surfactant deficiency, as evidenced by the rapid appearance of sufficient clinical illness to require mechanical ventilation and supplemental oxygen, are candidates for replacement therapy (Avery & Merritt, 1991). The treatment is expensive, averaging approximately $1,000 per dose and, typically, three doses are given into the trachea within the first 48 hours after birth. To date, the results are variable. It appears that surfactant-replacement therapy has a limited impact on overall mortality but does decrease morbidity and the incidence of chronic lung disease in babies weighing more than 1,000 grams. Fortunately, the majority of infants gradually recover to essentially normal lung function within a few weeks after birth. Few infants develop chronic lung changes that require intense life support therapy.

Aspiration

Aspiration refers to the physiological reactions to abnormal or foreign material that has gained access to the lungs (Avery, Fletcher, & Williams, 1981; Stahlman, 1981). The two most common substances aspirated around the time of birth are amniotic fluid and amniotic fluid containing meconium. When amniotic fluid is drawn into the lungs, proteins and cellular debris provoke an inflammatory reaction that resembles pneumonia. The subsequent course is variable and depends, in large measure, on the characteristics and amount of the fluid inhaled and its distribution within the lungs.

A more serious condition occurs when amniotic fluid containing meconium, a dark green sterile viscous material found in the intestine of the fetus, is aspirated (Gregory, Gooding, Phibbs, & Tooley, 1974). Approximately 5 percent of babies born after 34 weeks gestation have sufficient fetal distress to pass meconium reflexively. Severe complications may result. Normally, as we inhale, the airways expand, and as we exhale, they contract. If meconium is aspirated, air is passed beyond the thick material through the dilated airways, but then is trapped in the lung as the airways collapse in exhalation (Miller, Fanaroff, & Martin, 1992a). Such obstructions may progressively overdistend the involved portions of the lung, leading to rupture of alveoli. Subsequently, over a period of several days, the diverse components of meconium initiate severe injury to the lungs, with inflammation and excess lung fluid. More recent evidence has shown that free fatty acids from meconium interfere initially with surfactant function and then with surfactant production (Clark, Nieman, Thompson, & Bredenberg, 1987). Obviously, all of these changes interfere with the respiratory process.

Air Block Syndromes

There are three major types of *air block syndromes*. These syndromes involve conditions in which air collects in the chest and is unavailable for exchange of oxygen and carbon dioxide in the alveoli (Madansky, Lawson, Chernick, & Taeusch, 1979). The insult varies with the specific location of air in the chest, which can be determined by X-ray (Stahlman, 1981). *Pneumothorax* is a condition in which gas is located within the chest cavity, but is external to and compressing the lung. By insertion of a chest tube to drain the air, the lung can be reinflated. The second form of air blockage, *pneumomediastinum*, occurs when air is trapped around structures in the center of the chest. If this gas is under tension, the vessels returning blood to the heart may be compressed. Lastly, when air in the mediastinum is confined to the pericardium (the sac surrounding the heart), a *pneumopericardium* occurs. Under tension, a pneumopericardium does not permit adequate filling of the heart with blood and thus prevents cardiac output to circulate blood. Even with aggressive therapy, approximately 40 percent of babies with this condition die.

Among these air block syndromes, pneumothorax is seen with the greatest frequency, in as many as 5 percent of all newborns. Only approximately 1 percent of babies with pneumothorax are symptomatic, requiring medical or surgical intervention. Aside from the initial neonatal period when rapid expansion of lungs takes place, the various types of air block syndromes are manifested primarily in babies with acute respiratory diseases who require positive-pressure expansion of the lungs with mechanical ventilation.

Hemorrhage and Infection

Babies who have congenital heart disease or severe respiratory distress are at risk from overdistended, weak, pulmonary blood vessels that may rupture (Miller, Fanaroff, & Martin, 1992b). Pulmonary hemorrhage is seen often in neonates who experience significant perinatal asphyxia. With such illnesses, blood may fill the normally functioning lungs, thus preventing the exchange of gas. As with other forms of bleeding, enough blood may be lost to result in shock and death, despite aggressive intervention.

Typically, infection of the lungs (pneumonia) is seen when the membranes surrounding the baby have been ruptured for a prolonged period prior to birth (Hansen & Corbet, 1991a and 1991b). Under these conditions, bacteria and viruses ordinarily colonizing the mother's vagina may gain access to the amniotic fluid and, secondarily, invade the fetal lung. The clinical presentation of babies who are infected varies, with X-ray changes ranging from mild to severe and outcomes that are much less predictable than the prognosis of other acute respiratory diseases managed throughout the newborn period (Hanshaw & Dudgeon, 1978).

CHRONIC LUNG DISEASE

Several forms of chronic lung disease can be distinguished in the neonate. Each of these illnesses usually requires a long-term dependence on supplemental oxygen (Fox, Murray, & Martin, 1983). In addition, these conditions frequently are characterized by elevated blood carbon dioxide levels, resulting from inadequate surface area for gas exchange in the lung. In the very low birthweight infant (less than 1,000 grams), the most common problem is *chronic pulmonary insufficiency of prematurity* (CPIP) (Krauss, Klain, & Auld, 1975). In this condition, the alveoli are forced to grow and biochemically mature under the constant stress of the oxygen content of at least room air, which is approximately 6 times greater than that of the developing air sacs when the lungs are fluid-filled in utero. Lung growth, therefore, is delayed, leading to a long-term dependency on supplemental oxygen. Gradually, as the nutritional status of the baby improves, the alveoli grow and most children are weaned from oxygen within the first 6 months of life.

Bronchopulmonary dysplasia (BPD) is another variation of chronic lung disease that emanates from lifesaving, therapeutic maneuvers in the treatment of children with acute respiratory illnesses (Merritt, Northway, & Boyton, 1988). Although official definitions of BPD change every few years, current criteria indicate that a baby requires oxygen therapy 28 days after birth. The combination of supplemental oxygen (especially in amounts greater than 40 percent), positive pressure, and the trauma of mechanical ventilation inevitably leads to changes in the airways, which become thickened because of increased mucus production.

Surfactant production is decreased and alveolar growth is delayed in babies who have a prolonged oxygen requirement.

Babies with CPIP or BPD may have insufficient pulmonary repair and growth to sustain life. Those who do recover and are removed from supplemental oxygen continue to have diminished pulmonary reserve throughout the next several years of life. Hence, they are more susceptible to infection and often must be hospitalized again. Assuming no major intervening illness, however, the majority of survivors acquire relatively normal lung function by the time they reach kindergarten.

TREATMENT OF RESPIRATORY DISEASE

It should be obvious from our discussion of respiratory illness that the main goal of therapy is the maintenance of adequate blood oxygen and the concurrent control of blood carbon dioxide levels in order to prevent acidosis. Carbon dioxide diffuses more readily from blood vessels to the alveoli; therefore, the higher the blood carbon dioxide content, the greater the severity of pulmonary disease. Supplemental oxygen is given to maintain blood oxygen levels in a range of 50 to 80 millimeters of mercury. If adequate oxygenation cannot be maintained in 100 percent oxygen or if the blood carbon dioxide level exceeds 60 millimeters of mercury with poor respiratory effort, assisted ventilation is necessary. The first step in the therapeutic process is the use of constant positive airway pressure (CPAP). This treatment involves the infant's breathing against a low pressure, a process that stabilizes alveoli for gas exchange. If the newborn is unable to achieve adequate oxygenation, mechanical ventilation is used. There are many types of equipment for mechanical ventilation, and the concentration of oxygen delivered, respiratory rate, and inflation pressure are individualized to the child and are specific for the particular form of respiratory distress that is being treated.

Throughout the duration of therapy, general supportive care is important. Blood pressure must be carefully monitored, as well as the blood levels of the various minerals such as sodium and calcium. Nutrition is a high priority, but the baby is rarely able to feed adequately and, therefore, must receive intravenous nutrition. In addition, adequate temperature support is essential to conserve calories for growth and repair.

OUTCOME

While information on survival rates for newborns with respiratory distress is abundant, data on long-term development are more sparse. In general, the mild types of respiratory distress are associated with few and less persistent developmental delays. Babies with more severe illnesses, especially those requiring prolonged periods of ventilation are more apt to manifest developmental problems. At present, however, it is extremely difficult to distinguish the effects of the severity of disease from those related to intensity of intervention and associated medical complications such as lack of nutrition, intracranial hemorrhage, and infection, which may impinge on development.

BIBLIOGRAPHY

Avery, M.E. (1984). Hyaline membrane disease. In M.E. Avery & H.W. Taeusch (Eds.), *Schaffer's diseases of the newborn* (5th ed.) (pp. 133–147). Philadelphia: W.B. Saunders.

Avery, M.E., Fletcher, B.D., & Williams, R.G. (1981). Lung development. In M.E. Avery, B.D. Fletcher, & R.G. Williams (Eds.), *The lung and its disorders in the newborn infant* (4th ed.) (pp. 3–48). Philadelphia: W.B. Saunders.

Avery, M.E., & Merritt, T.A. (1991). Surfactant-replacement therapy. *New England Journal of Medicine, 324,* 865–869.

Bland, R.D. (1992). Formation of fetal lung liquid and its removal near birth. In R.A. Polin & W.W. Fox (Eds.), *Fetal and neonatal physiology* (6th ed.) (Vol. 1) (pp. 782–789). Philadelphia: W.B. Saunders.

Clark, D.A., Nieman, G.F., Thompson, J.E., & Bredenberg, C.E. (1987). Surfactant displacement by meconium free fatty acids: An alternative explanation for atelectasis in meconium aspiration syndrome. *Journal of Pediatrics, 110,* 765–770.

Fox, W.W., Murray, J.P., & Martin, R.J. (1983). Chronic pulmonary diseases of the neonate. In A.A. Fanaroff & R.J. Martin (Eds.), *Neonatal-perinatal medicine: Diseases of the fetus and infant* (3rd ed.) (pp. 467–476). St. Louis: C.V. Mosby.

Gregory, G.A., Gooding, C.A., Phibbs, R.H., & Tooley, W.H. (1974). Meconium aspiration in infants—A prospective study. *Journal of Pediatrics, 85,* 848–852.

Halliday, H.L., McClure, G., & McCreid, M. (1981). Transient tachypnea of the newborn: Two distinct clinical entities. *Archives of Disease in Childhood, 56,* 322–325.

Hansen, T., & Corbet, A. (1991a). Lung development and function. In H.W. Taeusch, R.A. Ballard, & M.E. Avery (Eds.), *Diseases of the newborn* (pp. 461–469). Philadelphia: W.B. Saunders.

Hansen, T., & Corbet, A. (1991b). Neonatal pneumonias. In H.W. Taeusch, R.A. Ballard, & M.E. Avery (Eds.), *Diseases of the newborn* (pp. 527–535). Philadelphia: W.B. Saunders.

Hanshaw, J.B., & Dudgeon, J.A. (1978). *Viral diseases of the fetus and newborn.* Philadelphia: W.B. Saunders.

Harwood, J.L. (1987). Lung surfactant. *Progress in Lipid Research, 26,* 211–216.

Hislop, A. (1986). Alveolar development in the human fetus and infant. *Early Human Development, 13,* 1–8.

Hodson, W.A. (1992). Normal and abnormal structural development of the lungs. In R.A. Polin & W.W. Fox (Eds.), *Fetal and neonatal physiology* (6th ed.) (Vol. 1) (pp. 771–782). Philadelphia: W.B. Saunders.

Jobe, A.H. (1992). The developmental biology of the lung. In A.A. Fanaroff & R.J. Martin (Eds.), *Neonatal-perinatal medicine: Diseases of the fetus and infant* (5th ed.) (Vol. 2) (pp. 783–800). St. Louis: C.V. Mosby.

Krauss, A.N., Klain, D.B., & Auld, P. (1975). Chronic pulmonary insufficiency of prematurity (CPIP). *Pediatrics, 55,* 55–58.

Madansky, D.L., Lawson, E.E., Chernick, V., & Taeusch, H.W. (1979). Pneumothorax and other forms of pulmonary air leaks in newborns. *American Review of Respiratory Disease, 120,* 729–737.

Merritt, T.A., Northway, W.H., Jr., & Boyton, B.R. (Eds.). (1988). *Bronchopulmonary dysplasia*. Boston: Blackwell Scientific.

Miller, M.J., Fanaroff, A.A., & Martin, R.J. (1992a). Meconium aspiration. In A.A. Fanaroff & R.J. Martin (Eds.), *Neonatal-perinatal medicine: Diseases of the fetus and infant* (5th ed.) (Vol. 2) (pp. 834–837). St. Louis: C.V. Mosby.

Miller, M.J., Fanaroff, A.A., & Martin, R.J. (1992b). Pulmonary hemorrhage. In A.A. Fanaroff & R.J. Martin (Eds.), *Neonatal-perinatal medicine: Diseases of the fetus and infant* (5th ed.) (Vol. 2) (pp. 839–840). St. Louis: C.V. Mosby.

Rawlings, J.S., & Smith, F.R. (1984). Transient tachypnea of the newborn. *American Journal of Diseases of Children, 138*, 869–872.

Reid, L. (1967). The embryology of the lung. In A.V.A. deReuck & R. Parker (Eds.), *CIBA Foundation symposium on development of the lung* (pp. 109–124). London: Churchill Livingstone.

Shapiro, D.L. (1992). Surfactant replacement therapy. In R.A. Polin & W.W. Fox (Eds.), *Fetal and neonatal physiology* (6th ed.) (pp. 1007–1014). Philadelphia: W.B. Saunders.

Stahlman, M.T. (1981). Acute respiratory disorders in the newborn. In G.B. Avery (Ed.), *Neonatology: Pathophysiology and management of the newborn* (2nd ed.) (pp. 371–397). Philadelphia: J.B. Lippincott.

Chapter 10

Nutrition and Metabolism

NUTRITION

Digestion and Absorption

Nutrition prior to birth is provided by the passage of nutrients from the mother via the placenta to the fetus. In turn, the waste products resulting from a high fetal metabolic rate (e.g., urea and bilirubin) are then returned to the mother for excretion. Once the infant is born, the intestine immediately must begin the complex process of converting breast milk or the complex components of formula into the simple nutrients that were previously provided by the placenta. Since many serious illnesses of the newborn limit the type and quality of feeding, the intravenous (IV) route of nutrition is often a necessity.

The intestinal tract of a full-term infant is approximately 100 to 110 inches long, and, at birth, most of the enzymes necessary to digest sugars, proteins, and fats are present (Moya, 1993). However, the more immature the infant, the greater the limitation of digestive capabilities. Despite increasing knowledge and sophistication in the nutrition of the newborn, IV nutritional therapy remains a poor alternative to a well-developed, properly functioning intestinal tract. Parenteral nutrition (IV nutritional therapy) is expensive, with many potential complications, and should be limited to situations in which it is absolutely essential.

The body composition of the full-term infant differs dramatically from that of a premature baby. In the full-term infant, approximately 12 to 15 percent of body weight is fat, and approximately 11 to 12 percent is protein (Clark, 1993). In premature infants, a much lower percentage of body weight is fat— as little as 1 percent at 28 weeks gestation. Conversely, a premature infant has a higher percentage of body weight as water—as much as 85 percent at 28 weeks gestation; the percentage subsequently decreases to a range of 70 to 75 percent at term. This difference in total body composition reflects the total energy reserve, which is much higher in the term newborn, who can modulate metabolism and has sufficient stored calories to maintain body heat and blood glucose level.

Each portion of the intestinal tract has a specialized function in digestion and absorption of nutrients (Grand, Watkins, & Torti, 1976). A mature newborn has a coordinated sucking and swallowing mechanism that is usually not found in a neonate less than 34 weeks gestation. Initially, the mature newborn has limited gastric volume, with delayed gastric emptying and decreased acid secretion. These may be important factors in allowing the early hormones, enzymes, and protective proteins of breast milk to gain access to the lower intestinal tract. In general, protein and fat digestion is initiated within the stomach, enhanced in the first portion of the small intestine (duodenum), and then completed through the remainder of the small intestine. Carbohydrate digestion is initiated in the mouth, and generally is completed within the first portion of the small intestine. Vitamins, minerals, water, and other vital nutrients are absorbed throughout the small and large intestines in various gradients.

Adequate digestion and absorption of nutrients within the intestine require continuous movement in the digestive system, from the mouth to the anus. This process is termed *intestinal motility* (Clark, 1993). The suck reflex is poorly coordinated in an infant younger than 34 weeks, and motility throughout the small and large intestines is limited. Many of the hormones secreted in the intestinal tract can modify digestive capabilities and increase or decrease motility of the intestine, promoting more efficient digestion. Dietary components themselves may influence intestinal motility. High fat meals and casein (the curd protein of milk) delay gastric emptying and slow intestinal movement. The slowing of intestinal motility presumably permits more time for the thorough digestion of fats and complex proteins.

The ability of kidneys to eliminate waste products in the newborn and to regulate electrolyte and water balance does not reach a mature level until 1 year of age. Renal blood flow and the filtration of the blood is lower in the preterm infant than in the term infant. Thus, a premature infant has a decreased ability to excrete an acid load and also is less able to dilute and concentrate the urine. Consequently, the premature baby or growth-retarded infant is more prone to dehydration or fluid excess if a proper fluid intake is not maintained.

Weight Gain and Energy Requirements

There are many obstacles to appropriate weight gain for premature and growth-retarded infants (Romero & Kleinman, 1993). In these newborns digestion, especially digestion of fats and carbohydrates, tends to be inefficient. Consequently, the number of calories available is less than the number consumed. Limited excretory function of both the liver and kidneys may decrease utilization of the amino acids and calories (sugars or fats) necessary for optimal growth and development.

In addition, in a premature infant, the need to maintain body temperature requires that calories be burned, thus sacrificing growth.

Although most infants are genetically healthy, some growth-retarded infants may have chromosomal anomalies such as trisomy 18 and trisomy 13. The poor suck and swallow also may be seen in these and other developmental syndromes in which neurological dysfunction is prominent.

Several illnesses may interfere with total caloric intake and utilization. One of the most common of these illnesses is surfactant deficiency, which causes respiratory distress, thus increasing the work of breathing and caloric consumption, while limiting the ability to feed. Intravenous glucose solutions may be the only caloric intake for the first several days of sickness. Intravenous infusion of lipids interfere with the ability to oxygenate the red blood cell hemoglobin; and exacerbates jaundice by binding to albumin and decreasing bilirubin transport to the liver. Therefore, lipid emulsions rarely are used in the first 3 to 4 days after birth. Other illnesses are caused by transplacental viral or parasitic infection, which may result in significant tissue disruption and subsequent growth retardation. Babies with such conditions often show central nervous system and hepatic involvement, with decreased ability to clear waste products of metabolism. Also, premature infants are prone to gastroesophageal reflux and malabsorption. The second most common killer of premature infants, necrotizing enterocolitis, is an inflammatory bowel condition seen more commonly in the premature infant born weighing less than 1,000 grams (Clark & Miller, 1990). In this condition, the intestine is so damaged that it cannot function. There may be sufficient destruction to require surgical resection of the intestine, resulting in short bowel syndrome, malabsorption, and limitation of intake.

Although weight gain in newborn infants is relatively easy to document, the composition of the weight attributed to tissue growth or edema is difficult to measure (Clark, 1993). Most full-term healthy infants receiving adequate calculated nutrition after birth recover birthweight within 7 to 10 days (Moya, 1993). Premature infants return to birthweight much more slowly because of limitations by caloric intake, excessive fluid loss, and increased caloric expenditure. The caloric requirements for premature and growth-retarded infants remain clearly defined and may be as little as 60 calories per kilogram per day or as much as 150 calories per kilogram per day (American Academy of Pediatrics Committee on Nutrition, 1985). Calories available for growth are those that remain after the various components of caloric expenditure have been subtracted. These components include digestion, metabolism at the basal metabolic rate, and spontaneous activity, all of which consume a moderate amount of calories.

Table 10–1 shows the distribution of caloric requirements in an active, growing, low birthweight infant. Unfortunately, despite the recent strides in knowledge of nutrition and growth, the approximation of intrauterine growth and development has not yet been accomplished. There remains a great debate as to whether

Table 10–1 Estimated Caloric Requirements in an Active "Growing" Low Birthweight Infant

Item	Caloric Requirement (kilocalories per kilogram per day)
Resting expenditure*	50
Specific dynamic action+	10
Fecal calorie loss	10
Intermittent activity	15
Growth allowance†	60
Total	145

*Includes calories for temperature maintenance.

+Difference between the resting caloric expenditure for the infant who has been fed and that for the fasted infant.

†Approximately 5 kilocalories per gram of tissue deposited.

neonatal growth paralleling intrauterine growth should be a goal and what the approximate composition of various body tissues should be. To best understand the appropriate nutrition, we need to separate the various components of nutrition into water, carbohydrate, fat, protein, minerals, and vitamins (Fomon, 1993).

Water

Dehydration is a common problem in the low birthweight infant because of the high water loss through the skin (Romero & Kleinman, 1993). A 1,000-gram, 28-week gestation infant has a cutaneous water loss 2 to 3 times that of a full-term infant. In combination with the limited ability of the kidney to concentrate urine, dehydration, especially with a high blood sodium level, becomes life threatening. On the other hand, the limited ability of the kidneys to excrete a water load may result in edema and congestive heart failure in the premature infant. Therefore, the range of total fluid that can be administered to the premature or growth-retarded infant is much narrower than that tolerated by the full-term baby. Critically ill newborns require extra fluids for many other reasons, including additional trans-cutaneous water loss from radiant warmers and phototherapy for jaundice (El-Dahr & Chevalier, 1990). Renal dysfunction following asphyxia and the presence of a patent ductus arteriosus with excess lung fluid are conditions that may require moderate fluid restriction, especially in the smaller (less than 1,500 grams) newborn.

Carbohydrates

Carbohydrates or sugars are the primary energy source and are the precursors of many metabolic pathways such as those for the formation of nucleic acids (DNA and RNA) and for bilirubin conjugation (Lifshitz, 1988). Dextrose, the right-handed isomer of glucose, is a monosaccharide used during intrauterine existence. The primary sugar of breast milk or infant formula is the disaccharide lactose, which is a compound of glucose and galactose. Enzymes involved in digestion of the complex sugars are present in the brush border in the surface villi of the intestine. The enzyme *lactase* is detected first at approximately 34 weeks gestation. Therefore, lactose digestion is limited in the preterm infant born before that time. In formulas for preterm infants, polymers of glucose have been substituted for up to 50 percent of the lactose content. These glucose polymers are readily digested, resulting in maximum glucose availability.

Undigested carbohydrates have been found in the stools of premature infants. These carbohydrates reach the colonic bacteria, which ferment them to produce compounds including organic acids and gases. Organic acids may be absorbed and metabolized, providing a recovery mechanism for some of the calories lost by inefficient digestion. However, should the organic acids accumulate in the terminal portion of the small intestine and colon, the increased acid concentration in the intestine is a prime factor in the induction of late-onset, feeding-associated necrotizing enterocolitis (Clark & Miller, 1990).

Fats

Lipids, which have diverse functions in humans, are vital for growth and development (Hamosh, 1988). Fats are the primary energy source of newborns and are essential for brain development. In the full-term newborn, body fat has increased 10- to 15-fold over that of the 28-week preterm infant. Approximately 10 percent of this fat is brown fat, which is found in the chest and axillae. Compared with other fat, this fat is more vascular, with a high density of mitochondria. Thus, it is responsive to the adrenal hormones that can rapidly mobilize it for an energy source.

The backbone of the fat molecule is glycerol, a three-carbon molecule attached to one, two, or three fatty acids (*monoglycerides, diglycerides,* or *triglycerides,* respectively) (Hamosh, Bitman, & Wood, 1985). Fat digestion requires that the pancreatic enzymes cleave fatty acids from the glycerol molecule. These fats are then absorbed and repackaged within the intestinal wall to form triglycerides by reattaching the fatty acids to the glycerol. These packages subsequently are transported via the bloodstream throughout the body. If not utilized as an energy source, they are placed in storage. The complete catabolism of glycerol and fatty acids yields energy, water, and carbon dioxide. This process can occur only if the fats can be delivered to the appropriate enzyme systems within the mitochondria of the cells. The process is dependent on carnitine, a tripeptide synthesized from two amino acids, lysine and methionine. Preterm infants may not be able to synthesize carnitine, so this tripeptide has been added to all the standard formulas for premature infants. Since a long-chain fatty acid may be less well metabolized by premature infants, approximately 50 percent of the fat content in preterm formulas is presented as medium-chain triglycerides—glycerol molecules that have attached fatty acids of medium chain length. Phospholipids are lipids with phosphate-containing portions and are critical components of the cell membrane. Pulmonary surfactant is a mixture of phospholipids that lowers the surface tension in the alveoli and helps prevent collapse at the end expiration. Fat metabolism may yield many other compounds such as the prostaglandins and leukotrienes, which are important in modulating blood flow at the tissue level.

Protein

Protein is the nutrient most essential for normal growth and development of both full-term and preterm infants (Raiha, 1989). Amino acids, derived from dietary proteins, are synthesized into cell membrane and transport proteins, enzymes, peptide hormones, immunoglobulins, coagulation factors, and neurotransmitters. The mature digestion of dietary protein is dependent on a series of enzymes found in the proximal duodenum and released from pancreatic secretions. By 20 weeks gestation, a preterm infant has developed gastric, intestinal, and pancreatic function for protein digestion and absorption. This function is limited; thus, several additional amino acids are essential in the nutrition of the preterm infant.

Total protein intake is limited by immature renal and hepatic function in the premature infant. Although over 90 percent of protein nitrogen is incorporated into tissue protein, the immature kidney cannot handle waste products of metabolism as efficiently as the placenta. Thus, premature infants fed over 6 grams of protein per kilogram per day have much higher urea nitrogen levels than full-term babies, which may cause growth retardation postnatally.

Digestion of the milk proteins is complex. The casein or curd proteins, which are found only in milk, are less readily digested than the whey proteins (Clark, 1993). Undigested caseins have been associated with delayed gastric emptying and lactobezoars, firm stomach masses that may require surgical removal (Miller, Witherly, & Clark, 1990). In addition, undigested proteins bind crucial minerals such as calcium, magnesium, and zinc. The casein proteins promote inflammation, by attracting and activating white blood cells. Over 95 percent of the whey protein fraction of milk is utilized, compared with 80 percent of the casein protein fraction.

Protein requirements for preterm and growth-retarded infants are thought to be approximately 2.5 to 4.0 grams per kilogram per day. Current formulas for premature infants have been adjusted to lower the casein fraction to 40 percent or less of the total protein content. Taurine, an amino acid derived from cysteine, is found in breast milk in high concentrations. This protein is important for growth and development of the central nervous system, especially the retina of the eye (Gault, 1989). All of the standard formulas now contain supplemental taurine in quantities approaching those in breast milk.

Minerals

The minerals important to body growth and development include calcium, magnesium, sodium, potassium, and iron, which frequently form complexes with phosphorus or iodine (Tsang, 1985). In addition, zinc, copper, manganese, chromium, fluoride, molybdenum, and selenium are considered to be important trace elements. Sodium and potassium are the primary minerals found in the body. Potassium is the major intracellular metal, and sodium is found in the extracellular fluid. The differential concentrations of these two minerals inside and outside of cells are crucial in maintaining the polarization (electrical activity) that moves nutrients into and waste products out of the cells. This polarity also facilitates transmission of electrical impulses throughout the nervous system, regulates muscular activity, and drives the beat of the heart.

Calcium and phosphorus are responsible for bone growth. Over 50 percent of the calcium content in the bones of a full-term baby is deposited in the last trimester. Therefore, infants born prematurely are more prone to abnormal bone growth, which is termed *osteopenia of prematurity* (neonatal rickets). The regulation of calcium and phosphorus absorption, metabolism, and deposition is accomplished by the parathyroid glands, the kidneys, and the liver. In addition to its crucial role in cellular growth, phosphorus is the base of many of the high energy compounds within the body, including adenosine triphosphatase (ATP).

Magnesium metabolism is closely linked to that of calcium. It is the second most common intracellular electrolyte in the body and is known to be important in many transport mechanisms and in enzyme function.

Iron is essential to the formation of hemoglobin. It is absorbed primarily in the first portion of the small intestine. Approximately 50 percent of iron from breast milk is absorbed, which is much greater than the amount absorbed from formulas. This situation exists because breast milk contains an iron-binding protein, lactoferrin, which enhances the transfer of iron across the intestinal surface. All newborns, including premature infants, have sufficient body iron at birth to supply their needs until their birthweight is almost doubled. Sick premature infants may develop iron excess as a result of receiving more iron in blood transfusions than is being lost from frequent blood sampling. Occasionally, a breast-fed low birthweight infant who receives no iron supplementation may develop iron-deficiency anemia. Symptoms include irritability, listlessness, inadequate growth, and feeding difficulties.

The need of premature infants for supplemental trace minerals has been well recognized (Mertz, 1985). Zinc deficiency may cause slowed growth, diarrhea, hair loss, and perianal skin lesions. Copper deficiency has been reported in infants with poor weight gain, edema, and decreased muscle tone. The precise need or deficiency state of the other trace elements is not well defined in preterm infants. Standard parenteral nutrition and routine formulas provide sufficient amounts of all of the known trace elements.

Vitamins

Vitamins can be classified as fat soluble and water soluble (Greene & Smidt, 1993). Few deficiencies have been demonstrated in the water soluble vitamins such as vitamin C and the B complex vitamins niacin, biotin, and pantothenic acid (Orzalesi, 1987). In contrast, the fat soluble vitamins may be linked to the absorption of fat. Deficiencies of vitamins A, D, and E have been linked to specific clinical findings in newborns. Vitamin A supplementation or replacement may be helpful for mitigating the severity of bronchopulmonary dysplasia. Supplemental vitamin D may be useful in limiting the osteopenia of prematurity. Vitamin E may reduce the severity of retinopathy of prematurity and may decrease the incidence of intraventricular hemorrhage.

Finally, vitamin K has long been recognized as critical for preventing hemorrhagic disease in newborns (Fomon & Suttie, 1993). All newborns are born deficient in vitamin K because this compound is synthesized by the intestinal bacteria. The large intestine is sterile at birth, and during the first week, the baby who has not received vitamin K is susceptible to hemorrhage. Only 1 to 2 percent of 1-week-old babies have hemorrhage, but the bleeding may be severe and involve the central nervous system, lungs, or adrenal glands.

Summary

Assuming a healthy intestine, the diet should contain sufficient calories distributed across the essential nutrients. For maximum infant growth, the intake of carbohydrates should be 35 to 45 percent of calories; fats, 30 to 55 percent; and protein, 7 to 16 percent. Breast milk and various newborn formulas all meet these requirements. Overall, breast milk remains the ideal feeding for healthy full-term infants, as well as for most neonates born after 34 weeks gestation. For the more premature infant, the lactose content of breast milk may not be appropriately digested and the fat may be too complex for the immature intestines and pancreas. Likewise, there may be insufficient minerals, especially calcium and sodium.

INBORN METABOLIC ENDOCRINE DISORDERS

Some metabolic diseases are fatal or currently have no therapy. There are inborn errors of metabolism that can be virtually corrected by elimination of a component of the diet or by specific simple therapy. To detect these conditions, Western countries have implemented screening programs that are cost-effective even though they are expensive (Theorell & Degenhardt, 1993). In each of these inherited diseases, a nutritional component cannot be handled properly by the cellular metabolism, usually because an enzyme deficiency blocks metabolism. This condition results in absorption of insufficient amounts of a substance critical for body growth and metabolism or the accumulation of an excessive amount of a substance that should be eliminated by the body. This energy deprivation or abnormal accumulation of a substance prevents the tissues from functioning properly. Many of these conditions are not amenable to therapy and result in severe mental retardation.

Although state programs vary, every state has routine metabolic screening of all newborns for the more common treatable inherited metabolic diseases. As Table 10–2 illustrates, New York State has one of the more extensive programs, but the incidence of even the most common of these conditions, hypothyroidism, is relatively low. These programs are cost-effective because the long-term medical and social care of an individual with severe mental retardation far exceeds the expenditures for screening and preventing these illnesses.

These metabolic defects do not interfere with development prior to birth because the excess materials can pass freely back to the mother via the placenta, and she can eliminate them and prevent toxicity to the fetus. Following delivery, however, these nutritional byproducts begin to accumulate in the body, resulting in damage to tissue, especially the brain. Three diseases are sufficiently common to warrant discussion: phenylketonuria (PKU), galactosemia, and hypothyroidism.

Phenylketonuria is the prototype of an inherited metabolic illness for which screening is justified (Berry, 1981). The impairment results from excess accumulation of phenylalanine (an amino acid), due to the absence or malfunctioning of

Table 10–2 Incidence of Metabolic Diseases in the New York State Metabolic Screening Program

Inherited Disease	Incidence
Adenosine deaminase deficiency	1/4,000
Hypothyroidism	1/16,700
Phenylketonuria (PKU)	1/73,000
Histidinemia	1/160,000
Homocystinuria	1/480,000
Galactosemia	1/600,000
Branched-chain ketonuria	1/1,200,000

Source: From "Newborn Metabolic Screening," *New York State Health Department Newsletter*, Fall 1982 (unpublished).

an enzyme that is normally produced in the liver. The body fails to convert phenylalanine to other amino acids. As a result, the excess phenylalanine accumulates within tissues and is especially disruptive to the central nervous system. Although there are several variations of this condition, restriction of phenylalanine in the diet within the first few weeks after birth and for several years has been effective in preventing most impairments. Phenylalanine cannot be totally removed from the diet, because it is an essential component of many proteins in the body.

Galactosemia results from inability to convert galactose to glucose, which can be utilized readily by tissues (Zinn, 1992). Glucose and galactose are the two simple sugars that combine to form the primary milk sugar lactose. As a consequence, galactose accumulates in the body and causes damage, initially to the liver (cirrhosis). Affected infants become jaundiced and bleed easily. Several months into the course of the disease, babies frequently develop cataracts from deposition of galactose in the lens. On the other hand, if lactose is removed from the diet, these newborns can grow and develop normally.

Congenital hypothyroidism has many causes; these include genetic disease, poor thyroid tissue formation, and environmental factors (Morishima, 1992). In each case, insufficient production of the thyroid hormone results in a general slowing of tissue metabolism throughout the body. Early hypothyroidism is characterized by a range of symptoms, including prolonged jaundice, poor sucking ability, decreased intestinal motility, lethargy, and respiratory insufficiency. The more classic manifestations of cretinism appear later, when progressive edema, enlarged tongue, hoarse cry, lethargy, and hypotonia are prominent. The diagnosis of hypothyroidism can be confirmed by assessing the serum level of thyroxine, a hormone produced by the thyroid gland. The type of hypothyroidism can be determined by more detailed tests that examine the hypothalamus and its relationship to thyroid function. Almost all forms of this illness can be treated inexpensively with oral thyroxine administration. Prevention of mental retardation has been closely associated with the early start of therapy. For example, Klein, Meltzer, and Kenny (1972) found that children treated before 3 months of age have substantially higher intelligence quotients (IQs) than those identified later. Given the individuality of families and variations of the disease, no firm predictions of excellent outcome can be made. Such babies need to be followed sequentially and their therapy should be monitored closely.

In summary, nutrition plays a major role in the adequate growth, development, and ultimate function of the various organ systems within the body. Growth disturbances, both in utero and after birth, should lead to detailed evaluations for possible occult metabolic illnesses that may be amenable to therapy. The ideal dietary composition for the preterm infant remains controversial, although breast milk is the "gold standard" for nutrition in the baby older than 34 weeks gestation. Further research will clarify the subtleties of nutritional needs and the vulnerabilities of these more fragile newborns.

BIBLIOGRAPHY

American Academy of Pediatrics Committee on Nutrition. (1985). Nutritional needs of low-birth-weight infants. *Pediatrics, 75,* 437–447.

Berry, H.K. (1981). The diagnosis of phenylketonuria. *American Journal of Diseases in Childhood, 135,* 211–213.

Clark, D.A. (1993). Nutritional requirements of the premature and small-for-gestational-age infant. In R.M. Suskind (Ed.), *Textbook of pediatric nutrition* (2nd ed.) (pp. 23–32). New York: Raven Press.

Clark, D.A., & Miller, M.J. (1990). Intraluminal pathogenesis of necrotizing enterocolitis. *Journal of Pediatrics, 117*(Suppl. 1, pt. 2), S24–S67.

El-Dahr, S.S., & Chevalier, R.L. (1990). Special needs of the newborn infant in fluid therapy. *Pediatric Clinics of North America, 37*(2), 323–336.

Fomon, S.J. (1993). Estimated requirements and recommended dietary intakes. In S.J. Fomon (Ed.), *Nutrition of normal infants.* Boston: C.V. Mosby.

Fomon, S.J., & Suttie, J.W. (1993). Vitamin K. In S.J. Fomon (Ed.), *Nutrition of normal infants.* Boston: C.V. Mosby.

Gault, G.E. (1989). Taurine in pediatric nutrition. *Pediatrics, 83,* 433–442.

Grand, R.J., Watkins, J.B., & Torti, F.M. (1976). Development of the human gastrointestinal tract. *Gastroenterology, 70,* 790–810.

Greene, H.L., & Smidt, L.J. (1993). Water soluble vitamins. In R.C. Tsang (Ed.), *Nutritional needs of the preterm infant.* Philadelphia: Williams & Wilkins.

Hamosh, M. (1988). Fat needs for term and preterm infants. In R.C. Tsang & B. Nichols (Eds.), *Nutrition during infancy* (pp. 133–159). Philadelphia: Hanley & Belfus.

Hamosh, M., Bitman, J., & Wood, D.L. (1985). Lipids in milk and the first steps in their digestion. *Pediatrics, 75,* 146.

Klein, A.H., Meltzer, S., & Kenny, F.M. (1972). Improved prognosis in congenital hypothyroidism treated before age three months. *Journal of Pediatrics, 81,* 912–915.

Lifshitz, C.H. (1988). Carbohydrate needs in preterm and term newborn infants. In R.C. Tsang & B. Nichols, (Eds.), *Nutrition during infancy* (pp.122–132). Philadelphia: Hanley & Belfus.

Mertz, W. (1985). Metabolism and metabolic effects of trace elements. In R.K. Chandra (Ed.), *Trace elements in nutrition of children* (pp. 1–13). New York: Raven Press.

Miller, M.J.S., Witherly, S., & Clark, D.A. (1990). Casein: A milk protein with diverse biologic consequences. *Proceedings of the Society of Experimental Biology and Medicine, 195,* 143–159.

Morishima, A. (1992). Thyroid disorders. In A.A. Fanaroff & R.J. Martin (Eds.), *Neonatal-perinatal medicine: Diseases of the fetus and infant* (5th ed.) (Vol. 2) (pp. 1199–1222). Boston: C.V. Mosby.

Moya, F.R. (1993). Nutritional requirements of the term newborn. In R.M. Suskind (Ed.), *Textbook of pediatric nutrition* (2nd ed.) (pp. 9–22). New York: Raven Press.

New York State Health Department (1982, Fall). Newborn metabolic screening. *New York State Health Department Newsletter* (pp. 1–3). (Unpublished newsletter.)

Orzalesi, M. (1987). Vitamins and the premature. *Biology of the Neonate, 52*(1), 97–112.

Raiha, N.C.R. (1989). Milk protein quantity and quality and protein requirements during development. *Advances in Pediatrics, 36,* 347–368.

Romero, R., & Kleinman, R.E. (1993). Feeding the very low-birthweight infant. *Pediatrics in Review, 14*(4), 123–132.

Theorell, C.J., & Degenhardt, M. (1993). Assessment and management of metabolic dysfunction. In C. Kenner, A. Brueggemeyer, & L.P. Gunderson (Eds.), *Comprehensive neonatal nursing* (pp. 480–525). Philadelphia: W.B. Saunders.

Tsang, R.C. (Ed.). (1985). *Vitamin and mineral requirements in preterm infants.* New York: Marcel Dekker.

Zinn, A.B. (1992). Inborn errors of metabolism. In A.A. Fanaroff & R.J. Martin (Eds.), *Neonatal-perinatal medicine: Diseases of the fetus and infant* (5th ed.) (Vol. 2) (pp. 1118–1151). Boston: C.V. Mosby.

Chapter 11

Abnormal Physical Development

Approximately 5 percent of all children have major birth defects and many others are delivered with minor variations of physical development. Although many researchers have contributed to our understanding of malformations, the late Dr. David Smith was preeminent in this field, devoting his life's work to describing the various etiologies of physical impairment. His schema, still generally accepted, includes three main categories of atypical development: deformations, disruptions, and malformations (Jones, 1988). While such distinctions may overlap in the same baby, they do help to clarify anomalies resulting from unusual in utero mechanical forces, genetic defects, infections, and toxic insults (Hoyme, 1990; Shepard, 1986). Thus, the present chapter is organized around these three classifications.

DEFORMATIONS

Deformations, the first major category of impairment, result from the impact of an abnormal mechanical force on tissue that initially was developing normally. The uterine pressure on the rapidly growing fetus in late stages of gestation is the primary cause of such abnormalities (Graham, 1988). Thus, deformations are found primarily in the individual parts of the body that are most malleable in utero, most commonly the head and extremities. Atypical physical growth of the head may include deformation of the nose, folding and ridging of the ears, asymmetry of the mandible, and variations in shape and symmetry of the skull. Deformations of the extremities usually affect the legs and may be demonstrable as equinovarus (a form of club foot), deformed toes, dislocated hips, and dislocated or recurved knees. In addition, if there has been prolonged compression of a peripheral nerve, paralysis may be seen in the muscles innervated by that nerve.

While several etiologies exist, one noteworthy and often catastrophic deformation sequence is precipitated by insufficient amniotic fluid (oligohydramnios), particularly in the late second and third trimesters (Thomas & Smith, 1974). This condition may result from maternal hypertension, severe toxemia of pregnancy, placental insufficiency, or inadequate flow of fetal urine, which is the major contributor to amniotic fluid in the late second and third trimesters. Another possible etiology of oligohydramnios is an early chronic leak of amniotic fluid. Under any of these circumstances, the fetus is compressed, limiting movement, and the umbilical cord is shorter, increasing the possibility of cord trauma and blood loss. Fetal compression may lead to multiple defects of hands and feet, usually with joint stiffness. The abdomen may be compressed, with subsequent limitation of movement of the diaphragm and chest wall, which interferes with adequate alveolar growth. Babies thus affected die from inadequate lung volume.

Apart from insufficient lung development, the prognosis for resolution of deformations is ordinarily favorable, given the fact that the problem results from compression of normal tissue rather than a true malformation. Therefore, once the infant is released from the uterus, growth and the judicious use of gentle mechanical force frequently shape the abnormality toward a more normal appearance and function.

DISRUPTIONS

Tissue disruptions that cause physical defects are likely to occur when the normal fetus is subject to a mechanical, infectious, or toxic insult. An example of mechanical insult is development of an amniotic band, which causes a portion of the amnion (the innermost membrane surrounding the amniotic fluid) to separate from the outer membranes and protrude into the fluid. This tissue then may wrap around any part of the body, constricting the blood supply, preventing further growth, and, in severe cases, resulting in amputation of the affected part. Transplacental infections such as toxoplasmosis, rubella, and cytomegalovirus can also adversely affect physical development (see Chapter 12).

MALFORMATIONS

In contrast with the insults described previously, which involve some alteration of normal processes of development, malformations emerge from poor tissue growth (Goldman, 1992). These problems may originate from abnormal numbers of chromosomes or genes (the fundamental structures of chromosomes), or they may have no identifiable genetic etiology (Warkany, 1971). In the evaluation of any child found to have a true defect, historical data are very important. The obstetrical background of the mother may provide valuable clues, especially if there is a history of frequent spontaneous abortions. The use of alcohol, illicit drugs, or medications may be important. In addition, data on the family may be useful in making a diagnosis, especially if there is a history of mental retardation, malformations, chromosomal abnormalities, or unexplained neonatal and infant illnesses.

Several principles should be kept in mind in assessment of infants with multiple defects. First, rarely is a single defect sufficient to make the determination of a specific syndrome. For example, there are many healthy individuals in the normal population who have a simian hand crease but do not have Down syndrome (Smith & Wilson, 1973). Second, among babies with identifiable conditions, there frequently is a great deal of variation. Slanted eyes and low muscle tone are evident only in 8 percent of newborns with Down syndrome. Also, in situations of intrauterine drug exposure, the timing, duration, and amount of exposure are critical factors influencing the severity of the defect. Third, adding to the complexity of the issue is the fact that similar features or malformations may arise from different etiologies. For instance, hydrocephalus has been associated with over 20 distinct syndromes. For these reasons, the evaluation of a malformed infant must be done carefully to include all possible anomalies. The constellation of findings then may be used, in combination with chromosomal analysis, to provide an explanation to the parents during genetic counseling.

It is well beyond the scope of this text to present a detailed discussion of the many types of physical impairment. Several excellent texts are available for in-depth information (Bergsma, 1979; Jones, 1988; McKusick, 1988). We will, however, describe several congenital malformations that emerge from chromosomal abnormalities, explain the various types of genetic inheritance, and discuss the most common disabilities.

Chromosomal Abnormalities

Normally, humans have 23 pairs of chromosomes, 46 in each cell of the body, with the only major difference of two X chromosomes in the female and an X and a Y chromosome in the male. Genes in these chromosomes determine the body structure in detail, but this determination may be modified by environmental influences. An excess or deficiency of chromosomes often causes poor tissue formation and, subsequently, recognizable malformations. The excess genetic material is most evident in the trisomy syndromes, in which there is an additional full chromosome. The most frequent condition is trisomy 21, with an additional chromosome 21. (Historically, this condition has also been termed *mongolism* or *Down syndrome*.) In this circumstance, an extra chromosome 21 is passed from the parents in the formation of the sperm or the egg; thus, two copies of chromosome 21 are transmitted by one of the parents, rather than one copy. It is well known that infants with Down syndrome generally are born to older women (more than 35 years old) (Cornel, Breed, Beekhuis, te Meerman, & ten Kate, 1993). Recently, it has been suggested that these older mothers are more likely to tolerate an abnormal fetus. Many different physical abnormalities have been associated with the trisomy 21 syndrome (Figure 11–1). The most prevalent features include hypotonia, poor reflexes, hyperflexible joints, excess skin, flattened face, slanted eyes, abnormal ears, atypical pelvis, and abnormalities in hand development. Virtually all of these children and those surviving to become adults have some degree of developmental disability. In addition, approximately 40 percent have serious cardiac defects, and abnormalities in the intestinal tract are found in increased frequency in comparison with those in the general population. In addition, growth retardation is common (Penrose & Smith, 1966).

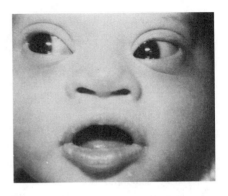

Figure 11–1 Facial characteristics of a baby with trisomy 21 syndrome

Trisomy 21 occurs with an overall incidence of 1 in 660 newborns; trisomy 18 occurs much less frequently, in approximately 1 in 3,500 infants. Trisomy 18 is manifested in the form of multiple malformations caused by the additional chromosome 18. Although the findings are somewhat variable, most babies are distinguished by low birthweight, a weak cry, abnormally shaped ears, a small mouth, undergrown fingernails, a short sternum (breast bone), an abnormal pelvis, syndactyly (fused toes) (Figure 11–2), clinodactyly (deviated fingers) (Figure 11–3), and decreased skeletal tissue, as expressed in "rocker-bottom" foot (Figure 11–4). These infants have a limited capacity for survival. Most have a very weak suck, making feeding extremely difficult. Thus, even with aggressive management, they often fail to thrive. The 10 percent who live beyond the first year invariably are severely mentally retarded (Jones, 1988; Smith, 1964).

Trisomy 13, which is caused by an inherited additional chromosome 13, is even less common, with an incidence of approximately 1 in 15,000 births. The most obvious characteristics are defects of the midface, including cleft lip and palate (Figure 11–5) and widely spaced eyes. These babies typically

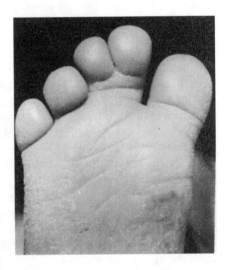

Figure 11–2 Syndactyly (fused toes) seen in babies with trisomy 18 syndrome

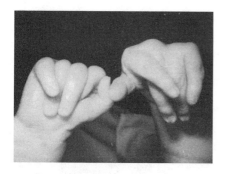

Figure 11–3 Clinodactyly (deviated fingers) of baby with trisomy 18 syndrome

have poor development of the internal structure of the brain. They may have skin defects on the scalp (Figure 11–6). The most common skeletal abnormalities are prominent heels and extra fingers and toes, often with fusion. Less than 20 percent of these severely retarded infants survive beyond the first year of life, and those who do have seizures and severe failure to thrive (Jones, 1988; Warkany, Passage, & Smith, 1966).

In contrast with malformations that arise from excess genetic material, monosomy defects are caused by the presence of too few chromosomes—a total of only 45 in each cell. Most fetuses thus affected die early in gestation. One example of this condition is Turner's syndrome, found in approximately 1 in 5,000 newborns and seen only in females, where one of the sex chromosomes is missing. These babies have small stature, a broad chest with widely spaced nipples, a low posterior hairline, webbing of the neck (Figure 11–7), and congenital edema of the extremities (Figure 11–8). Twenty percent of these children have cardiac defects. Unlike the syndromes already discussed, these infants do survive and many have relatively normal intelligence, with a mean tested IQ of approximately 95. Beyond the newborn period, they appear to be relatively healthy, with the exception of small stature and a tendency to become obese. Ovaries are underdeveloped, and the affected individuals are infertile and do not develop secondary sexual characteristics later in life. The occurrence of monosomy defects is thought to be sporadic, and there is no information on risk of occurrence in subsequent children of the same parents (Jones, 1988; Lindsten, 1963).

In numerous other chromosomal abnormalities, a portion of an individual chromosome may be missing (chromosomal deletion) or a portion of a given chromosome may have broken off and become attached to another (translocation). These events are much more rare.

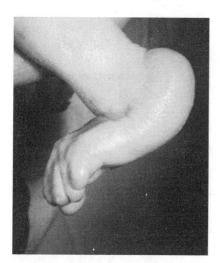

Figure 11–4 "Rocker-bottom" foot characteristic of babies with trisomy 18 syndrome

Although some specific associations have been reported, the amount of genetic material missing or duplicated leads to a wide variability of expression. The majority of these chromosomal defects are associated with abnormal brain development, mental retardation, and abnormalities of facial and limb development. Furthermore, since relatively few cases have been reported, it is difficult to make any broad generalizations with respect to the natural history of these syndromes (McKusick, 1988; Warkany, 1971).

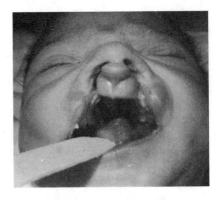

Figure 11–5 Severe bilateral cleft lip and palate in baby with trisomy 13 syndrome

Types of Inheritance of Genetic Disease

Genetic disease refers to inherited abnormalities that can be attributed to abnormal genes and have been shown to affect growth and development. Four patterns of gene inheritance have been well defined: autosomal dominance inheritance, autosomal recessive inheritance, X-linked inheritance, and polygenic or multifactorial inheritance (Jones, 1988; McKusick, 1988).

The 22 pairs of chromosomes that do not determine sex are *autosomes*. Therefore, an autosomal dominant gene is found on one of the non-sex chromosomes that, if present, affects a physical or developmental characteristic. There is no carrier state. If the gene is present, the individual is susceptible. Manifestations of an autosomal dominant gene may not be obvious in the newborn. Autosomal dominant inheritance usually emerges from a dominant gene passed from one parent to the child. Assuming that either the mother or father has the dominant gene, there is a 50 percent chance that any future child will be similarly affected. If neither parent has the dominant gene and the newborn shows indications that the gene is present, the condition is most likely the result of a new gene mutation. An example of an autosomal dominant illness that has variable manifestations is neurofibromatosis (von Recklinghausen's

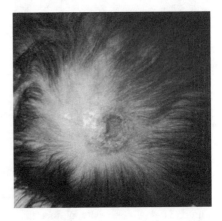

Figure 11–6 Scalp defect in newborn with trisomy 13 syndrome

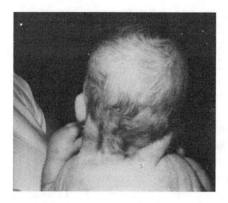

Figure 11–7 Webbing at neck of baby with Turner's syndrome

disease). Individuals with this disease have multiple cutaneous and connective tissue tumors that are fibrous and frequently contain nerve tissue. Over 90 percent of affected individuals have increased or decreased pigmentation of the skin. Although cutaneous lesions are the most common finding, nearly one-half of affected individuals develop some evidence of neurological impairment as a result of nerve compression. The estimated incidence is approximately 1 in 3,000 newborns. Approximately 50 percent of such infants are found to have a new gene mutation.

A second genetic condition, autosomal recessive inheritance, implies a less potent gene, which, though found in the non-sex chromosomes, must be present in a paired condition to result in an atypical state. Most diseases that have been defined as inherited have an autosomal recessive pattern of inheritance. Commonly, both parents are carriers and have no features of the illness. One-fourth of their offspring are completely normal genetically, one-half are carriers but have no obvious physical abnormalities, and one-fourth are affected. Examples of autosomal recessive inheritance include cystic fibrosis and virtually all of the inborn errors of metabolism such as phenylketonuria. Many autosomal recessive carrier states can now be detected, and these determinations are helpful for family planning (McKusick, 1988).

X-linked inheritance conditions have their origin with an abnormal gene present in one of the female X chromosomes. This gene is recessive and, therefore,

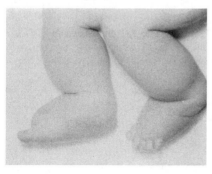

Figure 11–8 Edema of legs in baby with Turner's syndrome

the normal gene on the second X chromosome prevents expression of the disease. Every male has an X chromosome from his mother and a Y chromosome with relatively little genetic material from his father. If the male inherits his mother's X chromosome with the abnormal gene, he will be affected. Instances of such occurrence include adult-onset baldness, hemophilia (factor VIII deficiency), and Duchenne type muscular dystrophy. With each pregnancy, there is a 50 percent chance that a male child will have the inherited condition and a 50 percent chance that a female child will be a carrier capable of transmitting this gene to her offspring.

Thus far, we have discussed only combination genes in a single location, which result in an identifiable illness. In the event of polygenic (multiple gene) inheritance, several specific genes from both parents are necessary before the child will be affected. This type of inheritance has been associated with numerous malformations, including cleft lip and cleft palate, neural tube defects (meningomyelocele), and various congenital heart defects. If parents have a single child with a polygenetically inherited malformation, the risk of recurrence is approximately 5 percent. If a second child is affected, the risk effectively increases to approximately 15 percent (Smith & Aase, 1970). In utero, environmental insults may promote additional malformations in the fetus with a polygenic disposition. For example, in utero cytomegalovirus infection may increase the incidence of cleft lip and cleft palate. On the other hand, supplementation of mothers prior to the pregnancy with folic acid reduces the incidence and recurrence of neural tube defects.

In conclusion, numerous additional malformations may be present in the newborn. These include abnormalities of the intestine, abdominal wall, genitalia, kidneys, and extremities. The majority of these conditions are isolated instances, and there is no known genetic predisposition. On the other hand, as soon as any malformation or anomaly has been detected, a thorough examination of the child must be made. Beyond the routine normative data for weight, length, and head circumference by age, norms for measurements are also available for the hands, face, and other body parts. If a syndrome has been defined but the initial descriptions include very few examples, it is difficult to predict outcome in counseling a family. Therefore, cautious and continuing evaluation and conservative advice for parents generally is the best course of action.

BIBLIOGRAPHY

Bergsma, D.S. (1979). *Birth defects atlas and compendium* (2nd ed.). Baltimore: Williams & Wilkins.

Cornel, M.C., Breed, A.S., Beekhuis, J.R., te Meerman, G.J., ten Kate, L.P. (1993). Down syndrome: Effects of demographic factors and prenatal diagnosis on the future livebirth prevalence. *Human Genetics, 92,* 163–168.

Goldman, A.S. (1992). Pathophysiology of congenital malformations. In R.A. Polin & W.W. Fox (Eds.), *Fetal and neonatal physiology* (Vol. 1, pp. 36–46). Philadelphia: W.B. Saunders.

Graham, J.M. (1988). *Smith's recognizable patterns of human deformation* (2nd ed.). Philadelphia: W.B. Saunders.

Hoyme, H.E. (1990). Teratogenically induced fetal anomalies. *Clinics in Perinatology, 17,* 547–567.

Jones, K.L. (1988). *Smith's recognizable patterns of human malformation* (2nd ed.) (pp. 1–28). Philadelphia: W. B. Saunders.

Lindsten, J. (1963). *The nature and origin of X chromosome aberrations in Turner's syndrome.* Stockholm: Almquist & Wiksell.

McKusick, V.A. (1988). *Mendelian inheritance in man.* Baltimore: The Johns Hopkins University Press.

Penrose, L.S., & Smith, G.F. (1966). *Down's anomaly.* Boston: Little, Brown.

Shepard, T.H. (1986). *Catalog of teratogenic agents* (5th ed.). Baltimore: The Johns Hopkins University Press.

Smith, D.W. (1964). Autosomal abnormalities. *American Journal of Obstetrics and Gynecology, 90,* 1055–1059.

Smith, D.W., & Aase, J.M. (1970). Polygenic inheritances of certain common malformations. *Journal of Pediatrics, 76,* 653–659.

Smith, D.W., & Wilson, A.C. (1973). *The child with Down's syndrome.* Philadelphia: W.B. Saunders.

Thomas, I.T., & Smith, D.W. (1974). Oligohydramnios, cause of the nonrenal features of Potter's syndrome, including pulmonary hypoplasia. *Journal of Pediatrics, 84,* 811–814.

Warkany, J. (1971). *Congenital malformations.* Chicago: Year Book Medical.

Warkany, J., Passage, E., & Smith, L.B. (1966). Congenital malformations in autosomal trisomy syndromes. *American Journal of Diseases of Children, 112,* 502–517.

Chapter 12

Infection

Newborns may be infected by a variety of agents. Some of these infections may pass via the placenta from the mother to the baby during pregnancy, and others are acquired by exposure to organisms that are present in the vagina or in the environment after birth (Blanc, 1961; Cowles & Gonik, 1992). *Sepsis* is any viral, bacterial, or parasitic infection in the newborn. It occurs in approximately 1 in every 1,000 full-term births. Among infants born at less than 3 pounds, the incidence may rise as high as 15 percent. Infections may have profound effects on development early in the pregnancy and after birth, disrupting the normal formation of tissues and organs (Brown, 1970; Klein, Remington, & Marcy, 1983). Several risk factors for perinatal infection have been identified (Exhibit 12–1) (Klein & Marcy, 1990). In this last chapter dealing with newborn medical insult, we consider the diagnostic features of infections, discuss common conditions, and comment on prevention, treatment, and prognosis.

Exhibit 12–1 Perinatal Risk Factors for Infection

Premature rupture of the membranes (prior to onset of labor)
Prolonged rupture of the membranes (>24 hours)
Maternal fever, chorioamnionitis
Maternal urinary tract infection
Fetal distress or perinatal asphyxia
Prematurity
Low birthweight
Low socioeconomic status
Maternal drug use

DIAGNOSTIC FEATURES

The signs and symptoms of infection are diverse, and many can resemble or be disguised by other illnesses of the newborn. Although respiratory distress may be caused by infection, in premature infants, it more frequently results from retained lung fluid or a deficiency of surfactant. In newborns, irritability may arise from an inflammation of the membranes surrounding the brain (meningitis), but it is seen more often as a result of birth asphyxia, drug withdrawal, or hemorrhage into the central nervous system. Jaundice may result from the accelerated breakdown of red blood cells with infection; it can also be due to bruising during delivery and prematurity. Hypoglycemia, while evident with infection, more often is manifested in babies born preterm, growth retarded, or large-for-gestational age as a result of maternal diabetes. In short, many of the characteristics of infection are also common to other problems and illnesses of the neonate (Cowles & Gonik, 1992). If such complex and confusing patterns seem to predominate, what characteristics *do* serve as indicators? A few signs and symptoms are relatively useful in indicating the presence of infection (Exhibit 12–2) (Siegel & McCracken, 1981). These factors include poor temperature control and the early onset of apnea. Older children and adults generally respond to infection with a fever, and fever is very common among newborns. Typically, full-term babies have a decreased body temperature; premature infants, on the other hand, usually require intensive temperature support. Thus, if the effects of overheating and maternal medication can be ruled out as a cause of apnea in the first several days of life, the cause is commonly associated with infection (Mustafa & McCracken, 1992).

DECREASED RESISTANCE TO INFECTION

Prior to birth, the fetus has a limited capacity to ward off infection. For most babies, the intrauterine environment is sterile. Once delivered, however, newborns

---

Exhibit 12–2 Signs and Symptoms of Neonatal Infection

General	Central nervous system	Cutaneous
Temperature instability	Hypotonia, lethargy	Petechiae, purpura
	Irritability, seizures	Pustules
Cardiorespiratory	Poor suck	Jaundice
Apnea, tachypnea		
Intercostal retractions	**Gastrointestinal**	
Grunting	Emesis, gastric residuals	
Bradycardia, tachycardia	Abdominal distention, ileus	
Hypotension, pallor	Diarrhea, bloody stools	
Cyanosis		

are exposed to numerous viruses and bacteria with which they must cope. Moreover, the functions of the white blood cells and circulating blood proteins are critical to the ability to respond successfully to infection (Regelman, Hill, Cates, & Quie, 1992).

Basically, the white blood cells are divided into two subgroups, agranulocytes (without granules) and granulocytes (containing granules). The agranulocytes include small lymphocytes—small white blood cells that produce antibodies or proteins directed against infectious agents. The other primary agranulocyte is the monocyte, which enhances antibody production and is the prominent white blood cell involved in the clearing of the debris of infection. The granulocytes are white blood cells containing granules located outside the cell nucleus. Those that primarily fight bacterial infection are the *neutrophils*, which contain powerful enzymes (Miller & Stiehm, 1979). For bacterial infection to be managed effectively, the neutrophil must be attracted to the site of the infection, must be capable of ingesting the bacteria, and then must be able to destroy the bacteria. In the newborn, while the process of killing bacteria is similar to that in older children and adults, the mobilization of neutrophils to the site of an infection and subsequent ingestion of bacteria is somewhat restricted (Nelson, 1989).

Circulating blood proteins, primarily the antibodies (immunoglobulins), help in the process of neutralizing and eliminating bacteria and viruses. Immunoglobulin G (IgG) is a protein that can be transferred from the mother across the placenta to the fetus. If the mother has been exposed to an infection and has responded appropriately, some protection can be conveyed to the baby by these antibodies. This protection helps to explain the rarity of chickenpox, mumps, measles, and rheumatic fever in newborns. On the other hand, if the baby, after birth, is exposed to an organism that the mother has never coped with effectively, the infant is more likely to contract that disease. The few infants who become infected with agents their mothers have contracted usually have much milder illnesses. A second immunoglobulin, IgM, is a protein much larger than IgG and is the first antibody produced by the body in response to infection. IgM does not traverse the placenta in either direction, so that the maternal IgM is distinct from the baby's IgM. Thus, an elevated IgM level in the blood of the newborn suggests that the child has been exposed to an infectious agent and is responding (Bellanti & Boner, 1981).

A supplementary complex of proteins found in the blood, the complement system, aids the function of white blood cells in recognizing infection and of the immunoglobulins in fighting it. Unfortunately, this mechanism also may be deficient, especially in the premature infant (Regelman, Hill, Cates, & Quie, 1992).

In addition to these complications, babies are also more prone to infection after birth because of major differences in their anatomy compared with that of adults. In particular, their skin is thinner and, therefore, cutaneous infections are more common. Preterm infants frequently are unable to feed, and when a tube is placed into the stomach to provide adequate nutrition, the limited antibacterial and antiviral capabilities of the tonsils and adenoids are bypassed. Many invasive procedures, such as placement of a tube down the trachea for respiratory support and insertion of a catheter into a blood vessel, increase the risk of infection. One of the more common sites of infection, even in healthy full-term babies, is the navel, after the dried umbilical cord is shed.

TRANSPLACENTAL INFECTIONS

As we have indicated, the fetus can be infected prior to birth by a variety of organisms that initially infect the mother and are then passed transplacentally to the fetus. The most common diseases infecting the newborn have been designated as *TORCH* infections (Nahmias, 1974); this acronym represents the diseases toxoplasmosis (TO), rubella (R), cytomegalovirus (C), and herpes (H). Frequently, an *S* is added at the beginning to produce *STORCH*, with the *S* standing for syphilis. These organisms do not produce a homogeneous group of illnesses; they include agents with very different characteristics—three viruses (rubella, cytomegalovirus, and herpes), a parasitic infection (toxoplasmosis), and a parabacterial infection (syphilis) (Cowles & Gonik, 1992; Overall, 1992).

The list of organisms proven to cause congenital infections has grown rapidly so that the acronym *TORCH* is no longer inclusive. Two of the more pertinent transplacental viral infections are the human immunodeficiency virus (HIV) and hepatitis B.

Rubella

Rubella (German measles) is the prototype of viral infections. Much of the current information on this disease was obtained in the 1960s. This illness in the mother may be mild. Only maternal rubella with subsequent fetal infection in the first 4 months of gestation is likely to produce any abnormal physical finding or developmental disability. In the most severe situation, it is important to realize that infection prior to 4 months gestation is well established before the baby's own immune defenses are developed. Therefore, virtually every organ system of the body may be involved. Some of these effects may be transient; others may be long lasting (Overall, 1992).

The four most common persistent problems of newborns with rubella are hearing loss (in approximately 87 percent) (Miller, Rabinowitz, Frost, & Seager, 1969); visual problems, primarily cataracts and glaucoma (in approximately 34 percent); heart disease (in approximately 46 percent) (Cooper, 1985; Preblud & Alford, 1990); and mental retardation (in approximately 40 percent). Three decades ago, the national cost of the care of these infants was excessively high as a result of the combination of physical and developmental problems. A concerted effort in the late 1960s culminated in a rubella vaccine that was licensed in 1970.

Within several years of that accomplishment, the number of identifiable cases of both rubella and congenital rubella decreased by 80 percent.

The "classic" child with congenital rubella has low birthweight and bruising, a large liver and spleen, abnormalities of bone development, meningitis, hearing loss, cataracts, abnormal retinal development, various forms of cardiac disease, mental retardation, behavioral and language disorders, undescended testes, hernias, and microcephaly. Less commonly seen are jaundice, glaucoma, myopia, hepatitis, generalized enlargement of the lymph nodes, pneumonia, diabetes, thyroid dysfunction, seizures, and degenerative brain disease. Infected infants may excrete the virus for prolonged periods of time and as many as 10 percent still actively shed the organism in urine up to 1 year of age. These newborns are a potential source of infection to women of childbearing age (Cherry, 1990).

Although much has been done to elucidate the transmission and infection-induced malformations of rubella, there is, to date, no specific therapy to eradicate the illness in the newborn. Surgery may help to correct some of the cardiac and visual problems, but only early developmental evaluation and persistent follow-up can blunt the detrimental effects on the central nervous system. The immunization of children against rubella has greatly decreased fetal rubella infection (Hinman, 1985).

Cytomegalovirus

As the incidence of congenital rubella began to decrease with the introduction of immunization programs, a new virus—cytomegalovirus—rose to the top of the list of newborn infections (see Figure 12–1). This is one of the herpes viruses and, like all other members of the group, the infection, once acquired, remains throughout life. The individual may have no obvious symptoms, but in periods of decreased resistance, the organisms may be reactivated, much like the varicella herpes virus that causes chickenpox is reactivated in shingles (herpes zoster). Cytomegalovirus (CMV) may be passed transplacentally but also may infect the newborn as an infection ascending from the vagina (Alford, Stagno, & Pass, 1990). Manifestations of the virus in the newborn are similar to those of rubella. Infection in the mother, however, is much more difficult to recognize clinically, because she may evidence little more than flu-like symptoms. While maternal illness in the first trimester may produce fetal anomalies, later infection tends to produce much more subtle manifestations in the newborn. Hearing loss, secondary to a viral infection of the inner ear, may be one for the most subtle presentations of cytomegalovirus (Hanshaw, Dudgeon, & Marshall, 1985). No specific therapy for cytomegalovirus is available. Current research is focused on developing a reliable and safe immunization that can be used prior to pregnancy to prevent infection that might be passed to the fetus (Nankervis, 1985; Stagno, 1990).

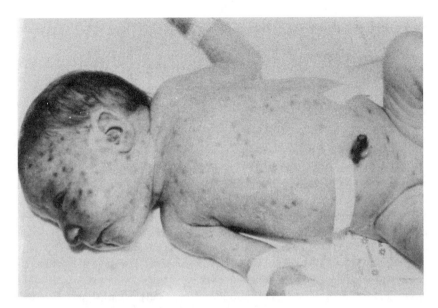

Figure 12–1 Infant with congenital cytomegalovirus infection

Toxoplasmosis

Toxoplasmosis differs from most of the other infections in that the *Toxoplasma* protozoan causing the disease is one of the few parasites that can be transmitted directly from the mother to the fetus. The mother usually is asymptomatic with this infection. Humans are aberrant hosts for this parasite, which primarily infects cats, but also may infect dogs. The small eggs produced by the parasite may be inhaled by the pregnant mother as she changes cat litter. Once in the human, the developing embryos complete their development within the intestinal tract and then seed to various organs throughout the body by means of the blood. Wherever a cyst forms, tissue disruption occurs (Feldman, 1968).

Mothers with infection in the first trimester of pregnancy tend to produce infants with severe congenital disease. Third trimester infections may be subclinical. Manifestations of the more severe conditions include microcephaly, deafness, retinitis, blindness, jaundice, seizures, large lymph nodes, pneumonia, and enlarged liver and spleen (Lee, 1988). Of greatest concern is the tendency of the parasite to travel to the baby's brain, with subsequent tissue disruption. The cysts may be seen by a simple X-ray of the skull, since they commonly calcify. Subtle cerebral cysts may be found by CAT (computerized axial tomography) scanning. Antibiotics are available to help limit the extent of the disease, but areas of the brain or other tissue that have been affected do not usually recover adequately. The neurodevelopmental outcome of babies who have toxoplasmosis is variable, depending on the distribution and number of parasites that infest the brain or other vital organs (Cowles & Gonik, 1992).

Syphilis

Neonatal syphilis is much less common than it was 30 years ago, as a consequence of the aggressive screening of mothers during pregnancy. The infectious agent *Treponema* is a worm-like microorganism that can invade and infect any organ of the body. The severity of the disease manifestation depends on tissue disruption and the host's response to the invasion of the organism (Taber & Huber, 1975). The typical presentations of congenital syphilis are a dry skin rash, bruising, large liver and spleen, hypotonia, jaundice, anemia, and a profuse rhinorrhea (Nabarro, 1954). The illness may show only subtle symptoms and thus go unrecognized. One of the more common characteristics of the disease is seen in the baby brought for medical care at several months of age who has joint swelling or limited movement of the extremities. Child abuse frequently is suspected. However, X-rays do not reveal fractures but, rather, an elevation of the outermost layer (periosteum) of the long bones, resulting from infection by the organism. Even with this relatively late presentation, if the disease is recognized and treated, long-term developmental disability may be minimal (Wendel, 1988).

Therapy for syphilis is comparatively simple. The disease is readily treated with penicillin or one of several other antibiotics. These medications must be given for a minimum of 10 days to assure minimal risk of recurrence. If there is involvement of the central nervous system, however, the treatment must be more aggressive and prolonged. Once infection is recognized in the child, the mother also should be examined and treated, and her sexual partners should be serologically tested and treated.

Human Immunodeficiency Virus

The human immunodeficiency virus HIV-1 is a member of the human retrovirus family. It is an RNA virus that can attach to a receptor on the surface of a helper T-cell lymphocyte. Once inside the helper lymphocyte, the virus can multiply rapidly and eliminate the lymphocyte's role in the immune system. T-cells promote the manufacture of antibodies by other lymphocytes (Fauci, 1988). In their absence, the child becomes vulnerable to many different infections.

Pregnancy does not appear to aggravate the severity of HIV infection in previously asymptomatic women, but HIV transmission from mother to infant can occur across the placenta, at the time of delivery or via breast-feeding or intimate contact with body secretions (Cowan, Hellman, & Chudwin, 1984; Gonik &

Hammill, 1990). The incidence of HIV infection in women in the childbearing age group is estimated at approximately 0.15 percent. However, the incidence of infection in pregnant women may be as high as 2 percent in some inner city populations. The typical profile of an infected pregnant mother is a poor young woman in the inner city who is an intravenous drug abuser or the sexual partner of an intravenous drug abuser. The rate of transmission from mother to child is approximately 15 percent to 30 percent (European Collaborative Study, 1991). Progression of HIV infection to acquired immunodeficiency syndrome (AIDS) is now the fifth leading cause of death among 1- to 4-year-olds.

In neonates, the most common clinical features of HIV infection that has progressed to AIDS are failure-to-thrive, hepatomegaly, and disseminated pneumonia. The average onset of severe immunodeficiency occurs at 5 to 10 months of age. The incubation period seems to be much shorter in children than in adults, and the disease course is much more aggressive, probably because of the immature immune function in combination with a larger infective initial dose of virus (Rubinstein, 1986).

At birth, most affected infants appear healthy (Hanson & Shearer, 1992). A few investigators have reported hypertelorism, a flat nasal bridge, long palpebral fissures, and other facial features, as suggestive of intrauterine HIV infection. Unfortunately, many of these characteristics overlap with clinical features of babies born to mothers who abuse drugs, especially alcohol.

The long-term prognosis is very poor (Mok, Giaquinto, & DeRossi, 1987). As many as 75 percent of children die within 1 year of the presentation of AIDS symptoms following HIV infection. The mothers and children need comprehensive social, medical, and supportive care. Any infant exposed to the HIV virus should have follow-up for 3 years to ascertain whether or not infection has occurred. All secondary infections, even minor ones such as a diaper rash, should be treated promptly. Immunizations with killed bacteria and inactivated viruses should be given. A live virus immunization should not be given to a symptomatic baby. AZT (zidovudine) is in clinical trials on pediatric populations by authorization of the U.S. Food and Drug Administration. Presently, it is available only by research protocol, while its efficacy, toxicity, and safety are being investigated.

Hepatitis B Virus

The hepatitis virus (HBV) is a large, double-stranded DNA virus. This virus can produce severe systemic illness, with jaundice, fever, and rash that can progress to chronic liver failure. The virus is common in Africa and Southeast Asia. Thirty-five to 40 percent of these populations are infected without overt symptoms (carriers).

The great influx of immigrants from underdeveloped countries has resulted in a greater risk of hepatitis B virus infection in the United States.

If a pregnant woman is infected with HBV, there is a 50 percent risk of the neonate acquiring HBV infection (Arevalo, 1989). The current recommendation from the Centers for Disease Control is that all newborns be vaccinated with the recombinant (synthetic) form of hepatitis B vaccine. Babies whose mothers are positive for hepatitis B surface antigen should also receive protective immunoglobulins. Since the HBV has a long incubation period (50 to 180 days), aggressive protection of the newborn can prevent a serious debilitating disease (Zeldis & Crumpacker, 1990).

Other Infections

Numerous other infections, primarily viral, can cross the placenta and infect the newborn (Amstey, 1984). Many of these illnesses have similar signs and symptoms which result in confusion about the diagnosis. The viruses that cause mononucleosis (Epstein-Barr virus), poliomyelitis, mumps, chickenpox, and influenza can infect the newborn after infecting the mother (Overall, 1992). In each case, an aggressive approach to the diagnosis is important, largely in order to counsel the parents and to prevent the spread of the infectious agent to other children in the facility caring for the child. Although many of the presenting symptoms of neonatal infections are similar, subsequent developmental disabilities differ with the types of viruses and their predilection for certain portions of the central nervous system.

ASCENDING AND NEONATAL INFECTIONS

Ascending infections are those that reach the fetus by passing through the cervix, generally after rupture of the membranes (Zeichner & Plotkin, 1988). The infant first may be exposed to these organisms in the process of vaginal delivery. *Neonatal infections*, on the other hand, are acquired after birth. These infections can be transmitted by family members, hospital personnel, or various materials used in the care of the baby.

Herpes

One of the most serious and virulent illnesses in the newborn, most often acquired as an ascending infection, is herpes (Whitley, 1990). There are several strains of the virus. Type 1 is predominantly an oral organism, responsible for cold sores and fever blisters. Type 2 herpes is primarily a genital organism. However, the sexual liberation of the last 20 years has led to an increase in type 1 oral infections and type 2 herpes genital infections.

The fetus or newborn may be affected by either form of the disease. The most frequent presenting symptom, found in approximately 80 percent of the cases, is lethargy. Respiratory distress is evidenced in approximately 60 percent. The typical rash of herpes is seen in less than 50 percent of affected newborns. Other signs of the disease are those usually evident with generalized infections of the newborn, including temperature instability, enlarged liver and spleen, poor coagulation of blood, and jaundice (Corey & Spear, 1986a and 1986b). Herpes, however, is an aggressive virus and what commonly appears to be localized infection may progress rapidly to systemic disease, especially targeted toward the central nervous system. The generalized form of the disease is devastating. Although survival is better with the localized form of the disease, as many as 40 percent of the survivors have serious sequelae, including seizures, mental retardation, and other forms of severe developmental disability (Nahmias, Keyserling, & Kerrick, 1983).

Although new antiviral agents are available, they are as yet no panacea for neonatal herpes. They are most beneficial when used in children who have localized disease, with the hope of preventing generalized disease and central nervous system disease. Furthermore, while the treatment of newborns with generalized illness has resulted in an increase in survival, many of the survivors still have serious sequelae (Brunell, 1980). It is difficult to prevent transmission of herpes from a mother to the newborn. Even though a mother who has had herpes may be asymptomatic at the time of delivery, the infant may become infected. If there are active herpes lesions in the mother, cesarean delivery may help limit the exposure of the baby and subsequent illness.

Gonorrhea

Gonorrhea is a sexually transmitted disease. Adult males usually have a penile discharge, whereas females may be asymptomatic. Babies born to mothers with active gonorrhea are at greatest risk for eye infection (Cowles & Gonik, 1992). Early in the 1900s in New York State, visual impairment resulting from neonatal eye infection was the most common single cause of loss of vision in children enrolled in schools for the blind. As a result, nearly all states now mandate eye prophylaxis against this infection.

Generally, the baby is exposed to the bacteria at the time of descent through the birth canal. Less commonly, after rupture of the membranes, the bacteria may ascend into the amniotic fluid surrounding the infant. In either case, the organism penetrates the anterior cell layer of the eye, and within 5 days a purulent infection results. If untreated, disease in the eye may progress to meningitis or other systemic infection. The disease may be treated with antibiotics. Unfortunately, although treatment may eradicate the organism, the damage has been done once the infection in the eye becomes purulent. Therefore, eye prophylaxis is very important. As we have discussed in Chapter 4 on typical newborn care, the most commonly used therapeutic agent is 0.1 percent silver nitrate solution. When this solution is instilled into each eye shortly after birth, it kills the organism. Treatment should not be delayed more than 30 minutes after birth, because after that time, the organism penetrates the outer layer of the eye and silver nitrate would thus be ineffective. Several topical antibiotics are now being used, including erythromycin and tetracycline. They are equally as effective as silver nitrate in killing the gonorrheal organism, but their cost is as much as 20 to 30 times greater.

Necrotizing Enterocolitis

Necrotizing enterocolitis is a disease that results in distention of the abdomen, feeding intolerance, and bloody stool. X-rays of the abdomen reveal distended intestine and, in the classic presentation, gas trapped in the bowel wall (pneumatosis intestinalis). Often, the clinical course culminates with hemorrhagic destruction of the intestine, metabolic acidosis, respiratory insufficiency, and infection progressing to death. While numerous epidemiologic associations have been suggested, only a few consistent underlying factors have been identified. These factors include prematurity, formula feeding, and bacteria within the intestine. In addition, outbreaks of neonatal illness suggest an infectious component. Autopsy analysis has shown that the intestines of babies with necrotizing enterocolitis contained sugar, protein, organic acids, and bacteria (Clark et al., 1985; Clark & Miller, 1990).

Infants who are fed formula are at greater risk for developing this disease than those receiving breast milk. The etiology of these differences is complex, but, in part, it may be attributed to a selective inhibition of the bacteria most capable of producing the organic acids that initiate inflammation in the lower intestinal tract. More specifically, as the pH in the intestine decreases, the mucosal barrier is broken and luminal proteins activate mast cells, which promote the secretion of various chemicals by cells lining the intestinal tract. Local changes take place in blood flow; and white blood cells, which fight infection, and platelets, which are involved in the blood clotting mechanism, are brought to the site of the initial insult. In many newborns, especially the more mature babies, this process suffices to repair the damage. In the more premature infant with an immature intestinal tract, the inflammation process may accelerate—even to the destruction of portions of the intestine. Bacteria may then gain access to the bloodstream, resulting in more generalized infection. Other etiologies of intestinal damage have been documented in newborns, including those who have not been formula fed or nursed. Most of these intestinal diseases arise after a period of inadequate blood flow to the intestine, again causing destruction and hemorrhage (Clark & Miller, 1990).

Outbreaks of necrotizing enterocolitis may be explained by slight differences in the metabolic capacities of bacteria that normally grow within the intestinal tract. Some of these bacteria are capable of fermenting carbohydrates such as lactose and move rapidly, thus producing excess acid which initiates intestinal inflammation. These bacteria may retain this ability for only a limited time (Carbonaro,

Clark, & Elseviers, 1988). The bacteria from babies who have necrotizing enterocolitis may be passed inadvertently from one infant to another in an intensive care nursery.

The primary therapy for neonatal necrotizing enterocolitis remains supportive. Feedings are stopped and intravenous infusions are begun, to provide sufficient fluid for the newborn. Cultures are taken, and the baby is given antibiotics to prevent a systemic infection originating in the intestine. Up to one-third of such newborns require surgical intervention to remove necrotic intestine. With medical or surgical management, approximately 50 to 60 percent of the afflicted newborns survive. The remaining group succumbs to the disease early, as a result of massive bowel destruction or surgical removal of the intestine. These babies may have an insufficient length of intestine for digestion, causing long-term failure-to-thrive and increased susceptibility to infection.

Systemic Infections

Any organism in the mother's vagina or in the baby's environment after birth may infect the newborn. The symptoms usually are those of systemic disease: temperature instability, respiratory difficulty, and other evidence of specific organ involvement. One common bacterial organism acquired, in some cases at birth and in other instances from family or hospital staff, is *Streptococcus*. There are many varieties of this bacteria. Group A *Streptococcus* is predominant with strep throat and also has been associated with rheumatic fever and severe kidney disease. It is rare for the newborn to be infected with this bacteria, since protective antibodies (proteins) from the mother that have crossed the placenta usually limit the bacterial proliferation. Group B *Streptococcus* infection, on the other hand, is a serious threat to the newborn (Baker & Edwards, 1990). Basically, it has two forms of presentation. The early type is marked by severe respiratory distress, simulating surfactant deficiency in the newborn (Ablow et al., 1976). Despite aggressive respiratory support and the use of antibiotics, the mortality rate remains high—up to 50 percent in many intensive care nurseries. A second, more subtle form of this infection is meningitis, generally caused by a different serotype of group B *Streptococcus*.

Typically, the illness is manifested 2 or 3 weeks after birth, but it may present as late as several months after birth. Early symptoms include poor feeding and lethargy. Fortunately, once identified, this form of infection is generally more amenable to therapy. Another bacteria with a similar pattern of neonatal disease is *Listeria monocytogenes*. There is an early respiratory form of infection and a late meningitic presentation. It can be treated with the same antibiotics (Mustafa & McCracken, 1992) used to treat streptococcal infections.

The most common environmentally acquired infection in the newborn is produced by *Staphylococcus* (Shinefield, 1990). Its mildest form is manifested as skin pustules that can be treated topically without the use of systemic antibiotics. The bacteria can infect any portion of the body, including the breast (abscess), umbilical cord (omphalitis), circumcision site, and lungs (pneumonia). One of the more severe manifestations of staphylococcal infection is the scalded-skin syndrome, which results from a toxin produced by a local colonization of the bacteria. In this disease, large patches of the skin are shed and there are major problems with fluid losses, much like those in burn patients. With aggressive supportive therapy, these infants generally survive.

There are many potentially harmful bacterial and viral infections. The most premature infants and those newborns requiring the greatest therapeutic intervention generally have the more serious manifestations.

PREVENTION AND TREATMENT

Prevention of neonatal infection resides largely with a high index of suspicion and concern among the health care team responsible for caring for the pregnant mother. She should be encouraged to avoid sexual contact with anyone with lesions or a discharge. Meat, a potential source of parasitic infections, should be cooked thoroughly. To prevent toxoplasmosis, the mother should avoid contact with feces of animals, especially kittens. In particular, she should avoid contact with kitty litter. She should be given no live vaccines such as those for rubella, poliomyelitis, or mumps during pregnancy. On visits to the health care team, the vaginal examination should include a surveillance culture for gonorrhea. Serologic testing for syphilis during the pregnancy is mandatory. If an infection is identified, it should be treated promptly to minimize the potential risk to the fetus.

Treatment of the neonate with infection is relatively straightforward. If the illness is bacterial, antibiotics for the specific organism should be used. If the child has signs and symptoms of the infection but no etiology is identified, the choice of antibiotic is then based on determination of the organism most likely to be infecting the baby (deLouvois & Harvey, 1988). Apart from general supportive therapy, transfusion with fresh frozen adult plasma or immunoglobulins may be useful (Baker, 1989). These therapies may offer essential elements that the baby has in short supply but needs to cope with infection.

The viral and protozoal infections are much more difficult to remedy. The antibiotics available for treatment are generally toxic and have limited application. For viral infections such as cytomegalovirus and rubella, no therapy is available.

The prognosis for any newborn with an infection is dependent on the responsible organism and its predilection for certain body organs. Overall, viral infections—especially herpes, cytomegalovirus, and rubella—tend to cause damage to the central nervous system and, therefore, are apt to produce more devastating developmental problems. Unfortunately, with many of the perinatal infections, much of the damage is irreversible, even if therapy is instituted immediately. Understandably, every child who has had an infection as a baby should be monitored closely for developmental delay.

BIBLIOGRAPHY

Ablow, R.C., Driscoll, S.G., Effmann, E.L., Gross, I., Jolles, C.J., Uauy, R., & Warshaw, J.B. (1976). A comparison of early-onset Group B streptococcal neonatal infection and the respiratory distress syndrome of the newborn. *New England Journal of Medicine, 294*, 65–70.

Alford, C.A., Stagno, S., & Pass, R.F. (1990). Congenital and perinatal cytomegalovirus infections. *Reviews in Infectious Diseases, 12*(Suppl. 7), 745–753.

Amstey, M.S. (1984). *Virus infection in pregnancy.* Orlando, FL: Grune & Stratton.

Arevalo, J.A. (1989). Hepatitis B in pregnancy. *Western Journal of Medicine, 150*, 669–674.

Baker, C.J., & Edwards, M.S. (1990). Group B streptococcal infections. In J.S. Remington & J.O. Klein (Eds.), *Infectious diseases of the fetus and newborn infant* (3rd ed.) (pp. 742–811). Philadelphia: W.B. Saunders.

Baker, C.J., & the Neonatal IVIG Collaborative Study Group. (1989). Multicenter trial of intravenous immunoglobulin (IVIG) to prevent late-onset infection in preterm infants: Preliminary results. *Pediatric Research, 25*, 275A.

Bellanti, J.A., & Boner, A.L. (1981). Immunology of the fetus and newborn. In G.B. Avery (Ed.), *Neonatology: Pathophysiology and management of the newborn* (2nd ed.) (pp. 701–722). Philadelphia: J.B. Lippincott.

Blanc, W.A. (1961). Pathways of fetal and early neonatal infection. *Journal of Pediatrics, 59*, 473–496.

Brown, G.C. (1970). Maternal virus infection and congenital anomalies. *Archives of Environmental Health, 21*, 362–365.

Brunell, P.A. (1980). Prevention and treatment of neonatal herpes. *Pediatrics, 66*, 806–808.

Carbonaro, C.A., Clark, D.A., & Elseviers, D. (1988). A bacterial pathogenicity associated with necrotizing enterocolitis. *Microbial Pathogenesis, 5*, 427–436.

Cherry, J.D. (1990). Enteroviruses. In J.S. Remington & J.O. Klein (Eds.), *Infectious diseases of the fetus and newborn infant* (3rd ed.) (pp. 325–366). Philadelphia: W.B. Saunders.

Clark, D.A., & Miller, M.J.S. (1990). Intraluminal pathogenesis of necrotizing enterocolitis. *Journal of Pediatrics, 117* (Suppl. l), S64–S67.

Clark, D.A., Thompson, J.E., Weiner, L.D., McMillan, J.A., Schneider, A.J., & Rokahr, J.E. (1985). Necrotizing enterocolitis: Intraluminal biochemistry in human neonates and a rabbit model. *Pediatric Research, 19*, 919–921.

Cooper, L.Z. (1985). The history and medical consequences of rubella. *Review in Infectious Diseases, 7*(Suppl. 1), 2–10.

Corey, L., & Spear, P.G. (1986a). Infections of herpes simplex viruses (Part I). *New England Journal of Medicine, 314*(11), 686–691, 749–757.

Corey, L., & Spear, P.G. (1986b). Infections of herpes simplex viruses (Part 2). *New England Journal of Medicine, 314*(12), 749–757.

Cowan, M.J., Hellman, D., & Chudwin, D. (1984). Maternal transmission of acquired immune deficiency syndrome. *Pediatrics, 73*, 382–386.

Cowles, T.A., & Gonik, B. (1992). Perinatal infections. In A.A. Fanaroff & R.J. Martin (Eds.), *Neonatal-perinatal medicine: Diseases of the fetus and infant* (5th ed.) (Vol. 1) (pp. 251–271). St. Louis: C.V. Mosby.

deLouvois, J., & Harvey, D. (1988). Antibiotic therapy of the newborn. *Clinics in Perinatology, 15*, 365–388.

European Collaborative Study (1991). Children born to women with HIV-1 infection: Natural history and transmission. *Lancet, 337*, 253–260.

Fauci, A.S. (1988). The human immunodeficiency virus: Infectivity and mechanisms of pathogenesis. *Science, 239*, 617–622.

Feldman, H.A. (1968). Toxoplasmosis. *New England Journal of Medicine, 279*, 1370–1375, 1431–1437.

Gonik, B., & Hammill, H.A. (1990). AIDS in pregnancy. *Seminars in Pediatric Infectious Disease, 1*, 82–88.

Hanshaw, H.B., Dudgeon, J.A., & Marshall, W.C. (1985). *Viral diseases of the fetus and newborn.* Philadelphia: W.B. Saunders.

Hanson, C.G., & Shearer, W.T. (1992). Pediatric HIV infection and AIDS. In R.D. Feigin & J.D. Cherry (Eds.), *Textbook of pediatric infectious diseases* (3rd ed.) (pp. 990–1011). Philadelphia: W.B. Saunders.

Hinman, A.R. (1985). Prevention of congenital rubella infection: Symposium summary. *Pediatrics, 75*, 1162–1165.

Klein, J.O., & Marcy, S.M. (1990). Bacterial sepsis and meningitis. In J.S. Remington & J.O. Klein (Eds.), *Infectious diseases of the fetus and newborn infant* (3rd ed.) (pp. 60–72). Philadelphia: W.B. Saunders.

Klein, J.O., Remington, J.S., & Marcy, S.M. (1983). Current concepts of infections of the fetus and newborn infant. In J.S.. Remington & J.O. Klein (Eds.), *Infectious diseases of the fetus and newborn infant* (3rd ed.) (pp. 1–26). Philadelphia: W.B. Saunders.

Lee, R.V. (1988). Parasites and pregnancy: The problems of malaria and toxoplasmosis. *Clinics in Perinatology, 15*, 351–364.

Miller, M.E., & Stiehm, E.R. (1979). Host defenses in the fetus and neonate. *Pediatrics, 64*, 705–833.

Miller, M.H., Rabinowitz, M.A., Frost, J.O., & Seager, G.M. (1969). Audiological problems associated with maternal rubella. *Laryngoscope, 79*, 417–426.

Mok, J.Q., Giaquinto, C., & DeRossi, A. (1987). Infants born to mothers seropositive for human immunodeficiency virus: Preliminary findings from a multicenter European study. *Lancet, 1*, 1164–1168.

Mustafa, M.M., & McCracken, G.H., Jr. (1992). Perinatal bacterial diseases. In R.D. Feigin & J.D. Cherry (Eds.), *Textbook of pediatric infectious diseases* (3rd ed.) (pp. 891–923). Philadelphia: W.B. Saunders.

Nabarro, D. (1954). *Congenital syphilis.* London: E. Arnold.

Nahmias, A.J. (1974). The TORCH complex. *Hospital Practice, 9*, 65–72.

Nahmias, A.J., Keyserling, H.L., & Kerrick, G.M. (1983). Herpes simplex. In J.S. Remington & J.O. Klein (Eds.), *Infectious diseases of the fetus and newborn infant* (3rd ed.) (pp. 636–678). Philadelphia: W.B. Saunders.

Nankervis, G.A. (1985). Cytomegaloviral infections: Epidemiology, therapy, and prevention. *Pediatric Review, 7*, 169–175.

Nelson, D. (1989). Cellular interactions in the human immune response. In E. Stein (Ed.), *Immunologic disorders in infants and children* (pp. 15–29). Philadelphia: W.B. Saunders.

Overall, J.C., Jr. (1992). Viral infections of the fetus and neonate. In R.D. Feigin & J.D. Cherry (Eds.), *Textbook of pediatric infectious diseases* (3rd ed.) (pp. 924–959). Philadelphia: W.B. Saunders.

Preblud, S.R., & Alford, C.A., Jr. (1990). Rubella. In J.S. Remington & J.O. Klein (Eds.), *Infectious diseases of the fetus and newborn infant* (3rd ed.) (pp. 196–240). Philadelphia: W.B. Saunders.

Regelman, W.E., Hill, H.R., Cates, K.L., & Quie, P.G. (1992). Immunology of the newborn. In R.D. Feigin & J.D. Cherry (Eds.), *Textbook of pediatric infectious diseases* (3rd ed.) (pp. 876–890). Philadelphia: W.B. Saunders.

Rubinstein, A. (1986). Pediatric AIDS. *Current Problems in Pediatrics, 16*, 361–409.

Shinefield, H.R. (1990). Staphylococcal infections. In J.S. Remington & J.O. Klein (Eds.), *Infectious diseases of the fetus and newborn infant* (3rd ed.) (pp. 866–900). Philadelphia: W.B. Saunders.

Siegel, J.D., & McCracken, G.H., Jr. (1981). Sepsis neonatorum. *New England Journal of Medicine, 304*, 642–646.

Stagno, S. (1990). Cytomegalovirus. In J.S. Remington & J.O. Klein (Eds.), *Infectious diseases of the fetus and newborn infant* (3rd ed.) (pp. 241–281). Philadelphia: W.B. Saunders.

Taber, L.H., & Huber, T.W. (1975). Congenital syphilis. In S. Krugman & A.A. Gershon (Eds.), *Infections of the fetus and newborn infant* (pp. 183–190). New York: Alan R. Liss.

Wendel, G.D. (1988). Gestational and congenital syphilis. *Clinics in Perinatology, 15*, 287–304.

Whitley, R.J. (1990). Herpes simplex viruses. In B.N. Fields & D.M. Knipe (Eds.), *Virology* (2nd ed.) (pp. 1843–1887). New York: Raven Press.

Zeichner, S.L., & Plotkin, S.A. (1988). Mechanisms and pathways of congenital infections. *Clinics in Perinatology, 15*, 163–188.

Zeldis, J.B., & Crumpacker, C.S. (1990). Hepatitis. In J.S. Remington & J.O. Klein (Eds.), *Infectious diseases of the fetus and newborn infant* (3rd ed.) (pp. 574–600). Philadelphia: W.B. Saunders.

Chapter 13

Substance Use and Abuse, Pregnancy, and the Newborn

Gail L. Ensher, David A. Clark, and Linda M. Yarwood

The youngest casualties of the current drug epidemic in the United States are the thousands of infants born each year who are exposed prenatally to drugs, alcohol, and cigarette smoking. Although the media have focused primarily on "crack" cocaine use by pregnant women, that attention ignores the immense number of expectant mothers who use and abuse one or more other legal and illegal substances. Unfortunately, the fact that substance abuse often involves more than one agent makes it exceptionally difficult to determine the effects of any particular agent in subsequent child development. Furthermore, the complexity of situations in which drug-using mothers live certainly contributes to the commonly observed developmental lags of children born into such circumstances (Miller & Hyatt, 1992). In many ways, prenatally drug-exposed children look much like other children who reside in similarly chaotic homes and neighborhoods and who exhibit behaviors that appear to be excessively negative. Unless prenatally drug-exposed children are referred by neonatal, perinatal, pediatric, or other medical professionals, their problems—subtle or overt—may go undetected for months and sometimes years.

PRENATAL EXPOSURE TO DRUGS, ALCOHOL, AND CIGARETTE SMOKING

Incidence and Prevalence

One of the most frequently cited national estimates of the number of drug-exposed infants is based on a 1987 nationwide survey of 36 hospitals conducted by the National Association of Perinatal Addiction, Research, and Education (NAPARE). At the time of this study, an approximate 11 percent of all newborns, or 375,000 neonates annually, had been exposed prenatally to drugs.

In 1988, a similar national survey of 18 hospitals (14 public and 4 private) in 15 large urban areas was conducted by the U.S. House of Representatives Select Committee on Children, Youth, and Families (Miller, 1989). This research disclosed that, at 15 of the 18 hospitals surveyed, deliveries of drug-exposed neonates had increased substantially since 1985. The survey further suggested that, at these 18 hospitals, the reported proportions of newborns exposed to substance abuse ranged from 4 to 18 percent. The statistics of this study represented infants whose mothers, during pregnancy, used not only crack, but also drugs such as heroin, methadone, cocaine, amphetamines, PCP (phencyclidine hydrochloride), and marijuana. Estimates of the use of cocaine, in particular, indicate that the popularity of this drug has escalated dramatically over the past decade (Lynch & McKeon, 1990).

Approximately 20 to 25 million Americans have experimented with the drug at least once, 4 to 6 million take the drug on a regular basis (Hoyme et al., 1990), and 2 to 3 million are compulsive users (Kelley, Walsh, & Thompson, 1991). Lynch and McKeon (1990) have noted that an additional 5,000 individuals daily try cocaine for the first time and that its use has risen most drastically among young people between the ages of 18 and 25—the childbearing years. Thus, these estimates of cocaine use approach 1 in every 10 women nationwide. Even higher rates are cited for some urban areas.

As startling as these statistics are, there is a strong likelihood that they actually understate the magnitude of the problem, which is largely a reflection of reporting modes and accessibility of information at lower income and educational levels of the public sector. Research by Chasnoff, Landress, and Barrett (1990) support this contention. Summarizing results of a study conducted in Pinellas County, Florida, on the prevalence and mandatory reporting of illicit drug or alcohol use during pregnancy, the authors concluded:

> Among the 715 pregnant women we screened, the overall prevalence of a positive result on the toxicologic tests of urine was 14.8 percent; there was little difference in prevalence between the women seen at the public clinics (16.3 percent) and those seen at the private offices (13.1 percent). The frequency of a positive result was also similar among white woman (15.4 percent) and black women (14.1 percent). Black women more frequently had evidence of cocaine use (7.5 percent vs 1.8 percent of white women), whereas white women more frequently had evidence of the use of cannabinoids [marijuana] (14.4 percent vs 6.0 percent of black women).
>
> During the six-month period we collected the urine samples, 133 women in Pinellas County were reported to health authorities after delivery for substance abuse during pregnancy. Despite the similar rates of substance abuse among black and white women in our study, black

women were reported at approximately 10 times the rate for white women ($P<.0001$), and poor women were more likely than others to be reported. (p. 1202)

The consumption of alcohol during pregnancy is a long-standing concern and continues to be a timely national problem of increasing magnitude (Giesbrecht, Krempulec, & West, 1993; Hansen, 1993; Klitzner, Stewart, & Fisher, 1993; Weiner & Morse, 1988). Duggan and colleagues (Duggan, Adger, McDonald, Stokes, & Moore, 1991) noted that "more than 15 million Americans are estimated to meet the *Diagnostic and Statistical Manual of Mental Disorders, Third Edition,* criteria for alcohol abuse or dependence, and about one in eight American children has a parent with a past or present drinking problem" (p. 613). Other experts have cited similar evidence, documenting a serious need for education and increased public awareness, especially among teens and women of childbearing ages. For example, Barbour (1990) stated that the incidence of alcohol-related birth defects are equal to that of Down syndrome and spina bifida—an estimated 1/1,000 to 3/1,000 children who are severely affected by intrauterine exposure to alcohol (p. 79). Moreover, prevalence among certain populations (e.g., Native American Indians) is even greater. Klitzner, Stewart, and Fisher (1993) have written:

> Several national epidemiologic studies have explored the extent of underage drinking. These include the Monitoring the Future and National Household Surveys sponsored by the National Institute on Drug Abuse (NIDA) and the Youth and Alcohol Surveys sponsored by the Office of the Inspector General of the U.S. Department of Health and Human Services. While the individual results of these surveys vary, all indicate that underage drinking is common and that a significant minority of underage youths are heavy, episodic drinkers. According to these surveys of American 12 to 18 year olds (1) between 50 and 80 percent have experimented with alcohol; (2) by high school graduation, the percentage of students who have used alcohol at least once approaches 90 percent; (3) about one-half of those surveyed had at least one drink in the past year; and (4) about one-third are heavy, episodic drinkers.
>
> Among high school seniors from the class of 1990 who were surveyed, about 10 percent reported drinking at grade 6 or earlier; about 4 percent reported getting drunk at grade 6 or earlier. (p. 13)

Rice (1993) has indicated that "The total economic costs of alcohol abuse and dependence for 1990 are estimated at $98.6 billion, a 40 percent rise during the 5-year period, 1985 to 1990" (p. 10).

Finally, despite the well-established and consistent association between low infant birthweight and maternal smoking, approximately 20 to 30 percent of American women of childbearing age continue to use cigarettes (Aaronson & MacNee,

1988). In addition, an estimated 5 to 34 percent of women in this country, depending on the populations studied, have used marijuana during the course of their pregnancies (Zuckerman, 1988).

Prenatal and Neonatal Problems

Evidence on the teratogenic effects of illicit drugs, alcohol, and cigarette smoking on fetal growth and development continues to grow, with little doubt about the adverse outcome (Chasnoff, 1988b). Research to date is far from complete and is still largely complicated by factors of poor maternal nutrition, inconsistent lifestyle and less than optimal parenting, use of multiple drugs, and poor health and prenatal care. All things considered, however, fetal exposure to specific substances has been associated with a number of serious prenatal and neonatal problems. Clinical research is accumulating data on the relationships between maternal abuse of cocaine and reductions in intrauterine growth (Bresnahan, Brooks, & Zuckerman, 1991; Kelley, Walsh, & Thompson, 1991; Phibbs, Bateman, & Schwartz, 1991); respiratory instability in neonates (Cassady et al., 1991; Chen et al., 1991); onset of early labor and delivery (Kelley, Walsh, & Thompson, 1991); a higher incidence of infectious diseases including hepatitis B, human immunodeficiency virus (HIV) infection, and other sexually transmitted diseases (Chasnoff, 1988b); circulatory problems (Phibbs, Bateman, & Schwartz, 1991); and a variety of neurobehavioral disturbances and disruption in organizational states (Miller & Hyatt, 1992; Peters & Theorell, 1991). In regard to organizational state, Chasnoff (1988a) has noted: "The majority of cocaine exposed infants could be classified as fragile infants with very low thresholds for overstimulation. These infants required a great deal of assistance from caretakers to maintain control of their hyperexcitable nervous systems" (p. 99).

Further influence of exposure to cocaine or combinations of illicit drugs has been demonstrated. Among these difficulties, premature rupture of membranes, preterm delivery, and diminished weight gain and head circumference have been noted among babies born to women addicted to heroin and maintained on methadone, as well as among mothers using cocaine and other opiates (Keith, MacGregor, & Sciarra, 1988). Significantly higher rates of spontaneous abortion and placental abruption (detachment) and higher incidence of stillbirth secondary to abruption (Nora, 1990) also are acknowledged complications of prolonged use of cocaine or its derivatives during pregnancy, either ingested intranasally or taken intravenously. Congenital anomalies such as skeletal or urogenital abnormalities are rare but have been observed, in part the suggested result of maternal hypertension, uteroplacental insufficiency, and hypoxia (Miller & Hyatt, 1992; Nora, 1990). Likewise, tachycardia, hypertension, and release of meconium into the amniotic fluid frequently are implicated side effects of active maternal cocaine abuse (Nora, 1990).

This accounting of fetal, neonatal, and maternal problems resulting from co-caine use should not be surprising in light of the fact the drug is a fat soluble substance that readily passes the blood-brain barrier and easily crosses the pla-centa to the fetus by diffusion (Lynch & McKeon, 1990). Due to the slow rate of metabolism of cocaine in pregnant women, there is delayed clearance of the drug and its metabolites, which remain in the urine of the expectant mother and the baby for as long as 4 to 7 days after use (Chasnoff, 1987). Further compromise of the fetus likely takes place as a result of the water soluble properties of cocaine, which inhibit transfer back to the mother across the placenta, thus slowing excre-tion in the urine (Chasnoff, 1987) and causing constant reingestion of cocaine-contaminated amniotic fluid by the fetus. In addition, studies of the association between exposure of males to cocaine and abnormal development of offspring now are underway. In a recent article published in the *Journal of the American Medical Association*, Yazigi, Odem, and Polakoski (1991) commented:

> There is now considerable evidence demonstrating that males ex-posed to drugs and other potentially toxic substances prior to mating have an increased incidence of offspring with abnormal development. These findings have been corroborated both in animal and human stud-ies but the mechanisms underlying this phenomenon remain unex-plained. Indirect evidence supports the view that the spermatozoa may have a role in the pathogenesis of such changes. For example, cocaine, a drug that has been related to neurologic abnormalities in the offspring born to exposed fathers, can decrease the count as well as the motility and increase the number of abnormal forms in spermatozoa from human users. These findings suggest an effect of cocaine on the male genital system and perhaps directly on the sperm. The possibility that the sperm may transport cocaine to the oocyte at the time of fertilization, affecting the normal development of the embryo, remains to be explored. (p. 1956)

Finally, variation in outcome among drug-abusing mothers and their neonates often is referenced in the literature. Again, such clinical findings probably are a function of many contributing factors, including the drug or drugs of choice, nutri-tional status of the mother, uniqueness in metabolic rates, and the time and dura-tion of substance use throughout the gestational period.

Short-Term and Long-Term Effects of Drug Abuse

Data on the immediate and long-term consequences of drug use for the infant are just emerging and are inconsistent. Similar to the problems of sorting out clear-cut relationships at prenatal stages of development, postnatal impact is compli-cated by variables such as family dysfunction, poverty, and environmental deprivation (Azuma & Chasnoff, 1993; Durfee & Tilton-Durfee, 1990; Gittler & McPherson, 1990; Howard, Beckwith, Rodning, & Kropenske, 1989; Tittle & St. Claire, 1989; Weston, Ivins, Zuckerman, Jones, & Lopez, 1989). Use of multiple drugs also is a major confounding dimension. Indeed, there is a compelling need for more rigorous studies to be conducted before definite conclusions can be reached about long-term effects. Nevertheless, research to date and clinical observations do indicate that drug-exposed babies run an increased risk of mortality or morbidity, with problems in both development and behavior (Bresnahan, Brooks, & Zuckerman, 1991; Eisen et al., 1991; Howard, Beckwith, Rodning, & Kropenske, 1989; Chasnoff, 1988a and 1988b; Janke, 1990; Miller, 1989; Peters & Theorell, 1991; Zuckerman et al., 1989).

Miller and Hyatt (1992) point out a particular complication of the research on drug effects on children: the present knowledge of prenatal drug exposure is based mainly on information gathered from lower socioeconomic groups who have poor social and family networks. While substance abuse during pregnancy cuts across all socioeconomic, educational, and ethnic groups, it is usually poor women and women of color who are identified, come to the attention of medical staff and service providers, and thus are included in research agendas. We do not know, for instance, whether outcome now attributed to drug use would be observed among more well-to-do families who, with additional resources, might be able to cushion the influence of drug exposure in their children.

Adding to the dilemma of evaluating the long-term effects of drug exposure are limitations of the tools available to assess child development, especially throughout the first 18 months of life. On the one hand, standardized measures may not be sensitive enough to detect subtle variations in learning and behavior of children exposed to drugs that later predict school-related difficulties. On the other hand, as many researchers (Azuma & Chasnoff, 1993) have suggested, even if differences are identified, we do not always understand the functional significance of such variance. In light of these complexities, we should expect to see disparities in data from studies purporting to address the same questions. However, given all cautions, some long-term consequences have been reported to be associated with the abuse of crack cocaine, marijuana, opiates, and other combinations of illicit drugs. Much of the research to this time has examined development through the age of 4 years, with a few studies looking at children through 7 years. Certainly, low birthweight, growth retardation in utero, and small head circumference, noted earlier in our discussion, are potential consequences of drug use during pregnancy and correlate with the risk of problems such as cerebral palsy, seizure disorders, and mental retardation—though not all infants develop such serious conditions (Chasnoff, 1988a; Howard, Beckwith, Rodning, & Kropenske, 1989).

Some researchers have speculated that damage to the central nervous system is the underlying cause of later developmental problems of children of mothers who used multiple drugs during pregnancy. These problems include irritability, tremulousness, and irregular sleep patterns. Also, with respect to behavior, even co-caine-exposed infants are not a homogeneous group, but seem to exhibit a cluster of behaviors. Immediately after birth, some infants are in great distress. Jittery and suffering tremors, they are irritable and sensitive to the mildest environmental stimulation (e.g., sound and light). They have a high-pitched cry and may show hyperextension of the joints and a prolonged persistence of early reflexes (Chasnoff, 1988a). Excitable and depressed cry characteristics, respectively, have been attributed to "neurotoxic effects and indirect effects secondary to intrauterine growth retardation" (Lester et al., 1991). Some infants do not fall asleep readily and, once asleep, are easily awakened. Their distress is obvious, and they are nota-bly unable to calm themselves. In contrast, other newborns born to mothers abus-ing cocaine sleep much of the time and appear to shut down in response to any environmental stimulations (Chasnoff, 1988a). While problems associated with motor development (e.g., high muscle tone and persistence of early reflexes) usu-ally diminish during the first year, irritability, sleep and feeding problems, and inability to calm easily may continue at least into the second year (Chasnoff, 1988a).

Two further observations of infants delivered by drug-abusing mothers are noteworthy. The first is the small increase in the rate of Sudden Infant Death syn-drome (SIDS) among neonates born to women using cocaine during pregnancy (Bresnahan, Brooks, & Zuckerman, 1991). Second, women taking opiates during pregnancy often have neonates showing symptoms similar to adult withdrawal from narcotics; e.g., high-pitched cry, tremulousness, sweating, excoriation of the extremities, and gastrointestinal disturbances.

Many studies concerning the long-term effects of maternal drug abuse during pregnancy are being carried out, but the findings to date are inconclusive. For instance, comparisons of toddlers who were drug exposed in utero and preterm infants from a similar prenatal environment have been done by Howard and her colleagues at the University of California, Los Angeles (Howard, Beckwith, Rodning, & Kropenske, 1989). The results show that developmental scores deter-mined in a structured setting were lower for the drug-exposed group than for the non-drug-exposed control group. In a free-play setting, the play of the drug-exposed toddlers was less age appropriate and more constricted and impulsive than that of other children. Those play patterns, characterized by throwing and batting objects, are not unlike those observed in children with neurological im-pairments. In addition, toddlers exposed prenatally to drugs appeared to be less securely attached to their caregivers than were the comparison group (Howard, Beckwith, Rodning, & Kropenske, 1989).

In another study, researchers in Chicago found that 30 to 40 percent of the prenatally drug-exposed children of toddler age had both language and behavioral problems, including delays in language development, lack of tolerance for frustra-tion, distractibility, and difficulties in organizing behavior (Chasnoff, 1988a).

These findings are similar to those of researchers in Amsterdam (van Baar, 1990), who studied children over the first 30 months of life. Specifically, a small sample of 30 children continued to test within the normal range on measures of psychomotor development. Many of the prenatally drug-exposed toddlers, however, had specific problems of early language development. Researchers working with a large Los Angeles Unified School District program for 3- and 4-year-olds exposed prenatally to drugs reported irritability, agitation, hyperactivity, speech and language delays, poor task orientation, emotional problems relating to difficulties with attachment and separation, passivity and apathy, aggression, and poor social skills. These behaviors were viewed as consequences of multiple risk factors, such as problems of trust and early "bonding" and of unstable home life and community environment, as well as parental abuse of drugs. Furthermore, the staff and program researchers cautioned that there was no *typical* profile of the child exposed prenatally to drugs; infants and toddlers revealed a continuum of impairments, ranging from mild symptoms in isolated areas to severe problems in multiple domains of development.

The complexity of issues is underscored again by Kelley, Walsh, and Thompson (1991), who have stated that:

> Child protective agencies are overwhelmed by increased numbers of abuse and neglect reports involving cocaine-dependent parents. A recent study of child abuse and neglect investigators conducted by the Massachusetts Department of Social Studies (1989) revealed the presence of illicit drug use and excessive alcohol use in 64% of cases involving Boston families. The drug most frequently identified was cocaine (42%). Cocaine use cases exceeded those where no substance abuse was identified (35%). Excessive alcohol was identified in 31% of the investigations, heroin in 6%, and other drugs, including methadone, were cited in 26% of the investigations.
>
> Ninety-two percent of the cases involving substance abuse involved single parents. Neglect was the type of maltreatment reported most frequently, followed by physical abuse. The severe and chronic neglect of young children associated with maternal cocaine use included lack of food in the home, medical neglect, extremely dirty living quarters, and absence of care and supervision of very young children. (p. 131)

Miller and Hyatt (1992) write of a similar scenario:

> . . . a substance-abusing mother may deliver an unstable irritable infant who interacts poorly with its environment. The infant may also have physical problems resulting from birth complications, making it more susceptible to fatigue and illness. This is further complicated by a lack of maternal support stemming from living in an unstable, drug-infested

environment. Often these women are also victims of poverty, with its lack of the basic necessities for survival. She may have ambivalence regarding her own parenting skills. Emotional scars from her childhood, as well as feelings of guilt over any maternal or neonatal problems resulting from the substance abuse, will play a role in her ability to parent. . . . This difficult triad of an unstable infant, environment, and mother sets up a vicious cycle that leads to dysfunctional parenting and child abuse. (p. 255)

Clearly, as these and numerous other authors have reiterated, the issue of long-term impact of drug abuse almost always is accompanied by a combination of events and living circumstances that add to the adversity of infants and young children (Azuma & Chasnoff, 1993). In that sense, the question of separating out "pure effects" of drug use becomes almost an impossible and perhaps irrelevant concern to resolve. Finally, we have not touched on the dimension of the exorbitant costs for medical care associated with fetal cocaine exposure. Some researchers (Phibbs, Bateman, & Schwartz, 1991) have estimated this cost at $500 million nationally for 1990, a figure that drives home the enormous need for treatment and multifaceted intervention programs.

Effects of Alcohol, Cigarette Smoking, and Marijuana Use

Alcohol

Experimental and epidemiologic research on the chronic abuse of alcohol has a long-standing history, dating back to the 1900s. Subsequent to that time, in the late 1960s and early 1970s, a pattern of neurological and physiological features was noted among infants born to mothers using alcohol (LeMoine, Harousseau, Borteyru, & Menuet, 1968) and later was termed *fetal alcohol syndrome* (FAS) by Jones and Smith (1973) (Figure 13–1). The characteristics of children with this syndrome sometimes mimic the features seen in other disorders, such as fetal hydantoin syndrome, which occurs in children born to women taking anticonvulsant drugs. Consequently, in 1980, the Fetal Alcohol Study Group of the Research Society on Alcoholism developed a minimum set of three criteria for diagnosis of FAS within the following categories:

1. prenatal and/or postnatal growth retardation (weight, length, and/or head circumference below the 10th percentile)
2. central nervous system involvement (signs of neurologic abnormality, developmental delay, or intellectual impairment)
3. characteristic facial dysmorphology with at least two of the following signs:

   a. microcephaly

b. micro-ophthalmia and/or short palpebral fissures

c. poorly developed philtrum, thin upper lip, or flattening of the maxillary area (Weiner & Morse, 1988, p. 128).

Over the past 15 years, the study of alcohol and its related prenatal and neonatal problems has been an active area of investigation, with important chemical evidence emerging relative to developmental outcome. For example, Aaronson and MacNee (1988) have noted that:

> Because alcohol passes easily through the placental barrier, concentrations found in the fetus are at least as high as those in the mother. Thus the rate at which alcohol is metabolized may affect the amount of fetal damage. Further, susceptibility to these effects may be genetic, or may depend on prepregnancy weight, parity, and possibly age. Therefore, results remain unclear as to which is critical in predicting outcomes: the duration of drinking or the interaction of drinking with other factors. (p. 283)

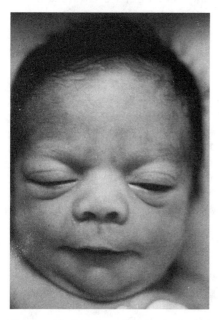

Figure 13–1 Baby with fetal alcohol syndrome

Some researchers have attempted to document a correlation between the degree of alcohol consumption and the number of physical anomalies present (O'Connor, Brill, & Sigman, 1986), even though other investigators have consistently pointed to the wide range of effects of alcohol, which depend on the timing and conditions of fetal exposure as well as the amount of alcohol consumed. Among the many consequences of prenatal exposure to alcohol for the developing child, several manifestations have been linked to heavy maternal drinking of alcohol—80 to 100 grams or 2.8 to 3.5 ounces daily (Aaronson & MacNee, 1988). These manifestations include disturbances in motor development (Barr, Darby, Streissguth, & Sampson, 1990), difficulties in state regulation of the infant (Sander et al., 1977), delays in language, hyperactivity, feeding problems, and perceptual difficulties.

Despite controversies over abstinence versus consumption of varying amounts of alcohol, most researchers and physicians today acknowledge the fact that there are no "safe" levels. Substantiating this conclusion are data on the more subtle but adverse effects of "modest" or "social" drinking by mothers during pregnancy— outcomes exhibited by children now identified as having *fetal alcohol effects* (FAE). Among the 100 neonatal features that have been associated with maternal alcohol abuse, children with FAE may present a variety of patterns including maladaptive behaviors, learning disabilities, speech and language problems, hyperactivity, and attention-deficit disorders (Barbour, 1990). Like children with FAS, those with FAE frequently are difficult to manage because of feeding, medical, and neurological problems. However, because these manifestations are more subtle in presentation, they may go unrecognized until later follow-up care or until school age (Barbour, 1990). Moreover, in addition to the teratogenic effects we have described, use of alcohol during the childbearing years has been reported to be associated with infertility, spontaneous abortion, stillbirth, and other medical, obstetric, and perinatal complications. Common among children with FAE and FAS are the heightened risks of postnatal parental abuse and neglect and failure of the infant to thrive (Barbour, 1990). As many authors reiterate (Klitzner, Stewart, & Fisher, 1993), addressing the enormous problems of drinking and its consequences will require efforts toward prevention and treatment on several fronts, including education prior to adolescence in the schools (Hansen, 1993) and communities at large (Giesbrecht, Krempulec, & West, 1993), with particular attention to targeting risk factors that appear to precipitate onset of these consequences.

Cigarette Smoking and Marijuana Use

Two inhaled substances—cigarette tobacco and marijuana—often are used in conjunction with drug and alcohol abuse. Since consumption is prevalent among young populations and pregnant women in particular, research, again, has been focused on questions of impact on fetal and neonatal growth and development.

With regard to the use of cigarettes during pregnancy, a substantial body of literature has documented, without question, the risks and adverse outcomes associated with smoking (Fried & Watkinson, 1990; Fried, Watkinson, Dillon, & Dulberg, 1987; Zuckerman, 1988). While structural defects such as those seen with alcohol abuse are not apparent, the smoking of cigarettes consistently has been correlated with reduced fetal growth, low birthweight, and increased complications of perinatal mortality (Fried & Watkinson, 1990). Moreover, when other variables are controlled, reductions in fetal and neonatal weight gain are directly proportional to the degree of cigarette use, ranging from a decrease of 40 to 430 grams (Zuckerman, 1988). Zuckerman summarized these data as follows:

> For white mothers, the incidence of low-birthweight babies ranges from 4.8% for women who do not smoke, to 8% for women who smoke 1–10 cigarettes per day, to 13.4% for women who smoke more than 20 cigarettes per day. For black women, the incidence of low-birthweight babies ranges from 8.3% for women who do not smoke, to 13.6% for

women who smoke 1-10 cigarettes per day, to 22.7% for women who smoke more than 20 cigarettes per day. (p. 84)

Additional observations and research findings, though not as clear-cut, have disclosed significant associations between prenatal exposure to cigarette smoking and lower language and cognitive scores at 36 and 48 months of age (Fried & Watkinson, 1990). Study results are not consistent, but some investigators have reported various associations between maternal cigarette smoking and neonatal congenital heart defects, lower Apgar scores, altered habituation and orientation to sound and voices, and hypertonicity with tremors (Fried, Watkinson, Dillon, & Dulberg, 1987). Finally, long-term follow-up of children exposed to smoking in utero suggest that early differences of general academic achievement and performance on measures of language, psychomotor, and cognitive skills are maintained, regardless of socioeconomic status.

Data on the effects of heavy marijuana use during pregnancy on prenatal and neonatal outcome are less well documented than the effects of cigarette smoking, and research findings are extremely inconsistent. As with the abuse of other substances, confounding variables may influence results and are difficult to separate. Like alcohol, cocaine, and other drugs, marijuana crosses the placenta and thus may have a direct impact on the developing fetus. In addition, this inhaled substance is known to cause elevated carbon monoxide levels in the blood and, as a result, hypoxia (Zuckerman, 1988). On the other hand, studies on the relationship between birthweight and marijuana use do not show uniform effects. Some studies have revealed evidence of lower birthweight, congenital anomalies, and depressed scores on developmental measures; other studies have found no predictive associations. Zuckerman (1988) has suggested that such inconsistent results may be a function of several factors, including differences in the content of marijuana, variations in the accuracy of maternal self-reporting, and incomplete identification of combinations of additional substances used.

In conclusion, because much of the available research suggests some adverse neonatal outcome with the smoking of marijuana, young women in their teens and childbearing years need to be educated about the potential consequences of abuse of this substance. Meanwhile, research should be pursued, with the goal of demonstrating more clearly the short- and long-term effects on growth and development.

INFLUENCE OF PRESCRIBED DRUGS

Prenatal Effects

During the early 1960s, obstetricians and pediatricians identified an alarming epidemic of congenital malformations associated with the use of the drug thalidomide. This substance was first synthesized in Germany in 1956 and was prescribed to control vomiting during pregnancy (Korf, 1991). Routine administration increased the incidence of newborn malformations of arms and legs, and approximately 10,000 neonates worldwide suffered anomalies associated with maternal use of the drug. This experience, which led to early disuse of the medication, kindled intense interest in the effects of such agents on the developing fetus and newborn.

Thalidomide is one of a few medications for which teratogenicity (capacity for inducing malformations) has been firmly established (Sucheston & Cannon, 1973). Similarly, methotrexate, a cancer chemotherapeutic agent, is well recognized as a risk factor for abnormalities in the fetus. Unfortunately, for most drugs, the information on teratogenicity is not as clear-cut as it is for thalidomide and methotrexate (Abdul-Karim, 1981). Data regarding possible changes in drug metabolism as a result of pregnancy are lacking for most medications. In addition, other side effects need to be considered, including fetal death, growth retardation, disturbance of fetal metabolism, disabilities that are manifested in later life, decreased longevity, predisposition toward malignancies, and drug dependence (Abdul-Karim & Clark, 1982).

There are many reasons why the risk of drug toxicity to a fetus cannot be readily estimated. Much of the work on drug effects has been done in animals, and no single animal species, including primates, can be used in research as an adequate substitute for the human. In addition, the impact of a drug varies widely with the amount given, as well as with the means and rate of administration. In general, the drug levels in the body are proportionate to the ability of the individual to metabolize and excrete the agent. If liver or kidney function is impaired, the severity of effects may be increased. For some drugs such as thalidomide, the substance itself is not the critical factor; the teratogenic agent is a breakdown product (metabolite) produced in the liver. The metabolic pathway that alters thalidomide is found only in rabbits and in humans and varies among individuals. A particular constellation of conditions ultimately was responsible for the resulting impairments: A pregnant mother received the medication, which was metabolized to the teratogenic metabolite at the critical embryonic developmental stage of 4 to 6 weeks gestation. Babies exposed to the breakdown product after 6 weeks into a pregnancy had no obvious developmental abnormalities (Aranda, Hales, & Gibbs, 1983).

Other difficulties in determining degrees of toxicity include the less obvious delayed effects of the medication. Behavioral or mental disorders that, theoretically, could arise from an early drug insult are difficult to quantitate. Virtually no animal model is adequate, and it is also impossible to determine the specific contributions of various factors such as genetics, perinatal history, and environmental and social deprivation. An additional concern is the prevalence of multiple-drug use during pregnancy. If vitamins and minerals are included, nearly all pregnant women receive one or more medications. Even if use of these substances is not a risk factor, the pregnant woman consumes many other prescribed and nonprescribed drugs that alone or in combination may be risk factors. These medications include antihistamines, analgesics (e.g., aspirin), antibiotics, tranquilizers, and antiemetics (to prevent vomiting) (Doering & Steward, 1978; Hill, Craig, Chaney, Tennyson, & McCulley, 1977). For the interested reader, several reviews examine the effects and potential risks of antibiotics, anticoagulants, and medications used to treat epilepsy (Cohlan, 1980; Hill, 1979).

In addition to medications that cause malformations, others are nonteratogenic but still may have marked negative consequences for the newborn. Analgesics may interfere with blood coagulation. Anesthetic agents may result in depressed respiration in the neonate. The antibiotic sulfonamides (sulfa drugs) may produce accelerated red blood cell destruction in certain suspectible newborns. Antihistamines may result in rapid heart rate, vomiting, and jitteriness, and diazepam (Valium), which crosses the placenta, may cause neonatal hyperthermia, irregular breathing, prolonged hypotonia, and a poor sucking reflex (Abdul-Karim & Clark, 1982; Hill, 1979).

In summary, medications administered to the mother in the first trimester have greater potential for producing fetal malformation. Medications given to the mother in the third trimester may produce a nonteratogenic effect in the newborn, most commonly, central nervous system depression with failure to adapt properly to extrauterine existence. The second most common effect is behavioral, including feeding difficulties, hypotonia, and withdrawal symptoms. There are relatively few data on subtle drug effects and, at present, these data are not easily obtained.

Drugs Used To Treat the Neonate

In the past, drug dosage for newborns was extrapolated from available information on rates of metabolism in adults and older children. However, such research failed to account for the delayed elimination of many medications in the newborn. Studies over the last decade have gone a long way toward providing a much better understanding of the diverse factors that can affect absorption, distribution, and excretion of drugs. As a result, safe and effective guidelines for medications in the neonate have been established.

The following discussion will afford the reader some appreciation of the delicate and subtle balance that needs to be maintained throughout the often long course of medical intervention with the high risk infant. For example, premature infants with restricted fat digestion and absorption generally are less able to absorb fat soluble vitamins (Bell, Brown, Milner, Sinclair, & Zipursky, 1979).

Once absorbed, drugs are distributed in the body. Some are primarily water soluble and others are basically fat soluble. Dosages in the infant vary, depending on the nature of the medication. In the newborn, who has a total body water content greater than that of an adult or older child, water soluble drugs have a greater volume of distribution and often must be given in larger amounts for therapeutic benefit. By comparison, the fat content of babies, especially preterm children, is lower, and therefore the lipid soluble drugs have a smaller volume of distribution, usually requiring reduced drug doses to maintain appropriate therapeutic levels (Marselli, 1976; Roberts, 1984).

Another set of concerns involves the liver and kidneys, major organs for the excretion of drugs. The liver in the newborn, for instance, has a restricted ability to metabolize medications such as Valium, and the rate of elimination is prolonged. On the other hand, phenobarbital induces the production of hepatic (liver) enzymes that rapidly increase the clearance of the drug. Understandably, such anticonvulsants must be monitored carefully to avoid subtherapeutic levels. Renal (kidney) function gradually improves after birth but does not reach an adult level until approximately 1 year of age. Therefore, medications for neonates must generally be given at lower doses to prevent toxic accumulation (Kauffman, 1981).

Basically, four major groups of drugs are used commonly in the newborn. These are antibiotics, cardiovascular medications, anticonvulsants, and medications to stimulate respiration. Each is used for a specific indication and only for a limited time, with careful attention to side effects and toxic effects. If adverse symptoms do arise, the drug is stopped and an alternative medication is prescribed. As is evident in the following discussion, all medications serve necessary purposes but have the potential to cause substantial impairment in the newborn.

Drugs classified as antibiotics are used to assist the immune defenses of the infant against bacteria (McCracken & Nelson, 1977; McIntosh, 1984). In general, they are divided into two groups: *bacteriostatic* and *bactericidal* medications. Penicillin and penicillin-like drugs such as ampicillin are bactericidal medications and serve the function of disrupting the cell walls of susceptible bacteria. In contrast, bacteriostatic antibiotics limit bacterial multiplication. Each of these groups has identified toxic effects. For instance, elevated blood levels of some of the bacteriostatic drugs may result in damage to the kidneys or the inner ear (cochlea).

Cardiovascular medications are a heterogeneous group of drugs used to control heart rate, improve cardiac function, and control blood pressure. The most commonly used form is digitalis; the specific variety used in children is called *digoxin* (Wettrell & Andersson, 1977). In neonates, the drug is short acting and is helpful in treating congestive heart failure and very rapid heart rates. Toxic effects of elevated blood levels of digoxin include vomiting, poor feeding, and arrhythmic heart patterns. Furthermore, for a number of the cardiovascular therapies, drug toxicity results in conditions that are the converse of problems being treated. For example, agents used for high blood pressure may produce an abnormally low blood pressure (Adelman, 1978), and medications for low blood pressure may have an opposite effect that is abnormal. Drugs prescribed to slow or speed the heart, in contrast, may create an opposing abnormal rhythm at toxic levels. For the most part, the majority of cardiovascular medications have no direct demonstrable impact on the central nervous system but indirectly may cause neurological complications by restricting adequate quantities of blood to the brain (Roberts, 1984).

Methylxanthine drugs are stimulants prescribed for apnea of prematurity; the two primary medications are theophylline and caffeine. Initially, these are given in small doses and then maintained while blood levels are monitored. Any beneficial effects of reducing the severity of apnea at premature birth are seen within 1 or 2 days after the medication is started. The most common side effects of each of these medicines are jitteriness and gastrointestinal symptoms, including abdominal distention and vomiting (Aranda, Grandin, & Sasyniuk, 1981).

Anticonvulsant drugs are given to control seizures during the newborn period. Because of its effectiveness and its rate of metabolism in the neonate, phenobarbital is the medication of choice for infants. Adequate blood levels and therapeutic ranges are relatively easy to achieve. The major detriment of acute phenobarbital excess is lethargy, sometimes associated with respiratory depression. Alternatively, Dilantin is a potent seizure medication, but the oral absorption of this drug is incomplete and somewhat unreliable. Other medications such as paraldehyde and Valium may be effective in the newborn but rarely are indicated and may have significant toxic effects on respiration (Johnson & Freeman, 1981; Roberts, 1984; Volpe, 1977).

BREAST-FEEDING AND DRUGS

Human milk is uniquely suited to the nutritional needs of the full-term infant. Within the past 20 years, however, numerous investigators have shown that maternal medications and environmental contaminants may pass into breast milk, resulting in harmful effects in the newborn. Thus, it is not always easy to decide whether or not a mother should nurse while she is taking a particular medication. Much of the information available regarding specific contraindications has been derived from individual case reports of affected infants. There are relatively few data on specific risks to a given infant when the mother is taking a particular drug.

Many factors determine the presence of a compound in a mother's milk. First, the drug level in the mother's blood, the time of administration of the medicine, the volume and time of feeding, and the breast milk composition all are important to the degree of absorption. Second, drug toxicity is influenced by the solubility of the drug, the size of the drug molecule, and its binding to the maternal proteins, both in the mother's blood and in her milk. Third, the intestinal tract of the newborn may limit the amount of drug that is metabolized (Anderson, 1979; Levy, Granit, & Laufer, 1977).

Few medications are absolutely incompatible with breast-feeding. Those that are incompatible include toxic drugs used in cancer chemotherapy and in the treatment of goiters. The antibiotic chloramphenicol, even in small concentrations, may produce an exaggerated response in which the bone marrow of the newborn fails to produce red blood cells. Isoniazid, a medication used to treat tuberculosis, is secreted into breast milk and may result in toxicity to the liver in the infant. A number of environmental chemicals, such as DDT (dichlorophenyltrichloro-ethane), PCBs (polychlorinated liphenyls), and PBBs (polybrominated biphenyls) may be concentrated in the milk and therefore pass to the baby. Lithium, a successful therapeutic agent for manic-depressive illness, can cause high blood levels in the infant, altering the sensorium (Abdul-Karim & Clark, 1982; Giacoia & Catz, 1979). Other medications that need to be used for the health of the mother should be given only with caution. These include sedatives and antipsychotic and anticonvulsive agents, which may produce decreased responsiveness in the newborn. In addition, aspirin in the breast milk can cause bleeding tendencies in the infant by interfering with platelet function, although this risk is minimized if the mother takes the medication just after nursing (Aranda, Hales, & Gibbs, 1983).

Several illicit drugs are under study, and data are accumulating relative to their very harmful effects in humans. Use of heroin or crack cocaine are contraindications for breast-feeding (Chasnoff, 1988a). Opiates are detectable in small quantities in breast milk, but it is unlikely that, in these amounts, they would produce addiction in the newborn (Abdul-Karim & Clark, 1982).

In general, drugs should be avoided during lactation. Medications are frequently prescribed for the nursing mother, with only marginal indications. If a maternal drug is necessary and there is a known hazard for the newborn, a more innocuous therapy can often be prescribed. Ultimately, the physician must consider every time a drug is recommended whether benefits to the mother outweigh dangers to the infant. Regrettably, problems arise inadvertently when mothers do not realize that they are pregnant. Also, although increasing numbers of elementary and high schools are instituting drug education programs, much more needs to be done to educate young people who are unaware of the devastating effects of drugs and alcohol.

BIBLIOGRAPHY

Aaronson, L.S., & MacNee, C.L. (1988). Tobacco, alcohol, and caffeine use during pregnancy. *JOGNN*, July/August, 279–287.

Abdul-Karim, R.W. (1981). *Drug usage during pregnancy*. Philadelphia: G.F. Stickley.

Abdul-Karim, R.W., & Clark, D.A. (1982). Drugs and pregnancy outcome. *Advances in Clinical Obstetrics and Gynecology, 1*, 75–94.

Adelman, R.D. (1978). Neonatal hypertension. *Pediatric Clinics of North America, 25*, 99–110.

Anderson, P.O. (1979). Drugs and breast-feeding. *Seminars in Perinatology, 3*, 271–276.

Aranda, J.V., Grandin, D., & Sasyniuk, B.I. (1981). Pharmacologic considerations in the therapy of neonatal apnea. *Pediatric Clinics of North America, 28*, 113–133.

Aranda, J.V., Hales, B.F., & Gibbs, J. (1983). Developmental pharmacology. In A.A. Faranoff & R.J. Martin (Eds.), *Neonatal-perinatal medicine: Disease of the fetus and infant* (3rd ed.) (pp. 150–173). St. Louis: C.V. Mosby.

Azuma, S.D., & Chasnoff, I.J. (1993). Outcome of children prenatally exposed to cocaine and other drugs: A path analysis of three-year data. *Pediatrics, 92*(3), 396–402.

Barbour, B.G. (1990). Alcohol and pregnancy. *Journal of Nurse-Midwifery, 35*(2), 78–85.

Barr, H.M., Darby, B.L., Streissguth, A.P., & Sampson, P.D. (1990). Prenatal exposure to alcohol, caffeine, tobacco, and aspirin: Effects on fine and gross motor performance in 4-year-old children. *Developmental Psychology, 26*(3), 339–348.

Bell, E.F., Brown, E.J., Milner, R., Sinclair, J.C., & Zipursky, A. (1979). Vitamin E absorption in small premature infants. *Pediatrics, 63*, 830–832.

Bresnahan, K., Brooks, C., & Zuckerman, B. (1991). Prenatal cocaine use: Impact on infants and mothers. *Pediatric Nursing, 17*(2), 123–128.

Cassady, G., Chasnoff, I.J., Clayton, E.W., Tan, S., Bandstra, E.S., Gerhardt, T., & Bancalari, E. (1991). Respiratory instability in neonates with in utero exposure to cocaine. *Journal of Pediatrics, 119*(1), 111–113.

Chasnoff, I.J. (1987). Perinatal effects of cocaine. *Contemporary Obstetrics and Gynecology, 29*, 163–179.

Chasnoff, I.J. (1988a). Cocaine: Effects on pregnancy and the neonate. In I.J. Chasnoff (Ed.), *Drugs, alcohol, pregnancy, and parenting* (pp. 97–104). Hingham, MA: Kluwer Academic.

Chasnoff, I.J. (1988b). Drug use in pregnancy: Parameters of risk. *Pediatric Clinics of North America, 35*(6), 1403–1411.

Chasnoff, I.J., Landress, H.J., & Barrett, M.E. (1990). The prevalence of illicit-drug or alcohol use during pregnancy and discrepancies in mandatory reporting in Pinellas County, Florida. *New England Journal of Medicine, 32*(17), 1202–1206.

Chen, C., Duara, S., Neto, G.S., Tan, S., Bandstra, E.S., Gerhardt, T., & Bancalari, E. (1991). Respiratory instability in neonates with in utero exposure to cocaine. *Journal of Pediatrics, 119*(1), 111–113.

Cohlan, S.Q. (1980). Drugs and pregnancy. In B.K. Young (Ed.), *Perinatal medicine today* (pp. 77–96). New York: Alan R. Liss.

Doering, P.L., & Steward, R.B. (1978). The extent and character of drug consumption during pregnancy. *JAMA, 239*, 843–846.

Duggan, A.K., Adger, H., Jr., McDonald, E.M., Stokes, E.J., & Moore, R. (1991). Detection of alcoholism in hospitalized children and their families. *American Journal of Diseases of Children, 145*, 613–617.

Durfee, M., & Tilton-Durfee, D. (1990). Prenatal substance abuse. *Children Today*, July/August, 3–7.

Eisen, L.N., Field, T.M., Bandstra, E.J., Roberts, J.P., Morrow, C., Larson, S.K., & Steele, B.M. (1991). Perinatal cocaine effects on neonatal stress behavior and performance on the Brazelton Scale. *Pediatrics, 88*(3), 477–480.

Fried, P.A., & Watkinson, B. (1990). 36- and 48-month neurobehavioral follow-up of children prematurely exposed to marijuana, cigarettes, and alcohol. *Developmental and Behavioral Pediatrics, 11*(2), 49–58.

Fried, P.A., Watkinson, B., Dillon, R.F., & Dulberg, C.S. (1987). Neonatal neurological status in a low-risk population after prenatal exposure to cigarettes, marijuana, and alcohol. *Developmental and Behavioral Pediatrics, 8*(6), 318–326.

Giacoia, G.P., & Catz, C.S. (1979). Drugs and pollutants in breast milk. *Clinics in Perinatology, 6*, 181–196.

Giesbrecht, N., Krempulec, L., & West, P. (1993). Community-based prevention research to reduce alcohol-related problems. *Alcohol Health and Research World, 17*(1), 84–88.

Gittler, J., & McPherson, M. (1990). Prenatal substance abuse. *Children Today*, July/August, 3–7.

Hansen, W.B. (1993). School-based alcohol prevention programs. *Alcohol Health and Research World*, *17*(1), 54–60.

Hill, R.M. (1979). *Perinatal pharmacology: Maternal drug ingestion and fetal effect* (pp. 1–18). Evansville, IN: Mead Johnson.

Hill, R.M., Craig, J.P., Chaney, M.D., Tennyson, L.M, & McCulley, L.B. (1977). Utilization of over-the-counter drugs during pregnancy. *Clinics in Obstetrics and Gynecology*, *20*, 381–393.

Howard, J., Beckwith, L., Rodning, C., & Kropenske, V. (1989). The development of young children of substance-abusing parents: Insights from seven years of intervention and research. *Zero to Three: Bulletin of the National Center for Clinical Infant Programs*, *IX*(5), 8–12.

Hoyme, H.E., Jones, K.L., Dixon, S.D., Jewett, T., Hansen, J.W., Robinson, L.K., Msall, M..E., & Allanson, J.E. (1990). Prenatal cocaine exposure and fetal vascular disruption. *Pediatrics*, *85*(5), 743–747.

Janke, J.R. (1990). Prenatal cocaine use: Effects on perinatal outcome. *Journal of Nurse-Midwifery*, *35*(2), 74–78.

Johnson, M.V., & Freeman, J.M. (1981). Pharmacological advances in seizure control. *Pediatric Clinics of North America*, *28*, 179–194.

Jones, K.L., & Smith, D.K. (1973). Recognition of the fetal alcohol syndrome in early infancy. *Lancet*, *2*, 999–1001.

Kauffman, R.E. (1981). The clinical interpretation and application of drug concentration data. *Pediatric Clinics of North America*, *28*, 35–45.

Keith, L.G., MacGregor, S.N., & Sciarra, J.J. (1988). Drug abuse in pregnancy. In I.J. Chasnoff (Ed.), *Drugs, alcohol, pregnancy, and parenting* (pp. 17–46). Hingham, MA: Kluwer Academic.

Kelley, S.J., Walsh, J.H., & Thompson, K. (1991). Birth outcomes, health problems, and neglect with prenatal exposure to cocaine. *Pediatric Nursing*, *17*(2), 130–136.

Klitzner, M., Stewart, K., & Fisher, D. (1993). Reducing underage drinking and its consequences. *Alcohol Health and Research World*, *17*(1), 12–18.

Korf, B.R. (1991). Congenital anomalies. In H.W. Taeusch, R.A. Clark, R.D. Ballard, & M.E. Avery (Eds.), *Schaffer and Avery's diseases of the newborn* (6th ed.) (pp. 159–191). Philadelphia: W.B. Saunders.

LeMoine, P., Harousseau, H., Borteyru, J.P., & Menuet, J.C. (1968). Les enfants de parents alcoholiques: Anomalies observees a propos de 127 cas. [Children of alcoholic parents: Anomalies observed in 127 cases]. *Ques. Med.*, *21*, 476–482.

Lester, B.M., Corwin, M.J., Septoski, C., Seifer, R., Peucker, M., McLaughlin, S., & Golub, H.L. (1991). Neurobehavioral syndromes in cocaine-exposed newborn infants. *Child Development*, *62*(4), 694–705.

Levy, M., Granit, L., & Laufer, N. (1977). Excretion of drugs in human milk. *New England Journal of Medicine*, *297*, 789.

Lynch, M., & McKeon, V.A. (1990). Cocaine use during pregnancy: Research findings and clinical implications. *JOGNN*, *19*(4), 130–136.

Marselli, P.L. (1976). Clinical pharmacokinetics in neonates. *Clinical Pharmacokinetics*, *1*, 81–86.

McCracken, G.H., & Nelson, J.D. (1977). *Antimicrobial therapy for newborns: Practical application of pharmacology to clinical usage*. New York: Grune & Stratton.

McIntosh, K. (1984). Bacterial infections of the newborn. In M.E. Avery & H.W. Taeusch (Eds.), *Diseases of the newborn* (5th ed.) (pp. 729–747). Philadelphia: W.B. Saunders.

Miller, G. (1989). Addicted infants and their mothers. *Zero to Three: Bulletin of the National Center for Clinical Infant Programs*, *IX*(5), 20–23.

Miller, G. (April 27, 1989). Born hooked: Confronting the impact of perinatal substance abuse. Unpublished opening statement to the Select Committee on Children, Youth, and Families, U.S. House of Representatives, Washington, DC.

Miller, W.H., Jr., & Hyatt, M.C. (1992). Perinatal substance abuse. *American Journal of Drug and Alcohol Abuse, 18*(3), 247–261.

National Association of Perinatal Addiction Research and Education (NAPARE) (1989). Innocent addicts: High rates of prenatal drug abuse found. *ADAMHA News,* October.

Nora, J.G. (1990). Perinatal cocaine use: Maternal, fetal, and neonatal effects. *Neonatal Network, 9*(2), 45–52.

O'Connor, M.J., Brill, N.J., & Sigman, M. (1986). Alcohol use in primiparous women older than 30 years of age: Relation to infant development. *Pediatrics, 78,* 444–450.

Peters, H., & Theorell, C.J. (1991). Fetal and neonatal effects of maternal cocaine use. *JOGNN, 20*(2), 121–126.

Phibbs, C.S., Bateman, D.A., & Schwartz, R.M. (1991). The neonatal costs of maternal cocaine use. *JAMA, 266*(11), 1521–1526.

Rice, D.P. (1993). The economic cost of alcohol abuse and alcohol dependence: 1990. *Alcohol Health and Research World, 17*(1), 10–11.

Roberts, R.J. (1984). Principles of neonatal pharmacology. In M.E. Avery & H.W. Taeusch (Eds.), *Diseases of the newborn* (5th ed.) (pp. 950–968). Philadelphia: W.B. Saunders.

Sander, L.W., Snyder, P.A., Rosett, H.L., Lee, A., Gould, J., & Ouellette, E. (1977). Effects of alcohol intake during pregnancy in newborn state regulation: A progress report. *Alcoholism: Clinical & Experimental Research, 1*(3), 233–241.

Sucheston, M.E., & Cannon, M.S. (Eds.). (1973). Thalidomide syndrome. *Congenital malformations* (pp. 233–239). Philadelphia: F.A. Davis.

Tittle, B., & St. Claire, N. (1989). Promoting the health and development of drug-exposed infants through a comprehensive clinic model. *Zero to Three: Bulletin of the National Center for Clinical Infant Programs, IX*(5), 18–20.

van Baar, A. (1990). Development of infants of drug dependent mothers. *Journal of Child Psychology and Psychiatry, 31*(6), 911–920.

Volpe, J.J. (1977). Neonatal seizures. *Clinics in Perinatology, 4,* 43–63.

Weiner, L., & Morse, B.A. (1988). FAS: Clinical perspectives and prevention. In I.J. Chasnoff (Ed.), *Drugs, alcohol, pregnancy, and parenting* (pp. 127–148). Hingham, MA: Kluwer Academic.

Weston, D.R., Ivins, B., Zuckerman, B., Jones, C., & Lopez, R. (1989). Drug-exposed babies: Research and clinical issues. *Zero to Three: Bulletin of the National Center for Clinical Infant Programs, IX*(5), 1–17.

Wettrell, G., & Andersson, K.E. (1977). Clinical pharmacokinetics of digoxin in infants. *Clinical Pharmacokinetics 2,* 17–25.

Yazigi, R.A., Odem, R.R., & Polakoski, K.L. (1991). Demonstration of specific binding of cocaine to human spermotozoa. *JAMA, 266*(14), 1956–1959.

Zuckerman, B. (1988). Marijuana and cigarette smoking during pregnancy. In I.J. Chasnoff (Ed.), *Drugs, alcohol, pregnancy, and parenting* (pp. 73–89). Hingham, MA: Kluwer Academic.

Zuckerman, B., Frank, D., Hingson, R., Amaro, H., Levenson, S.M., Kayne, H., Parker, S., Vinci, R., Abragye, K., Fried, L.E., et al. (1989). Effects of maternal marijuana and cocaine use on fetal growth. *New England Journal of Medicine, 320,* 762–768.

Chapter 14

Ethical Issues and the High Risk Infant

The practice of medicine requires that a physician acquire a vast sum of scientific knowledge and information that applies to the clinical and therapeutic decision-making process. Unfortunately, this is a flawed process since the scientific database is neither perfect nor complete, and "correct decisions" often are not obvious. Physicians and other health care professionals are guided by the first rule of practice, "primum non nocere": First of all, do no harm. Advances in the sciences and technology, promoting the complex world of intensive care nurseries, have led to the identification of key questions in areas such as prenatal evaluation, intrauterine intervention, withholding or withdrawing life support, donation of fetal or neonatal tissues for transplantation, and maternal versus fetal rights. The purpose of this chapter is to highlight some of the major ethical issues surrounding fetal and neonatal care.

HISTORICAL PERSPECTIVES

When a family turns to health care professionals—obstetricians, pediatricians, neonatologists, or nurses—the family members have certain expectations regarding nonscientific aspects of care. First and most obvious is the belief that the health care professional is acting on behalf of the best interests of the child. In recent years, this responsibility has been broadened in the intensive care nursery to the anticipation that the health care professional is acting in the best interests of both the child and the family. Sometimes inappropriately, this expectation presupposes that these professionals, as individuals and as team members, are capable of making unbiased, objective decisions without regard to the social or economic status of the family. The deliberations and care rendered are supposed to be confidential and are assumed to be based on societal concepts of moral and ethical standards. This situation raises many difficult questions with respect to the use of technology. In particular, it is easy to initiate, and charge for, the use of technological systems (e.g., for life support), but it is sometimes extremely difficult to withhold or withdraw such systems, even from neonates with obviously irreversible fatal illness, when individuals in the society often expect "everything be done."

BASIC PRINCIPLES

The ethics of decision making have been defined by four primary principles: autonomy, nonmalfeasance, beneficence, and justice (Beauchamp & Childress, 1983). All other ethical rules are derived from the principles of accountability, responsibility, truth, integrity, and confidentiality.

Autonomy is the ability of an individual to make decisions, free from the influence or constraints of others. The individual is at liberty to accept or reject plans of medical management. Although the fetus or neonate is incompetent to comprehend responsible choices and therefore cannot act independently, health care professionals must provide information adequate for the informed consent of the family members responsible for the child. There are four key elements of such informed consent on behalf of the newborn:

1. disclosure of accurate information
2. comprehension of the information by the individuals who will make a decision
3. voluntary acceptance of recommended therapy, without coercion
4. individual competence to make an independent decision.

In the case of a newborn, obviously only the first three apply, the fourth being reserved to the responsible parties.

In the intensive care nursery setting, decisions regarding care of the newborn are often made quickly. Informed consent is obtained from the family in a general way; the family is frequently informed after therapy has been initiated, and consent is obtained tacitly rather than actively.

According to the second basic principle, *nonmalfeasance,* it is the responsibility of the health care team not to inflict harm. The issue involved is the ongoing analysis of risk versus the benefit of any therapy administered to the patient. The likelihood of death or severe morbidity must be weighed against the potential benefits of intervention and the risk of the therapy, which is intended to neutralize or blunt the threat of a specific medical condition. For example, mechanical ventilation and the administration of oxygen to treat respiratory distress is clearly beneficial to maintaining adequate blood oxygen and proper function in the body, even though this procedure may result in complications such as pneumothorax, infection, or chronic lung disease.

Beneficence is the process of promoting good, while preventing or eliminating harm. This process requires a careful balance between acting on behalf of an individual who is unable to make an autonomous decision (the newborn) and making a decision that may have a result in conflict with another party's interest (Weil, 1989b). For example, although fetal surgery may be technically possible, is it in the best interest of the mother, who obviously also must undergo surgery? Beneficence requires consideration of the fact that withholding or withdrawing treatment actually may be in the best interest of the child. Is it appropriate to prolong the life (or death) of a 400-gram, extrauterine fetus at 24-week gestation who has suffered a severe intracranial hemorrhage and is neurologically nonresponsive?

The last of the four guiding principles is *justice*—giving what is due to the entitled individual. Even in the United States, resources have become more scarce and precious than generally is imagined by the populace. Is society (i.e., the tax-payer) willing to pay for care of the 1,000-gram premature infant, born to the 13-year-old inner-city mother with no resources, at the same level of technical expertise that is routinely available in facilities providing care to well-insured individuals in affluent suburban areas? On a daily basis in the United States, access to advanced technology is frequently being denied on the basis of the inability of the poor to pay.

Superimposed on these ethical principles are the complexities of the law. Laws differ from state to state. Malpractice judgments and court rulings, along with rules and regulations of state and federal health agencies, have greatly complicated the decision-making process. An ethical decision may not be legal and, conversely, a decision may be legally sound but morally bankrupt.

PRENATAL PROBLEMS

The incidence of multiple births has increased dramatically because of the aggressive therapy of families with problems of infertility. In vitro fertilization and gamete transfer commonly result in two or more fetuses. An excess number of fetuses stresses the mother physiologically. Moreover, most multiple gestations result in preterm infants, and greater prematurity is associated with the increased number of fetuses. Firstborn twins rarely are delivered beyond 36 weeks gestation and preterm triplets usually are delivered prior to 32 weeks gestation. In addition to the obvious morbidity and mortality associated with prematurity in its various conditions, the financial consequences of multiple long-term hospitalizations may be overwhelming. One solution currently promoted is the selective reduction (termination or abortion) of some of the fetuses by lethal cardiac injection (Selective fetal reduction, 1988). Usually, two fetuses are spared so that if anything should happen to one, a single baby might still be born alive.

These practices lead to some obvious possibilities. For instance, the sex of the fetus may be accurately determined via ultrasound or chromosome analysis, and selective reduction could allow the parents to abort a baby that is unwanted because of gender. Beyond such decision, families have been given other options such as the instance in which one twin with trisomy 13 has been selectively eliminated, leaving the normal twin to develop. Obviously, such circumstances present moral dilemmas and no simple solutions.

INTRAUTERINE THERAPY

Fetal therapy such as intrauterine blood transfusions for erythroblastosis fetalis—a condition with rapid destruction of red blood cells—has been accepted as standard, effective treatment for over 40 years (Fetal therapy, 1988). Another medical condition of the fetus amenable to intrauterine therapy is paroxysmal tachycardia, an abnormally rapid heart beat, which often responds to digitalis—a drug that can be given to the mother in sufficient doses to medicate the fetus in utero.

More recently, the accurate and early diagnosis of structural defects that may be amenable to therapy has been accomplished. For example, early in utero repair of diaphragmatic hernia may allow more appropriate fetal lung development. In babies with this defect, the lack of diaphragm motion, along with the movement of intestine into the chest, interferes with lung development.

Although there has been much publicity and a great deal of enthusiasm about intrauterine therapy, few fetal defects are amenable to prenatal surgery. The benefits and risks to both the fetus and the mother must be considered. Among others, risks to the mother include the threat of premature labor, infection, hemorrhage, and the experimental nature of the proposed intervention.

Obviously, fetal therapy must involve some risk to the mother. The diagnosis of in utero conditions is not foolproof, even in the hands of an experienced perinatologist and ultrasonographer, and all therapies that might benefit the fetus also have risk to both the fetus and the mother. Do society and the health care team have the right to over-ride the mother's autonomy in order to improve the outcome for the fetus? This question extends far beyond the issue of surgical correction of a fetal anomaly; it also applies to the treatment of other health problems in the mother that may adversely affect the fetus. Can society compel the mother with syphilis to use antibiotics? Can a mother's self-destructive behavior (e.g., alcoholism, cocaine abuse, or cigarette smoking) be curtailed forcefully? Even more troublesome is the issue of voluntary versus mandatory therapy. The mother has the right to refuse experimental treatment for her fetus, even if it might be extremely beneficial. She also can refuse standard treatment for herself. Does society have the right to insist on testing and treatment, and is it willing to pay for such intervention in order to detect a few abnormal pregnancies?

WITHHOLDING AND WITHDRAWING LIFE SUPPORT

Most ethicists would agree that there is no significant difference, morally, between not initiating use of life support systems and withdrawing them (President's Commission for the Study of Ethical Problems in Medicine and Biomedical and

Behavioral Research, 1983). Depending on the jurisdiction, however, there may be significant distinctions legally. Failure to initiate a form of therapy may be considered neglect, but aggressive withdrawal of a therapy may be interpreted severely as second degree murder.

Considerations

In this arena, the choices are not simple, the relationships are complex, and the problems are numerous. There are four major considerations: dependency of the patient, uncertainty of therapeutic outcome, risks of treatment, and expense.

Dependency of the Patient. The decision regarding the appropriateness of care must be made by parties other than the newborn—families and health care professionals. On the side of the family, the decision is extremely emotional, with superimposed guilt, fear, and anger. Everyone involved wants the best possible outcome, but guarantees cannot be given. Adding to the difficulty of the decision-making process are the myriad moral, ethical, religious, and other individual beliefs of all the concerned parties, including the health care professionals (Harrison, 1986).

Uncertainty of Therapeutic Outcome. The severity of the disease process rarely can be estimated with accuracy (Rhoden, 1986). Even with Down syndrome (trisomy 21), there is considerable variability of congenital defects and a wide latitude of eventual mental capacity. Many treatments have become standard therapy before they were adequately studied. Furthermore, the true benefits cannot be ascertained because controlled, randomized, prospective studies cannot be performed. Such uncertainty regarding therapeutic outcome is compounded by the unique, individual responses of patients; for example, not all preterm infants who have surfactant deficiency will respond to surfactant-replacement therapy. In addition, rapid advances in technology may provide several treatment options, and the benefits of therapy may depend substantially on the training, skill, and experience of the practitioners.

Risks of Treatment. Most treatments administered to critically ill neonates have risks as well as benefits. For instance, antibiotics, which are crucial for ameliorating an infection, may cause renal insufficiency or hearing damage.

Expense. Care of the critically ill neonate remains very expensive. The high cost of technology and prolonged hospitalizations often is underestimated by public and private insurance programs (Weil, 1989a). There seems to be great willingness to fund the triple bypass cardiac surgery of a 70-year-old man, but a reluctance to care for the 1,000-gram premature infant, even though the chance of good *long-term* outcome is far better in the preterm infant. Moreover, the cost amortized over the remainder of life expectancy also favors the premature baby. Nevertheless, few of the nursery survivors are irreversibly disabled, physically and developmentally, and need resources and services that frequently are available only in larger metropolitan areas.

Consensus

Taking all of these concerns into account, the current consensus is that treatment is not mandatory but can be denied or withdrawn in the following situations:

1. The child is dying and treatment will not significantly prolong life.
2. The infant is totally unresponsive to environmental stimuli and is likely to remain so permanently even with treatment.
3. The treatment is highly unlikely to be beneficial and will be excessively burdensome to the family and child.

In conclusion, withholding treatment frequently is not discussed with the family, whereas withdrawing a treatment almost always is discussed. Prolonging death has a profound emotional and economic impact on the family, in addition to the burden of suffering for the baby. However, the fear of the complexities of withdrawing therapy may result in failure to initiate therapy in some extremely low birthweight infants who might benefit.

ANENCEPHALIC AND FETAL TRANSPLANT DONATIONS

Anencephaly is a severe form of the neural tube defects in which the fetus never has developed functional cortical tissue. The only recognizable portion of the brain is the brainstem, which for a time after birth can support heartbeat and respiratory effort. The incidence is approximately three anencephalic fetuses for every 10,000 pregnancies. Over 95 percent of anencephalic fetuses are aborted, once discovered. Approximately two-thirds of the remainder are stillborn, and many are premature or low birthweight. If all of these factors are taken into account, only approximately 70 to 80 anencephalic babies per year would be available for organ donation, following parental consent. The three major organs for transplantation would be kidneys, hearts, and livers. There are sufficient numbers of babies with anencephaly to provide for nearly all of the 7 to 10 infants needing livers and the 12 to 15 babies needing hearts per year. Approximately 25 to 30 kidneys per year are needed by infants, but there is an extremely poor success rate of kidney transplants from anencephalic donors.

Beyond the technical aspects of transplantation of these potentially available organs lie a series of difficult philosophical, legal, and moral decisions with respect to salvaging organs from infants with anencephaly (Davis, 1988). The philosophical issues center on three questions (Botkin, 1988): (1) Do these babies truly have life as we understand it? (2) What is a person? (3) Who decides whether or not these organs should be made available—individuals, parents, the electorate, or other subsections of society? Legally, the Uniform Determination of Death Act does not apply to these infants. Although severely impaired, these babies are human and alive and, therefore, need protection under our legal concepts of personhood (Harrison, 1986).

Even more complex ethical issues arise in the area of fetal tissue donations (Council on Scientific Affairs and Council on Ethical and Judicial Affairs, 1990). There are numerous medical conditions with potential for benefit from transplantations of fetal tissue, which often is well tolerated and may grow in the recipient. Hematologic and immune deficiencies may benefit from fetal bone marrow transplants. Diabetes mellitus may be ameliorated by transplantation of fetal pancreatic tissue. Other genetic and metabolic diseases, including Parkinson's disease, might be treated with fetal tissue that could replace a missing neurotransmitter or provide enzymes for a metabolic pathway that previously was blocked (Fetal therapy, 1988).

There are, however, obvious ethical concerns. The primary concern is the possible motivation of a woman to maintain a pregnancy until there is sufficient fetal tissue to donate, perhaps for profit. Another concern is the possible participation of physicians and researchers in an ever-aggressive attempt to gain funding and fame, which could result in commercialization of the termination of pregnancies. Individuals at all levels of the government have waffled on taking a position regarding such ethical concerns. The Clinton administration, however, appears to be reopening these issues with little constraint.

It is clear that neither aborted fetuses nor anencephalic babies clearly qualify for the category of the brain-dead tissue donors. For organs and tissues to be donated, there must be absence of brain function as a result of an irreversible condition with an identified cause; the patient must be comatose and apneic. In addition, there must be absence of brainstem function, which can be documented by a sophisticated examination of the eyes, eye movements, and various cranial nerve reflexes. The patient cannot be hypotensive or hypothermic and must have no spontaneous or induced muscle movement. The observation period must be at least 7 days and include two formal examinations and at least two electroencephalograms, separated by at least 48 hours showing no activity. A supplemental test, cerebral angiography, should demonstrate no evidence of blood flow to the brain.

The majority of babies who might be considered brain dead according to these criteria have suffered severe perinatal asphyxia and damage to the organs of greatest importance to the transplant physician. Most neonates who die are premature infants who have been treated for several days and die of severe acidosis and hypotension. The small size of the organs and organ tissue necrosis and destruction, frequently with associated infection, preclude their usefulness for transplantation.

MATERNAL VERSUS FETAL RIGHTS

The development of high technology for fetal diagnosis and treatment has led to a conflict between the interests of the mother and those of the fetus or newborn (Strong, 1987). In the majority of pregnancies, the babies are wanted, and most mothers will agree to treatment that will benefit the unborn child without exposing themselves to unreasonable harm.

The substance for conflicts between maternal and fetal rights and the resolutions of these conflicts depend on the relationship and understanding of the mother in cooperation with her health care practitioner. In some situations, the maternal health is the most important consideration and fetal welfare is secondary. Under other circumstances, the fetus is considered a child and the mother is an obligate support system for its development. Under the best circumstances, the mother and practitioner together commit to the best possible outcome, a healthy full-term baby, but not survival without regard to outcome. Several points must be considered in resolving conflicts between maternal and fetal rights (Southwell & Archer-Duste, 1993):

1. reliability of predicting fetal harm relative to the magnitude of benefit to the fetus
2. advocacy for fetal therapy
3. personhood status of the fetus
4. encroachment on maternal autonomy
5. consequences of coerced maternal consent to fetal therapy.

In summary, ethical decisions in medical practice were far easier in the era of simple technology. As the issues and technology become increasingly complex, the health care practitioner must anticipate ethical issues and actively intervene for the best possible outcome for the family. Prolongation of therapy for profit, misadventures in research for fame and funding, and disregard of the needs of the family cannot be tolerated. The cutting edge of science and technology must be integrated with the soft touch of philosophy and the humanities to keep the environment of the neonatal intensive care unit sane and functional.

BIBLIOGRAPHY

Beauchamp, T.L., & Childress, J.B. (1983). *Principles of biomedical ethics.* New York: Oxford University Press.

Botkin, J.R. (1988). Anencephalic infants as organ donors. *Pediatrics, 82,* 250–256.

Council on Scientific Affairs and Council on Ethical and Judicial Affairs (1990). Medical applications of fetal tissue transplantation. *JAMA, 263,* 565–570.

Davis, A. (1988). The status of anencephalic babies: Should their bodies be used as donor banks? *Journal of Medical Ethics, 14,* 150–153.

Fetal therapy: Ethical considerations (1988). *Pediatrics, 81,* 898–899.

Harrison, H. (1986). Neonatal intensive care: Parent's role in ethical decision making. *Birth, 13,* 165–175.

President's Commission for the Study of Ethical Problems in Medicine and Biomedical and Behavioral Research (1983). *Securing access to health care.* Washington, DC: U.S. Government Printing Office.

Rhoden, N.K. (1986). Treating Baby Doe: The ethics of uncertainty. *Hastings Center Report, 16*(4), 34–42.

Selective fetal reduction. (1988). *Lancet , 2*, 773–775.

Southwell, S.M., & Archer-Duste, H. (1993). Ethical aspects of perinatal care. In C. Kenner, A. Brueggemeyer, & L.P. Gunderson (Eds.), *Comprehensive neonatal nursing* (pp. 14–35). Philadelphia: W.B. Saunders.

Strong, C. (1987). Ethical conflicts between mother and fetus in obstetrics. *Clinics in Perinatology, 14*, 313–328.

Weil, W.B., Jr. (1989a). Allocation of resources. *Current Problems in Pediatrics, 19*(12), 637–639.

Weil, W.B., Jr. (1989b). Conflict of interest. *Current Problems in Pediatrics, 19*(12), 655–659.

Chapter 15

Assessing Infants and Preschool Children within a Family Context

The advent and implementation of Public Law (PL) 99–457 have ushered in a new decade of long-term and far-reaching changes for the theory and practice of early childhood assessment. Historically, the evaluation of infants and preschool children has been an ill-defined process, often wanting in application to educational intervention. Identifying risk, describing behavior, and estimating the prognosis for future development are integral steps in the assessment of young children, leading to the culmination of programatic plans and implementation. Often, these primary goals have been far from adequately addressed, particularly within the context of family values and priorities. Some difficulties have evolved by nature of the populations served; some have been the result of imprecise techniques of evaluation; still others have surfaced as a result of misguided interpretations. Though parents and professionals have searched long for accurate indicators of competence and developmental delay in infants, untimely and/or inappropriate predictions sometimes have caused both children and families more harm than benefit. Given the inevitable limitations of assessment, sensitive and carefully applied evaluations with new initiatives in the field now offer the potential for resolving many of the troubling dilemmas of the past.

Strategies and techniques for screening and diagnosis in the years ahead will reflect marked departures from known and accepted convention. Increasingly, professionals are becoming more clinically astute, more eclectic, and less comfortable with plan-for-plan measures. Time, follow-up, direct parent participation, and a range of natural settings are becoming routine in the course of evaluation, and the use of multiple criteria with a spectrum of behavioral and developmental measures is becoming common practice rather than the exception. Finally, professionals are learning that the real task of screening and assessment lies in the disclosure of competence (of both parents and children) rather than deficiency and that this goal is carried out most wisely with a realistic and unavoidable, but healthy, uncertainty. This chapter focuses on recent trends and growth in these directions.

SCREENING, DIAGNOSIS, AND ISSUES OF PREDICTION

Identifying Risk

It is well documented that conditions of risk and impairment leading to later developmental delay are difficult to identify, track, and assess in infancy and the preschool years (Aylward, 1988; Gordon & Jens, 1988; Keogh & Koff, 1978; Kopp & Parmelee, 1979; Teti & Gibbs, 1990). With the passage of PL 99–457, states have been given the challenge and incentive to provide services for the very youngest populations, from birth to 2 years of age. This mandate includes children who had clearly defined problems at the time of delivery, as well as infants considered to be at risk for later developmental delay.

There are ever-increasing numbers of newborns exposed prenatally to the products of maternal substance abuse and neonates delivered at the edge of viability at 24 to 25 weeks gestation. The complexities of sorting out and offering helpful and accurate information to parents early in the survival and later, during the development of these infants, is a difficult task for health care and education specialists alike. For example, it is not unusual to find that newborns with substantial medical insult, given the advantage of caring home environments, will later reflect those benefits in the evidence of far fewer problems than were initially predicted. By the same token, it is a familiar scenario that infants with mild symptoms of distress after birth nonetheless manifest unexpected delays at 12, 18, or 24 months of age, as observed in follow-up clinics. Indeed, researchers continue to hold to the view, reinforced by a substantial base of data, that parent education is one of the most accurate indicators of developmental outcome for both typical and high risk neonatal populations (Gordon & Jens, 1988). At the same time, such findings, when applied to groups, often break down with closer examination of the qualitative differences among families and their offspring. Thus, for all children, without exception, educational ability is a function of continuous and cumulative vulnerabilities and advantages that interact either to depress or enhance intellectual abilities. Aylward (1988) has stated the issue as follows: ". . . findings support the transactional model, as well as the risk route approach to follow-up, which underscores the dynamic, interactive and cumulative effects of medical/biologic, environmental/psychosocial, and behavioral/developmental influences on outcome" (p. 307).

One of the most thorny and elusive problems confronting professionals responsible for screening and assessment of infants and preschoolers at risk is the duration and type of follow-up necessary to determine outcome. Several problems contribute to this difficulty, and researchers and clinicians continue to struggle with issues that appear to lead either to overestimation or underestimation of long-term outcome. Clearly, short-range concerns are much more easily and accurately identified. Parents, however, ultimately always want to know the full range of implications of early delivery and/or medical complications for their child in the

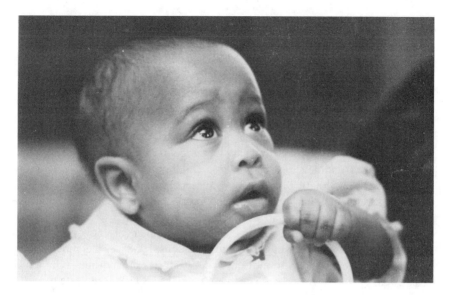

Figure 15–1 Serena, born at 27 weeks gestation, holds rattle at 8 months

future. Several questions are common in discussions with families. When will I know that my baby is all right? What does an early delivery mean? Will the hospital stay hurt my baby emotionally? What are some of the early signs of learning disabilities?

Years of follow-up in perinatal clinics have enabled us to respond to some, though not all, of these concerns. Most researchers today recommend follow-up for at least 3 years for children who meet specified criteria that in the past have been associated with less positive outcome; e.g., birthweight less than 1,500 grams and/or delivery at 24 to 30 weeks gestation; the presence of severe respiratory conditions requiring extended mechanical ventilation; evidence of intraventricular hemorrhage (grade 3 or 4); evidence of maternal substance abuse; or other conditions predisposing the child to neurological insult prior to or during delivery and the perinatal period. Typically, revisits are scheduled two to three times during the first 12 to 18 months of life and at least once or as needed during the 2nd and 3rd years.

In cases of early delivery, preterm infants are usually evaluated according to their adjusted age, with correction for the number of weeks of prematurity. This adjustment factor is, in no way, an accurate indicator in terms of degree or type of developmental delay. The concept is most helpful during the first 12 to 18 months but is less relevant as children enter their 2nd and 3rd toddler years, when the influences of environment and experience play a more significant role. In addition, the yardstick of corrected age may be problematic at either end of the continuum of prematurity. Throughout their 1st and 2nd years of life, infants delivered at 24 to 30 weeks gestation often present with developmental delays well beyond expectations, based solely on correction of age for prematurity. Similarly, an increasing number of newborns (especially boys) delivered at 35 to 36 weeks, who may have had acute respiratory distress and received mechanical ventilation are surfacing as developmentally delayed when they enter kindergarten programs, with attentional disorders, auditory processing disabilities, or other subtle behavioral problems. According to criteria applied in past years, such newborns were predicted to be relatively free from later learning difficulties. Professionals tracking the learning and development of these children frequently have referred to such transient, fluctuating, or changing determinations as "sleeper" effects, whereby development may appear to be appropriate at one age, only to be identified at a later stage as having areas of delay.

Due to the surfacing of such latent effects, researchers are now calling for a "dynamic conceptualization of risk" (Gordon & Jens, 1988)—a theoretical model that allows for "individuals to move out of or into risk at any time" (Gordon & Jens, 1988, p. 281). More specifically, Gordon and Jens (1988) indicate that:

> The Moving Risk Model . . . provides for assessment of the risk status of individual children at several times during the period of early development, and assesses risk in several areas at each time. In addition, the Moving Risk Model considers measures of risk status as both dependent (status resulting from prior events) and independent (the basis for future events) variables. As such, each time of assessment may be considered a measure of current outcome as well as a measure of future risk. (pp. 281–282)

Carefully established criteria and prudent decisions are critical to the feasibility, benefit, and success of any risk model or screening program. In high risk populations, the main goal is identification of infants and families in greatest need and jeopardy. Consequently, the concept of *levels of risk or vulnerability* is useful. Consistent with the Moving Risk Model, infants may progress up the ladder of service, receiving more frequent and comprehensive evaluations and intervention programming as necessary and appropriate to their needs and those of their families. Likewise, they move down the cascade of services, having had their early, most intense needs met, their primary disabilities addressed in normalizing educational programs, and secondary disabling conditions prevented altogether. Full development of this concept and cautious implementation on a widespread basis could resolve many problems of screening, identification, and diagnosis that continue to thwart efforts of early intervention. In addition, such a plan is entirely consistent with the charge and imperatives of PL 99–457 and PL 102–119, which mandate delivery of services to groups of high risk children from birth to 2 years of age.

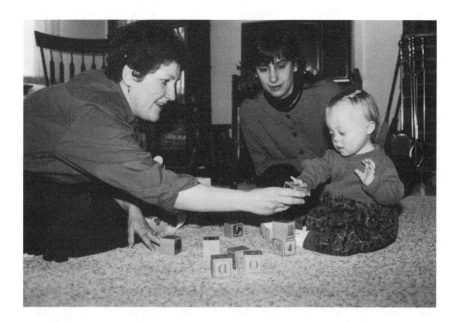

Figure 15–2 Assessment of an infant in a home-based setting with mother and teacher working together

At best, the task of identifying accurately those newborns who may later develop school-related problems is a formidable one. To the present time, developmental screening techniques for newborns and infants have yielded *general estimations* of current functioning and have largely fallen short of the goal of predicting greatest impairment or future potential.

Many children leaving intensive care nurseries have eluded identification but have later manifested moderate to severe disabilities. These findings, consistently supported in follow-up clinics, also point to the fact that any valid risk indices appropriate to the newborn period and shortly thereafter must encompass both biomedical criteria relative to the child and environmental conditions surrounding the family and community. In terms of the magnitude of impact, it is obvious that certain factors are more important at particular stages than others and that the relative influence of these factors changes over time. For example, closer to the newborn period, initial medical factors, not surprisingly, have a more substantial bearing on performance. Later into the toddler and preschool years, the interplay with environment becomes a more dominant variable. In addition to the continuing maturation of the neurological system throughout the early months following delivery, this shift in significant influences is one of the major explanations for the variable patterns observed in the development of all young children in their earliest years. These variable patterns are especially apparent in preterm populations.

In part, this shifting continuum of "caretaking casuality" also accounts for the familiar observation that premature children may appear to "catch up" and close the gap in motor development, while, at the same time, revealing new discrepancies of language and social-emotional delays.

As we noted earlier, there is no substitute for astute clinical acumen. Carefully drawn criteria within a flexible conceptual model are essential, but applied without attention to individual child and family characteristics, they may prove to be of little benefit. In short, whatever the differentiated criteria, there are few absolutes in terms of the presence, absence, or extent of disability. Some children, because of the nature of their medical course and home environment, need to be observed more often with hands-on evaluations. Others do not require such frequent follow-up. The final decision-making model needs to take into consideration all of these issues and possibilities if it is ultimately to serve a useful purpose within the context of divergent and changing populations.

Implications of PL 99–457 and PL 102–119 for Assessment

Now and in the future, the implementation of PL 99–457, in particular Part H, has changed and will continue to change many conventional practices in the assessment of young children (Barnett, Macmann, & Carey, 1992; Neisworth & Bagnato, 1992). The institution of the Individual Family Service Plan (IFSP) alone has introduced sweeping modifications in the ways in which early childhood special education programs conduct business. No longer are children the sole targets of the assessment process; families are at the heart of this new legislation in terms of their priorities, needs, and expressed desires. No longer will assessment take place out of context and unconnected to intervention programing goals and implementation (Bailey & Wolery, 1992). Moreover, Part H of the new legislation has introduced a clear distinction between the terms *evaluation* and *assessment* (Campbell, 1991). This differentiation lays out the continuum of screening and diagnostic contact that must infuse every process of interaction between professionals, child, and family. In particular, the parameters are spelled out as follows:

> *Evaluation* means the procedures used to determine a child's initial and continuing eligibility for services and to describe performance in a variety of developmental areas. *Assessment* means the use of ongoing procedures throughout the period during which services are provided to identify a child's unique needs, the family's strengths and needs in relation to enhancing the child's development, and the nature and extent of early intervention services needed by the child and family. (Campbell, 1991, p. 36)

Meisels (1991) has delineated further the various dimensions of *assessment*. At the initial stages, developmental and health screening is essential in identifying individual children who are at high risk for later developmental problems. Typically, such infants and preschoolers have been recognized on the basis of three factors:

1. conditions at birth that, in the past, have been associated with developmental delay (e.g., Down syndrome)
2. a history of family risk factors that historically have been linked to less advantageous outcome (e.g., substance abuse)
3. a significant medical history surrounding the prenatal and/or perinatal period (e.g., prolonged period of mechanical ventilation).

Such children are often scheduled for follow-up at the time of discharge from a Level One newborn nursery if they have been hospitalized or at the time of discharge from a Level One newborn nursery if they have been identified as being at risk.

In other cases, these children may receive periodic follow-up by public health nurses assigned prior to or at the time of hospital discharge. One of the most widely used standardized instruments at this initial stage of identification is the *Denver Developmental Screening Test (DDST)* (Frankenburg, Dodds, Fandal, Kazuk, & Cohrs, 1975), revised in 1989 as the *Denver II.* The first edition of this instrument, like other screening measures, has been severely criticized because of a lack of sensitivity (Bailey & Wolery, 1989; Ensher & Clark, 1986) in either over-referring or under-referring children within major risk populations.

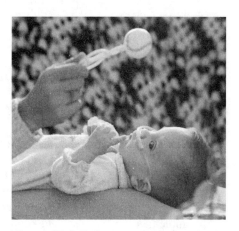

Figure 15–3 Follow-up assessment in the home with a 7-month infant on oxygen

Given the constraints of available resources, screening programs vary in their individual components in terms of personnel and setting. To ensure best practice, models should include certain fundamental qualities, as outlined by Bailey and Wolery (1989). These characteristics include use of:

> . . . (a) reliable tests and reliable administration, scoring, and interpretation; (b) measures that have concurrent validity with current development or can predict later outcomes; (c) economical procedures; (d) tests and procedures that can be administered quickly and easily; (e) measures that are comprehensive and appropriate to the population; (f) measures and procedures that are acceptable to the population; (g) procedures that can be used repeatedly; (h) screening procedures to provide

parents with training and information; and (i) regular program evaluation. (p. 130)

Assessment should be a natural extension of the screening and eligibility phase. Again, though the specific interpretation and translation into practice inevitably will vary from county to county and state to state, Section 677 of the regulations describing the components of the IFSP are specific relative to particular requirements. As detailed by McGonigel, Kaufmann, and Johnson (1991), a written plan must include the following components:

- A statement of the child's present level of physical development (including vision, hearing, and health status), cognitive development, language and speech development, psychosocial development, and self-help skills, based on acceptable objective criteria
- A statement of the family's strengths and needs relating to enhancing the development of the family's handicapped infant
- A statement of the major outcomes expected to be achieved for the child and family; the criteria, procedures, and timelines used to determine the degree to which progress toward achieving the outcomes is being made and whether or not revisions of the outcomes or services are necessary
- A statement of specific early intervention services necessary to meet the unique needs of the child and family, including the frequency, intensity, and method of delivering services
- The projected dates for initiation of services and the anticipated duration of the services
- The name of the case manager (from the profession most immediately relevant to the child's or family's needs) who will be responsible for implementing the plan and coordinating with other agencies and persons
- The steps to be taken supporting the child's transition to Part B preschool services, if appropriate. (p. 47)

At first glance, these requirements appear to be specific and clearly defined. In reality, however, they raise many issues relative to implementation, including concerns about cultural diversity, intrusiveness, the nature of assessment of the family, and the processes for establishing family outcomes (Beckman & Bristol, 1991; Lynch & Hanson, 1992). For example, although preschool programs throughout the United States often include a significant number of families of varying ethnic, cultural, and economic backgrounds, the values and goals often projected in programs are most reflective of middle class, upper income, cohesive, America-speaking parents (Lynch & Hanson, 1992). Failure to recognize such differences and the specific impact of diversity that may even slightly affect every step of the service delivery process from screening to assessment and planning to program implementation will lead to erroneous conclusions (Beckman & Bristol,

1991) and likely will jeopardize meaningful access to and work with many families.

Equally important and serious is the question of how the needs of families are to be determined or "assessed." The ecological concept of offering services to young children within the context of their communities and family units is one that few scholars or researchers would disagree with, in principle. Without special precautions, however, the risk of intrusion is exceedingly high. Put in another way, the thought of "assessing families" in the traditional-historical sense

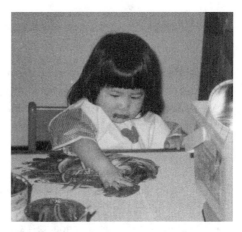

Figure 15–4 Ana painting, a wonderful task for informal, play-based assessment

runs counter to the primary intent of PL 99–457 to create a network that is supportive and conducive to healthy family functioning. Thus, within the genuine spirit of this new legislation, both the process and content of screening and assessment endeavors will need to change. For example, questions asked of caregivers will need to focus directly on issues relevant primarily to developmental outcome for the child. In addition, observations of family-child interactions will need to be centered on ways in which to enhance the inclusion and behavior of young children in their respective homes, rather than on value judgments of particular lifestyles that represent departures from conventional living patterns. Moreover, if "being family-focused in the assessment process" is genuinely recognized in the decade ahead, professionals will be required, at a minimum, to build into the sequence of service delivery a degree of flexibility that has not been evidenced to date in the evaluation process. This flexibility will have to be reflected in the settings for assessment, the persons involved, and the time apportioned for delivery of services.

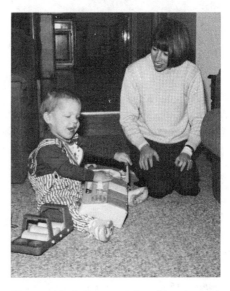

Figure 15–5 Home visit with physical therapist, a member of the initial and continuing assessment-intervention team

Stages of Assessment

PL 99–457 and PL 102–119 inevitably will impact on the processes or stages of evaluation, as well as on the content or substance of what professionals do. While situations will and should vary from child to child and from family to family, certain guidelines ought to be adopted as part of best practice in working with young populations. At a minimum, these guidelines should include the following components for gathering information:

- statement of reason for referral
- record of family and child history
- establishment of screening and assessment goals and parameters
- observation and work with child
- development of recommendations and implementation plan
- maintenance of ongoing evaluation plan.

Statement of Reason for Referral. The statement of the reason for referral is the first step in the assessment process and should document clearly the concerns and questions being raised. Although issues may exist relative to the family, the focus should be centered directly on the child, within the context of the home, community, and school environments, as appropriate. In addition, though multiple dimensions may surface during the course of the evaluation, the referral statement is especially important in setting the initial parameters of the screening and diagnostic process.

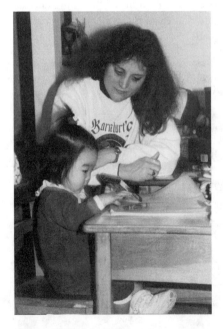

Figure 15–6 Merrick drawing, as Mom watches. Direct involvement of caregivers is a new and crucial part of family-centered assessment.

Record of Family and Child History. Prior to implementation of the new early childhood legislation, the process of recording the family and child history was often one of the most intrusive components of the evaluation. Frequently, parents or caregivers have been asked personal questions about their family lives and those of their children that were completely unrelated to the issues and questions at hand, with little or no recourse but to respond. With the family-focused orientation of PL 99–457, such practice will change.

From the caregiver's perspective, the information given needs to be complete and related to the reason for referral, as well as preparatory for the assessment to follow. Important areas to be covered are information about the child's development and behavior, family priorities for the evaluation, child functioning within the family unit, medical information that includes identified conditions of the child, and basic information surrounding prenatal care and delivery. The psychoeducational team involved in the assessment also should take care to retrieve and document any prior records or evaluations, medical or developmental. Also it is essential to obtain the caregiver's or parent's view of the child's current level and quality of learning and functioning, gains that have and have not been made, and areas of greatest need. In securing such information, the team should be able to keep to a minimum the serious differences between parent and professional goals that are often observed and that may cause discord, which is difficult to resolve during the later process of evaluation. Finally, at the close of the assessment, the team needs to ask the caregiver whether behavior observed during the screening and diagnostic sessions represented typical patterns for the child.

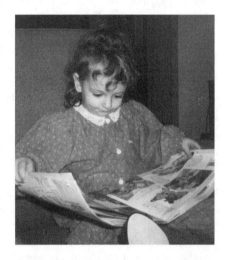

Figure 15–7 Allison at 2½ years, enjoying a book. Observations of toddlers with such material offer teams valuable insight about language, cognitive, and perceptual development.

Establishment of Goals and Parameters of Screening and Assessment. Based on information obtained from the reason for referral and child-family history, the team should be prepared to establish the goals and parameters of the screening-assessment process. Major questions to be answered should be raised, and these should serve as the primary guide to selection of methods and measures used during the evaluation.

Observation and Work with Child. Depending on the complexity of a given child's learning and behavioral patterns, the time devoted to observation and work with the child may range from two to three or more sessions with the psychoeducational team. *Never* should this phase be based on one opportunity alone for observing and working with the child. Instead, this stage should be broadly representative of the places where and significant people with whom the infant, toddler, or preschooler spends the majority of his or her time. Both formal and informal, standardized and nonstandardized, measures are appropriate for use in gathering data. The critical criterion for using certain instruments and strategies is their relationship and relevance to the goals of the evaluation.

Again, the most helpful approach is the identification of typical patterns within the family context, where the infant's or young child's development and learning are primarily grounded during the first months and years of life. With the passage and implementation of PL 99–457, professionals have been offered a much needed flexibility in measurement, as long as the tests and strategies utilized are effective in documenting the need for intervention services. As we have noted, the professionals involved should build special precautions into this stage of the assessment to ensure that caregivers or parents—in isolation from the child—do not become the target of the evaluation, with all of the surrounding judgments that may accompany such practices. Diversity needs to be welcomed and respected across varying lifestyles and cultures, which should be appreciated and understood for their fundamental contributions and value to the child.

At the conclusion of the observation and diagnostic phase, which also may include preliminary screening, the team should be prepared to describe a comprehensive, holistic picture of the child within his or her family, community, and school environments, detailing strengths as well as areas of need. This report subsequently becomes the foundation for developing an initial set of recommendations and the implementation plan.

Development of Recommendations and Implementation Plan. The fifth and next to final stage in the assessment process needs to embrace both home and community/school environment and needs to establish the critical goals that will be followed in the plan for implementation. In addition, it comprises another entry point where caregiver/parent input is essential. Historically, the writing of educational recommendations for the child has been a task assumed entirely by the team responsible for evaluation. The mandate and primary intent of PL 99–457 adds another important step to this process. In particular, prior to the finalizing of any recommendations and plans for implementation, the child's caregiver needs to be involved directly in the basic formulation of goals in order to assure a coherent and meaningful transition to delivery of services.

Maintenance of an Ongoing Evaluation Process. Once a child and family are receiving services, the final stage of maintaining an ongoing process for feedback and evaluation needs to be set in place. This mechanism subsequently provides an essential means for dialogue and exchange between family and professionals for the duration of programming and intervention and empowers caregivers to question, discuss, and bring about change in the implementation of services.

APPLICATIONS

Standard Approaches

In recent years, much research on infant and preschool assessment has concentrated on more natural approaches, whereas developmental evaluation in pediatrics and education has continued to rely heavily on standardized, traditional practices. Frequently, the screening and assessment of young children have been based

on brief visits, with parent and child in strange situations, with unfamiliar professionals, under sometimes strained and difficult circumstances. The net result has
been a less than optimal response from caregiver and child. Moreover, formal
assessment has historically almost always involved standardized instruments,
sometimes informal measures, and rarely, systematic data-based observations.
Ideally, best practice in evaluation combines all three techniques, and this strategy
is now receiving greater recognition in the various fields of developmental and
child psychology, as well as in the clinical-educational disciplines.

It is important to identify and describe a child's characteristics in relation to
those of other infants and young populations that are determined on the basis of
normative measures. Yet, developmental screening and assessment have routinely
fallen short of including the substantial basic information that is most closely related to the planning and implementation process; e.g., the quality of responses.
Reinforcing this point, researchers in human development, the social sciences, and
special education over the past decade have endorsed the need for more dynamic
and process-oriented approaches toward understanding families and their infants
and young children (Berkeley & Ludlow, 1992; Neisworth & Bagnato, 1992).
Such an approach is essential in situations of social and cultural diversity that have
continued to escape definition in large groups of children across the United States.
In addition, genuine concern about the inappropriateness of conventional tests
widely used with developmentally delayed and high risk infants and preschoolers
(Barnett, Macmann, & Carey, 1992; Neisworth & Bagnato, 1992) should not be
dismissed lightly. This position is reflected in contemporary efforts to create new
measures of infant and preschool development in such areas as play, cognition,
temperament, the organization of behavior, and speech and language abilities
(Ensher et al., 1994; Wetherby & Prizant, 1993).

It has long been a familiar theme in early childhood special education that problems of test interpretation arise, not from the nature of standardized or norm-referenced instruments, but from the ways in which these measures have been used.
There are myths and truths on both sides of the controversy. Despite the enormous
contributions of Piaget, Bruner, Erickson, and other theorists to the understanding
of child development, much of our knowledge and research on learning and behavior in the early years has remained, in practice, unconnected to planning, methodology, and procedures of evaluation. This limitation is especially apparent in
measures for evaluation of severely impaired children that consist of infinite
minute steps and tasks with little resemblance to approximations and expectations
for typical growth and development. In point of fact, instruments such as the
Bayley Scales of Infant Development (Bayley, 1969) and Cattell's *Scale of Infant
Intelligence* (Cattell, 1940) have a long tradition of use with groups of typical
children. However, the static nature of these instruments and the restricted range
of behavior and development examined do not begin to meet the challenge of
assessing today's children within the ecological context of their social, emotional,
family, and community environments. In addition, many such instruments appear

to lack a degree of flexibility and appeal in presentation and administration that seems absolutely crucial to age-appropriate work with infants and young children.

Unfortunately, with few exceptions, traditional approaches to infant and preschool evaluation have assumed a unidimensional rather than a problem-solving model of behavior and learning. For instance, while many norm-referenced tests and scales have included diverse items for motor, language, cognitive, and behavioral development, rarely do they provide tasks for observation within the context of varying situations of social interaction with familiar and unfamiliar persons, the use of familiar and unfamiliar materials, and the use of alternative testing procedures and modalities for response (see Figures 15–1 through 15–7). Moreover, parallel information about home and school environments that might confirm or invalidate test findings and expand on test results with the soliciting of caregiver input has seldom been pursued, because of the exclusive adoption of more traditional practice and intelligence testing. Experience and expertise with vulnerable and developmentally disabled young populations consistently show strong evidence that all of the variables we have discussed deeply affect the quality of responsiveness of such children and that, without planned variability and a more natural setting for assessment, many youngsters are severely penalized. Neisworth and Bagnato's summarizing statement makes the point so well:

> We can do no better than to close with Stephen Gould's (1981) lament that there are "few injustices deeper than the denial of an opportunity to strive or ever hope, by a limit imposed from without, but falsely identified as lying within" (p. 28). (1992, p. 17)

New Thinking about Assessment

Assessment is a progressive and rapidly growing scene. Over the past 5 or 6 years, there has been a recognition of the diversity and changing quality of infant and preschool behavior, and this recognition holds important implications for the types of measures now needed for appropriate assessment. Most researchers, educators, and clinicians involved in delivering assessment services today would agree that multiple techniques should be used. Present thinking on the selection and decision-making processes is largely driven by con-

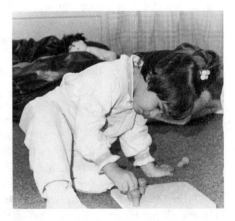

Figure 15–8 Lindsey at 28 months, playing with pegboard

scious efforts to link evaluation directly to subsequent stages of intervention (Barnett, Macmann, & Carey, 1992). In our view, the absence of this connection has been one of greatest sources of criticism of past assessment practices.

Virtually hundreds of scales, criterion-referenced measures, norm-referenced instruments, naturalistic observational strategies, interview guides, and ecobehavioral analysis systems are presently available to professionals for use in obtaining information relevant to understanding children within their various environments. Choosing appropriate assessment strategies from among such options needs to be guided by several underlying considerations, including the following concerns:

- Do strategies allow for a sufficient sampling of behavior and learning over time?
- Are strategies sensitive to cultural diversity, so that the strengths of children and families are heightened and problematic areas are identified?
- Can instruments and strategies be used in diverse settings?
- Do instruments and strategies allow for cross-confirmation of information obtained from work with the child and information obtained from primary caregivers?
- Are measures and strategies valid and reliable over time?
- Do measures and strategies address issues related to teaching the child?
- Do measures and strategies address issues connected to the child's everyday functioning and behavior at home and in the community?
- Do strategies and measures lead to a genuine breadth of understanding functional as well as developmental aspects of the child's learning and behavior?

In our judgment, all of the various *types* of measures are valid tools for use in the effort to fully comprehend the complexity of young children, their diverse styles of learning, and appropriate accommodations that may be necessary in order to achieve optimal educational opportunities. This statement, by no means, is intended to justify the selection and use of techniques that fall short of the criteria we have listed. Indeed, many measures used today unfortunately continue to serve the sole purpose of singling out and isolating children, focusing almost exclusively on their departures from "the norm." Ideally, assessment measures need to offer a means toward obtaining data that will encourage and allow teachers and clinicians to see and seize possibilities for connecting children to their peers and family members, rather than emphasizing differences. Accordingly, we are suggesting that assessment efforts in the future will need to move increasingly toward an *integrated* approach, in which different measures provide important pieces of the total information-gathering process. Toward this goal, the following methods may fulfill different functions that are critical to responsive and meaningful evaluation:

- naturalistic observations
- norm-referenced measures
- criterion- and curriculum-based assessment
- judgment-based assessment
- ecological and behavioral techniques.

Naturalistic Observations

The strategy of naturalistic observation is one of the most helpful to both team members and caregivers for recording and subsequently interpreting what is happening in significant settings where a given child spends the majority of his or her time. These observations may be carried out in home, program, and community settings over specific periods of time, and they afford essential information about peer and adult interaction and overall functional, adaptive, and behavioral skills. Some of the events and situations that may be tapped with this approach are opportunities for observing children during play, in the course of interacting with siblings, caregivers, and peers, during structured and unstructured activities, during mealtimes, and during transitions between activities (see Figures 15–8 through 15–13).

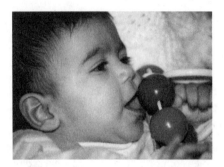

Figure 15–9 Lindsey at 5 months, bringing rattle to mouth

Several methods can be used in gathering information through naturalistic observations (Bailey & Wolery, 1992, pp. 105–106). These include:

- a running account or record of all child behaviors for a specified period
- event sampling, in which the frequency and duration of particular behaviors are recorded
- category sampling, in which types of behaviors of particular interest are noted.

Naturalistic observations are one of the primary ways in which professionals, firsthand, can gather information over several days and thus accommodate the "natural" changes of temperament and behavior that are characteristic of young children. In particular, this approach is a safeguard against making immediate judgments based on less familiar and short-term situations. In addition, this format may be adapted to new and contemporary variations of *transdisciplinary, play-based assessment* (Linder, 1993), in which observational guidelines are provided to professional team members and parents for data gathering and interpreting of selected areas of child development (i.e., cognitive, social-emotional, communicative, and sensorimotor). As described by Linder (1993), the advantages of this type of assessment (TPBA) are several:

> TPBA is implemented by a team. The team, consisting of the parents and representatives of disciplines who are knowledgeable about all areas of development, observes the child for an hour to an hour and a half during play activities with a play facilitator, the parents, and a peer. Developmental level, learning style, interaction patterns, and other relevant behaviors are analyzed based on the TPBA guidelines. Communication between the parents and other team members, prior to and during the assessment, is the key to ongoing dialogue that will continue throughout the child's involvement in an intervention program. (p. 1)

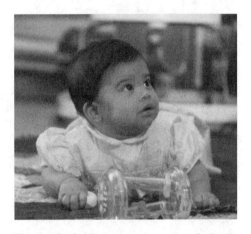

Figure 15–10 Kimberly at 6 months, playing in prone position

Norm-Referenced Measures

Norm-referenced measures constitute the type of assessment that has received the most severe criticism from early childhood special educators in recent years (Neisworth & Bagnato, 1988, 1992). As indicated earlier in this chapter, the *Bayley Scales of Infant Development* (Bayley, 1969) have been renormed and revised (*Bayley II*). These scales have been one of the most widely used instruments during the infant and toddler years.

Despite the precedence of history, however, the degree to which this instrument and similar measures should be used with children who have special needs or who are at risk for delayed development continues to be a paramount issue for several reasons. First, the current edition of the *Bayley Scales of Infant Development* is designed to obtain a holistic view of intellectual and developmental performance in isolation from affective, social, and emotional functioning. Such dimensions are, in fact, almost invariably a critical part of realistic and meaningful evaluations of infants and preschoolers with any kind of disability or condition of risk. Second, the *Bayley Scales* or similar types of measures have often been used as predictive instruments, rather than being interpreted as a means toward understanding current functioning. In particular, questions have been raised regarding the reliability and validity of such tools for assessment during the first 6 to 12 months of life. Third, there is little doubt that the use of the current *Bayley Scales* is inappropriate for children who have moderate to severe sensory, intellectual, and/or neuromotor impairments. For years, professionals and parents alike have expressed concern about the major disadvantages placed on children who are unable to respond in the conventional ways specified by "standard" procedures. In addition, while deficits usually are massively apparent with the use of this type of measure, rarely are strengths, special talents, and abilities highlighted or cultural values recognized. In the future, should professionals and parents decide that key pieces of information might be gained with the administration of measures like the new version of the *Bayley Scales*, these instruments or tests might be better utilized at the conclusion of the evaluation as a confirmatory strategy, rather than at the outset of the assessment process. Finally, this type of instrument should never be used as the sole basis for decision making.

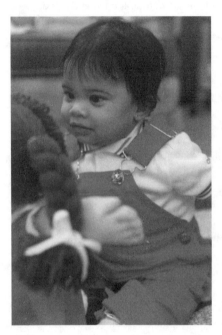

Figure 15–11 Kimberly at 8 months, sitting

Criterion- and Curriculum-Based Assessment

Criterion- and curriculum-based assessment is one of the most rapidly growing, state-of-the-art approaches in early childhood special education, and it offers a clear alternative to some of the major shortcomings and controversies raised with respect to "traditional" norm-referenced instruments. As described by Neisworth and Bagnato (1988), curriculum-based assessment (CBA):

... tracks individual child performance on specific program objectives; in essence, each child's current performance is compared to past performance in order to monitor progress and learning. The foundation of CBA is the sequence of developmental objectives that constitute a program's curriculum. Objectives may vary from general 'landmark' goals in each developmental domain (e.g., walks independently) to finely graded sequences of prerequisite behaviors that constitute a given skill-objective (e.g., turns head 30° to search for an auditory stimulus). CBA enables the teacher or diagnostic specialist to determine the specific breakdown of skills that a child has or has not acquired within the developmental task analysis. The scope, quality, and extent of individual learning can be described by profiling ranges of absent (-), fully acquired (+), and emerging (±) capabilities which then provide curriculum entry points for instruction and treatment . . . . The primary strength of curriculum-based assessment is its direct synchrony between testing and teaching. (pp. 27–28)

Several frequently used assessment measures exemplify the criterion- and curriculum-based approach to assessment in the early years. These include the *Learning Accomplishment Profile (LAP)* (Sanford & Zelman, 1981), *Hawaii Early Learning Profile (HELP)* (Furuno et al., 1979), *Carolina Curriculum for Infants and Toddlers* (Johnson-Martin, Jens, Attermeier, & Hacker, 1991), *Carolina Curriculum for Preschoolers with Special Needs* (Johnson-Martin, Attermeier, & Hacker, 1990), and the *Battelle Developmental Inventory* (Newborg, Stock, Wnek, Guidubaldi, & Svinicki, 1984).

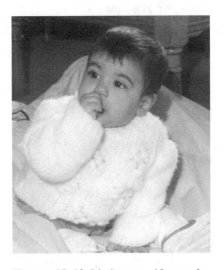

Also defined as a criterion-referenced instrument is a newly developed measure entitled the *Syracuse Scales of Infant and Toddler Development (SSITD)* (Ensher et al., 1994). These scales are currently being standardized with a national sample of infants and toddlers. Historically, the *Syracuse*

Figure 15–12 Lindsey at 10 months, forward propping

Scales came into being in response to the need for a new and different approach to the assessment of learning and behavior of high risk and developmentally disabled children from birth to 36 months of age and in response to the need for acknowledging the priorities of families in natural home and school settings. This measure seeks to offer cross-disciplinary teams of educators, physicians, nurses, psychologists, other clinical specialists, and parents a fundamentally integrated tool that directly connects programming for intervention and the mandate for professional-parent collaboration specified in PL 99–457. With use of a levels-of-assistance strategy, the *Syracuse Scales* have been designed to provide information, in a play-based format, about the quality and process of response and interaction. Such information is critical to the understanding of behavior and development in infants and toddlers and of the most intense needs of their parents as they move through the course of evaluation, transition, and participation in intervention programming.

Taken as a whole, the *Syracuse Scales* afford a comprehensive assessment-education package for working with very young populations and their families from the point of early identification to screening, in-depth diagnosis, and ongoing monitoring of progress. In addition, this instrument includes materials for training competent examiners to accomplish these goals (pp. 3–4). A detailed caregiver guide for initial and follow-up visits and a caregiver report of home and program environment complement the child-focused, developmental portions of the instrument, which are organized into four early play and three toddler scenarios. Items throughout the *SSITD* represent task activities across five primary developmental and adaptive behavior areas including neuromotor, sensory-perceptual, cognitive, communicative, and social-emotional skills. To be developed is a screening instrument, which will be especially helpful to clinical and medical staff interested in follow-up of infants and toddlers at risk for or suspected of having various developmental delays. The extensive research agenda for the *Syracuse Scales* includes not only the collection of standardization data for the development of norms, but also a series of special studies with selected groups including extremely premature and moderately premature infants and toddlers; children exposed prenatally to drugs or alcohol because of maternal substance abuse; children with diverse sensory and neuromotor impairments; and youngsters at high risk for or having developmental delay who represent various cultural groups, with matched control subjects in the standardization sample.

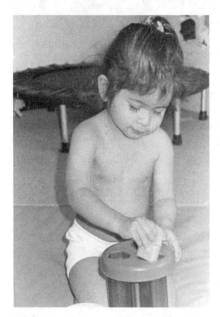

Figure 15–13 Ali playing with shape sorter

Overall, the design of this new assessment package is a signal to professionals that behavior and development of infants and toddlers should be viewed holistically and interdependently, rather than in terms of pure isolated abilities and skills. The instrument has a substantial degree of flexibility of administration, directly incorporates natural settings, and involves primary caregivers throughout the entire evaluation process. Last, the *SSITD* includes the critical quality of offering to children several response options, a feature that has, to date, been clearly absent from norm-referenced tests.

Judgment-Based Assessment

The term *judgment-based assessment (JBA)* was first used by Neisworth and Bagnato (1988). As described by several contemporaries writing about early childhood special education assessment, this approach holds much promise as a data-gathering strategy (Fleischer, Belgredan, Bagnato, & Ogonosky, 1990; LeLaurin, 1990; McCloskey, 1990). Specifically, Neisworth and Bagnato (1988) have described this structured clinical process as follows: "Judgment-based assessment (*JBA*) collects, structures, and usually quantifies the impressions of professionals and caregivers about child environmental characteristics" (p. 36).

In their subsequent discussion, Neisworth and Bagnato (1988) comment on several advantages of utilizing "*JBA* scales," which allow for the evaluation of "ambiguous traits and behaviors that are not gauged by more objective instruments" (p. 37). The authors cite various possibilities for assessing reactivity, consolability, temperament, motivation, muscle tone and tension, reinforcement behavior, play style, attention, self-control, and self-esteem, as well as the "traditional assessment domains such as language, motor ability, self-care, and social competence" (Fleischer et al., 1990, p. 15).

In addition, *JBA* measures are immensely helpful because they incorporate corroboration of data obtained from other more formal instruments and rely on the impressions and observations of individuals who have continuous or frequent contact and relationships with the child within the context of his or her natural environment. Finally, as Fleischer and associates note (Fleischer et al., 1990, p. 16) this assessment method affords an important means toward:

- facilitating communication between parents and professionals in different disciplines,
- aiding in program planning and evaluating intervention programs, and
- bringing to light both congruency and discrepancy between individuals' perceptions of a child.

Two instruments representing the *JBA* approach were developed by Neisworth and Bagnato: the *Perceptions of Developmental Status (PODS) Scale* (Bagnato & Neisworth, 1987) and the *System to Plan Early Childhood Services (SPECS)* (Bagnato & Neisworth, 1990). The revised form of the *PODS Scale* samples 18 developmental and behavioral qualities of children from 2 to 6 years of age, including seven major clusters within the areas of communication, sensorimotor, physical, self-regulation, cognition, self-social, and general development (Neisworth & Bagnato, 1988, p. 36). Based on this earlier work, *SPECS* allows team members and caregivers to rate, on a scale of 1 to 5, 19 dimensions of child behavior and development within the six domains of communication, sensorimotor, physical, self-regulation, cognition, and self-social abilities. Although the *JBA* approach is retrospective, it has the added asset of helping various members of the psychoeducational team, including parents, to sort out differences in perspective and, accordingly, to make adjustments of personal or professional views of the child. *JBA* is an excellent supplement to assessment of many of the behaviors and abilities included in the *Syracuse Scales of Infant and Toddler Development* that we have described, such as self-calming abilities, attention-gaining behaviors, initiation of play, interactive abilities with familiar and unfamiliar adults, turn-taking abilities, and other developmental and self-adaptive skills, that traditionally are not sampled by norm-referenced instruments.

Ecological and Ecobehavioral Techniques

Overlapping some of the strategies we have described is another cluster of instruments and strategies that fall under the category of ecological and ecobehavioral assessment. An underlying basic premise of such measures is the criterion of data gathering within the natural environment of the child. Highlighting the benefits of this kind of evaluation, Barnett, Macmann, & Carey (1992) have written:

> Ecobehavioral analysis focuses on natural systems such as families, classrooms, schools, and communities (McEvoy, 1990; Rogers-Warren, 1984). Ecobehavioral analysis establishes a broad context for understanding adjustment and planning interventions by requiring multiple perspectives for each stage of problem solving (Cantrell & Cantrell, 1985) . . . . Thus assessment plans can be directed to the identification of (a) a range of treatment options based on research and functional analysis; (b) naturally occurring parent or teacher intervention strategies that are likely to be successful (either as implemented or with modifications, guidance, and feedback); or (c) interventions that may be adapted to individual styles of parenting or teaching. (pp. 35–36)

Two existing and widely used instruments that tap home and community environments are the *Home Observation for Measurement of the Environment (HOME)* (Caldwell & Bradley, 1978) and the *Early Childhood Environment Rating Scale (ECERS)* (Harms & Clifford, 1980), which focuses on the classroom setting. In addition as we have noted, the *Syracuse Scales of Infant and Toddler Development* are designed specifically to provide for evaluation and caregiver self-reporting along these dimensions.

Focusing more broadly on the overall strategy of ecobehavioral assessment, Barnett, Macmann, and Carey (1992) have discussed the potential for numerous measures to be included within the fold of this type of evaluation for young children. Observations, problem-centered interviews, and criterion-based measures all qualify. From the perspective of these authors, the basic criterion for use rests with the contribution that any given measure might make to the fundamental intervention design. In a comprehensive work entitled *Family Assessment in Early Intervention* (1988), Bailey and Simeonsson also have described a myriad of strategies and instruments that can be utilized to obtain information pertaining to the child within the family-community environment. Indeed, the ecological-ecobehavioral perspective has attracted the interest of a cadre of supporters, and rightfully so, in light of the critical importance of mediating interactive influences of the family and of significant others to the well-being and healthy development of the child.

Team Models for Implementation

Basic to every dimension of the PL 99–457 and PL 102–119 is the tenet of an interdisciplinary approach, and assessment is a prime example of how this fundamental guideline can be implemented. Depending on the number of people involved in the actual evaluation and later delivery of services, various terms have been used to describe the actual team process. As discussed by Bailey and Wolery (1989):

> The *multidisciplinary team* contains members from multiple disciplines, but each remains relatively independent and is affected very little by the actions of other team members. The *interdisciplinary team* involves greater interactions among team members, with each member relying on the others for important information and suggestions. The final product is an integrated plan of services that involves significant cooperation between disciplines. The *transdisciplinary team* is one in which multiple disciplines work together in the initial assessment, but the provision of services is conducted by one or two team members. (p. 15)

Within the past 10 years, another collaborative approach involving both parents and professionals has increasingly been adopted; i.e., *arena assessment,* a term first described by Wolery and Dyk (1984). Accordingly,

> A temporary facilitator, generally the team member with the most expertise in the child's area of need, is assigned prior to the actual assessment activities. The facilitator serves as the primary assessor while other team members and parents sit away from the child and record observations and score portions of assessment tools relevant to their discipline. As the assessment progresses, team members may ask the facilitator to administer certain items relevant to the observer's discipline. Occasionally, an observer may assist the assessor or administer the items directly. Parents are present during the assessment to provide information, administer items if necessary, and validate the child's performance. (pp. 231–232)

Many factors influence the appropriateness and selection of any given approach, which essentially constitute variations of a common theme. Among these considerations are the specified preferences of caregivers, the individual styles of children who may work better with one person versus several unfamiliar persons, and the ease of cross over among professional team members representing different disciplines. If it is realistic and feasible, a degree of flexibility needs to be built into the process to make it genuinely responsive to individual situations, issues important at the time of assessment, and the richness of different cultures and ethnic backgrounds. Pursuit of particular models without regard to these variables represents less than "best practice" in all of the disciplines of the professionals involved in assessment.

BEST PRACTICE: INTERACTION OF FAMILY, CHILD, PROFESSIONALS, AND COMMUNITY

In conclusion, observing behavior and analyzing competence in high risk and developmentally disabled infants and young children is a process that has prompted much study and debate, reflecting significant progress toward more balanced views and strategies for implementation in recent years. Having examined a few of these issues in detail, we close this discussion with some speculations and suggestions about future directions in this important area of early childhood education.

We are convinced that all aspects of evaluation in the early years—screening, diagnosis, and ongoing monitoring and observation—must reflect interactions of child, family, professional, and setting. Selections of methodology and process need to be governed less by individual preference, availability, and ideology and more by a genuine sense of immediate problems and dynamics. Furthermore, innovative measures must survive the rigor of valid and reliable standardization with widely divergent populations for whom they are intended, in addition to exploring new qualities of child learning and development that previously have been outside the realm of traditional instruments and assessment. At a minimum, instruments should assess behaviors such as child endurance, temperament, various aspects of play, attention-gaining and self-calming abilities, responsiveness to new tasks and unfamiliar situations, unstructured discovery, spontaneous activity, levels of frustration and irritability, and primary modes for responding. Some strategies should be defined to set limited ranges of expected behavior; others ought to be open-ended, allowing for response and novelty beyond the information given. Finally, professionals committed to a genuine understanding of infants and young children must adhere tenaciously to the goal of achieving a more natural, integrated, and flexible approach to evaluation.

BIBLIOGRAPHY

Aylward, G.P. (1988). Issues in prediction and developmental follow-up. *Developmental and Behavioral Pediatrics, 9*(5), 307–309.

Bagnato, S.J., & Neisworth, J.T. (1987). *Perceptions of developmental status: A system for planning early intervention.* University Park, PA: Penn State University.

Bagnato, S.J., & Neisworth, J.T. (1990). *System to plan early childhood services (SPECS).* Circle Pines, MN: American Guidance Service.

Bailey, D.B., Jr., & Simeonsson, R.J. (1988). *Family assessment in early intervention.* Columbus, OH: Merrill.

Bailey, D.B., Jr., & Wolery, M. (1989). *Assessing infants and preschoolers with handicaps.* Columbus, OH: Merrill.

Bailey, D.B., Jr., & Wolery, M. (1992). *Teaching infants and preschoolers with disabilities* (2nd ed.). New York: Merrill.

Barnett, D.W., Macmann, G.M., & Carey, K.T. (1992). Early intervention and the assessment of developmental skills: Challenges and directions. *Topics in Early Childhood Special Education, 12*(1), 21–43.

Bayley, N. (1969). *Bayley scales of infant development.* New York: Psychological Corp.

Beckman, P.J., & Bristol, M.M. (1991). Establishing family outcomes. *Topics in Early Childhood Special Education, 11*(3), 19–31.

Berkeley, T.R., & Ludlow, B.L. (1992). Developmental domains: The mother of all interventions; or The Subterranean early development blues. *Topics in Early Childhood Special Education, 11*(4), 13–21.

Caldwell, B.M., & Bradley, R.H. (1978). *Home observation for measurement of the environment.* Little Rock, AR: University of Arkansas, Center for Child Development and Education.

Campbell, P.H. (1991). Evaluation and assessment in early intervention for infants and toddlers. *Journal of Early Intervention, 15*(1), 36–45.

Cattell, P. (1940). *The measurement of intelligence of infants and young children.* New York: Psychological Corp.

Ensher, G.L., & Clark, D.A. (1986). *Newborns at risk: Medical care and psychoeducational intervention.* Gaithersburg, MD: Aspen Publishers.

Ensher, G.L., Gardner, E.F., Bobish, T.P., Michaels, C.A., Butler, K.G., & Meller, P.J. (1994). *The Syracuse scales of infant and toddler development* (research edition). Chicago: Riverside.

Fleischer, K.H., Belgredan, J.H., Bagnato, S.I., & Ogonosky, A.B. (1990). An overview of judgment-based assessment. *Topics in Early Childhood Special Education, 10*(2), 13–23.

Frankenburg, W.K., Dodds, S.B., Fandal, A.W., Kazuk, E., & Cohrs, M. (1975). *Developmental screening test: Reference manual* (revised). Denver: LADOCA Project and Publishing Foundation.

Furuno, S., O'Reilly, K.A., Hasaka, C.M, Inatsuka, T.T., Allman, T.L., & Zeisloft, B. (1979). *Hawaii early learning profile.* Palo Alto, CA: VORT.

Gordon, B.N., & Jens, K.G. (1988). A conceptual model for tracking high-risk infants and making early service decisions. *Developmental and Behavioral Pediatrics, 9*(5), 279–286.

Harms, T., & Clifford, R.M. (1980). *Early childhood environmental rating scale.* New York: Teachers College Press.

Johnson-Martin, N.M., Attermeier, S.M., & Hacker, B. (1990). *The Carolina curriculum for preschoolers with special needs.* Baltimore: Paul H. Brookes.

Johnson-Martin, N.M., Jens, K.G., Attermeier, S.M., & Hacker, B. (1991). *The Carolina curriculum for infants and toddlers with special needs.* Baltimore: Paul H. Brookes.

Keogh, B.K., & Koff, C.B. (1978). From assessment to intervention: An elusive bridge. In F.D. Minifie & L.L. Lloyd (Eds.), *Communicative and cognitive abilities—Early behavioral assessment* (pp. 523–547). Baltimore: University Park Press.

Kopp, C.B., & Parmelee, A.H. (1979). Prenatal and perinatal influences on infant behavior. In J.D. Osofsky (Ed.), *Handbook of infant development* (pp. 29–75). New York: John Wiley & Sons.

LeLaurin, K. (1990). Judgment-based assessment: Making the implicit explicit. *Topics in Early Childhood Special Education, 10*(3), 96–110.

Linder, T.W. (1993). *Transdisciplinary play-based assessment: A functional approach to working with young children* (rev. ed). Baltimore: Paul H. Brookes.

Lynch, E.W., & Hanson, M.J. (1992). *Developing cross-cultural competence.* Baltimore: Paul H. Brookes.

McCloskey, G. (1990). Selecting and using early childhood rating scales. *Topics in Early Childhood Special Education, 10*(3), 39–64.

McGonigel, M.J., Kaufmann, R.K., & Johnson, B.H. (1991). A family-centered process for the individualized family service plan. *Journal of Early Intervention, 15*(1), 46–56.

Meisels, S.J. (1991). Dimensions of early identification. *Journal of Early Intervention, 15*(1), 26–35.

Neisworth, J.T., & Bagnato, S.J. (1988). Assessment in early childhood special education: A typology of dependent measures. In S.L. Odom & M.B. Karnes (Eds.), *Early intervention for infants and children with handicaps: An empirical base* (pp. 23–49). Baltimore: Paul H. Brookes.

Neisworth, J.T., & Bagnato, S.J. (1992). The case against intelligence testing in early intervention. *Topics in Early Childhood Special Education, 12*(1), 1–20.

Newborg, J., Stock, J.R., Wnek, L., Guidubaldi, J., & Svinicki, J. (1984). *Battelle developmental inventory.* Chicago: Riverside.

Sanford, A.R., & Zelman, J.G. (1981). *The learning accomplishment profile.* Winston-Salem, NC: Kaplan.

Teti, D.M., & Gibbs, E.D. (1990). Infant assessment: Historical antecedents and contemporary issues. In E.D. Gibbs & D.M. Teti (Eds.), *Interdisciplinary assessment of infants: A guide for early intervention professionals.* Baltimore: Paul H. Brookes.

Wetherby, A., & Prizant, B. (1993). *Communication and symbolic behavior scales.* Chicago: Riverside.

Wolery, M., & Dyk, L. (1984). Arena assessment: Description and preliminary social validity data. *Journal of the Association for the Severely Handicapped, 3,* 231–235.

Part III

Intervention: Process and Practical Application

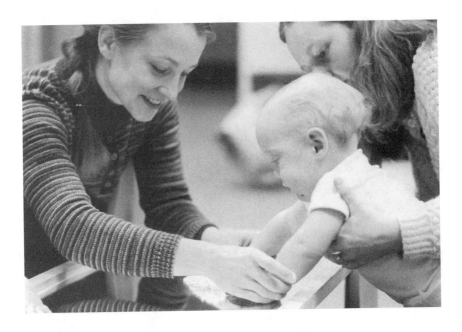

Perhaps in no other era of education have professionals witnessed the magnitude of interest and change that has been so evident over the past 25 to 30 years in early childhood education. Some intervention projects continue to pursue the precedent of the 1970s, emphasizing prevention of disability among low income, less educated, and under-represented groups. However, Public Laws 99–457 and 102–119 have now introduced into the public sector a new dimension to service delivery. Today, efforts are more broadly based and integrated, offering to high risk and disabled infants and their families programs that start at the earliest ages. Current models, too, reflect genuine attempts at collaboration and cooperation across a range of professional disciplines and caregivers. Put to rest are more general questions of the effectiveness of interventions, with contemporary researchers examining more specific issues of with whom, when, and under what conditions services are most beneficial to both children and families.

Chapter 16

Intervening in Intensive Care Nurseries

Mary Jo Hayes and Gail L. Ensher

Concerns today for high risk infants do not center solely on medical treatment. While improved survival rates have required the use of aggressive, highly technological therapies, professionals over the past 25 years simultaneously have pursued a keen interest in the developmental environments of newborns hospitalized for extended periods. Among those infants born prematurely in the United States every year, most acutely ill babies continue to be especially vulnerable to the stressful influences of neonatal intensive care, as a result of their neurological immaturity and physiological instability. As we examine the care that now is available for these tiniest infants, it is apparent that medical technology can provide intervention for conditions affecting virtually every organ system. However, these amazing contributions to the preservation of life have concurrently presented us with very real new challenges.

GOALS OF INTERVENTION IN THE NEONATAL UNIT

When we refer to the high risk infant, we need to remember that the concept of "risk" applies not only to the newborn's chance of survival. As a result of life threatening medical events (Barb & Lemons, 1989; Catlett & Holditch-Davis, 1990; Colditz, 1991; Field, 1990; Gunderson & Kenner, 1987; Lott, 1989), the infant admitted to the intensive care unit has also experienced major physiological and environmental conditions that may well interfere with or compromise typical development. Thus, as we address medical needs, so too should we respond to developmental, psychosocial, and family concerns. Accordingly, there are at least two basic goals for intervention in intensive care:

1. to reduce adverse and potentially detrimental stimuli to the lowest possible level
2. to create supportive and developmentally appropriate environments for both newborns and their families (Bass, 1991; Lott, 1989; Harrison & Woods, 1991; Schultz, 1992).

227

Three broader objectives are critical to achieving these goals. The first involves education of both nursery and professional staff who are involved with infants in the neonatal intensive care unit (NICU) and of the parents who will assume caregiving when the child is ready to go home. Educators, child development specialists, and medical personnel are acknowledging the strong interaction among physiological, environmental, and developmental processes that determine the well-being of the premature infant (Lester & Tronick, 1990). Consequently, NICU staff need to have an awareness and knowledge of the types of stimulation or protection most beneficial to the newborns they care for, as well as techniques to optimize interactions with such infants.

Parents likewise must learn about their babies who have been born early or are otherwise at risk. Most importantly, they should understand the many behavioral responses that newborns may evidence and should be able to interpret what these mean. For example, if parents can identify early signs of stress or avoidance or engagement cues, they can respond more appropriately to their baby. In addition, they need to be prepared for many "typical" problems that they may encounter with an early delivery, such as excessive irritability, mixed wake and sleep cycles, difficulties with feeding, and slow attention patterns. In working with and educating parents, nursery staff can encourage mothers and fathers to touch, hold, and care for their infants in ways that, hopefully, will facilitate attachment and decrease anxiety in the NICU and in the transition to home.

The second component of the process for developing more appropriate nursery environments is the monitoring and assessment of the infant states, including attention to muscle tone, reflexes, regulation of behavioral state, neurobehavioral responses, and feeding issues. In an effort to gain baseline information about an infant's neurological status, it is important to remember that newborns are differentially sensitive and responsive to various types of stimulation, depending on their conceptual age, illness, and individual neurophysiology and temperament (Lester & Tronick, 1990). On the basis of this ongoing process of behavioral observation and assessment, hospital staff can apply various types of intervention and strategies for environmental protection that seem to be indicated.

The final aspect of intervention for the high risk infant and the family is the provision for a smooth transition to home and for services after discharge. Ideally, this planning process is not limited to family education in the NICU; it should begin when the baby is admitted, involve the family with a primary care team, and subsequently continue in follow-up until the child reaches preschool or school age. Included in the discharge and postdischarge programs are the basic training for home care by the parents, information about equipment, and referrals for home- or community-based intervention, which need to be set in place before the infant leaves the NICU. An essential feature of this process is the development of a method for maintaining contact with families after discharge to facilitate the transition from hospital to home and to address any concerns in a timely manner. Research findings have reinforced further development of such hospital-to-home approaches for low birthweight newborns, demonstrating improved outcome as a result of this kind of programing (Gennaro, Brooten, & Bakewell-Sachs, 1991). Indeed, support for parents of high risk children, beginning in the NICU, has emerged as one of the most promising strategies for enhancing the growth and development of young children.

THE VULNERABLE BRAIN

Basic to any discussion of specific developmental intervention with hospitalized newborns is a fundamental understanding of the changes that take place when an infant is born several weeks or months early. Simply stated, the brain develops through a continuous process, which begins in utero and proceeds beyond birth until approximately 2 years of age (Bellig, 1989). Preterm infants are delivered before in utero stages of brain development are completed, a condition that places them at risk for potential abnormal brain growth and development (Barb & Lemons, 1989).

As described by Barb & Lemons (1989, p. 8), brain development can be classified into four categories.

1. *Neuronal proliferation* is a process that involves the rapid and repeated production of neurons, which are made up of the axon, cell body, and the dendrite. Neuronal production initially occurs between 2 and 4 months gestation and is followed by development of the glial cells (supportive tissue of the central nervous system) at approximately 5 months gestation.

2. *Migration* refers to the movement of nerve cells from their site of origin to the area they eventually occupy within the mature central nervous system. Migration occurs primarily between 3 and 5 months gestation.

3. *Organization* involves several changes including: (a) the alignment and layering of the cortex, (b) further development and expansion of the axons and dendrites, (c) establishment of synaptic contacts, (d) selective elimination via cell death of neuronal processes, and (e) additional differentiation and proliferation of the glial cells. Organization takes place primarily in the third trimester and establishes the elaborate network of the central nervous system.

4. *Myelinization* is the development of the myelin sheath covering the axon, which enhances conduction of impulses in the nervous system. This process begins at 20 weeks gestation and continues into adult life.

Thus myelinization within the cortex parallels the development of associated brain function and associated skills (Mastropaolo, 1992).

As noted above, in the preterm infant much of the brain growth and maturation that normally occurs in utero takes place in an extrauterine environment that is characterized by a variety of medical insults during the perinatal period. Conditions such as hypoxia, acidosis, infection, and inadequate nutrition may lead to intraventricular hemorrhage or other cerebral insults, which may have serious consequences for immediate and later brain development. Increasingly, researchers are focusing on the physiological changes and responses of the premature newborn to pain and the long-term detrimental effects of exposure to pain (Brown, 1987; Colditz, 1991; Tichy, Braam, Meyer, & Rattan, 1988). Thus, despite extraordinary and extremely successful efforts to improve prenatal, perinatal, and neonatal care, some infants sustain neurological damage and developmental problems. This issue, which has become more critical with the survival of smaller and smaller babies, brings us to two questions directly related to the potentials of NICU intervention: What can be done on the side of prevention? When damage does occur, can predictable delays be attenuated?

The human brain exhibits powerful, plastic capabilities that allow the central nervous system to cope with a variety of conditions including damage, aging, and an ever-changing environment (Spinelli, 1990). Fundamentally, the structure of the cortex is determined by genome (genetic make-up), but ongoing changes in the brain are possible because the full configuration of the cortex takes place after birth, basically guided and promoted by stimuli, information, and challenges of any given environment (Spinelli, 1990, p. 77). Spinelli has noted that the primary task for the premature infant is the achievement of homeostasis despite the fact that a substantial cohort of stimuli bombard a nervous system not yet ready for exposure and intervention. Spinelli writes, "These stimuli are permanently changing, for better or worse, the actual structure of the brain. The caregiver is unavoidably a brain shaper, one who has a very large impact in determining the future of the infant" (p. 81). If the environment and care that we offer to premature newborns is as vital as Spinelli and other researchers suggest, professional caregivers and parents must be vigilant in their observations of infant behavior in response to environmental change and intervention.

INFANT BEHAVIOR

Infants communicate through the windows of their behavior. They offer clues as to what they need, how much they need, and when they need it (Cole, 1985, p. 24). If we are sensitive in our observations of and work with the preterm baby, behavioral cues can be integrated into daily routines and treatment as important, appropriate, individualized interventions (Cole, 1985). Premature infants differ considerably from their full-term counterparts and from each other in their overall capacities to respond to their environments—variables that are largely dependent on gestational age and status of recovery and health (Cole, 1985). Als (1986) has provided a meaningful framework for understanding individual differences through her description of five subsystems and related behavioral manifestations of the preterm newborn.

1. The *autonomic system,* or physiological functioning, is observed behaviorally in patterns of respiration, heart rate, color changes, and visceral signals such as bowel movements, gagging, and hiccoughing.

2. The *motor system* is manifested behaviorally in the posture, tone, and movements of the baby. Lott (1989) states that the premature infant moves little, activity is jerky and irregular, and underlying muscle tone often is low.

3. *State organization* is seen behaviorally in the states of consciousness available to the newborn, ranging from periods of sleep to arousal to alert wakefulness; in patterns of state transition; and in the clarity and definition of states. Six conditions of arousal are available to the infant:

   a. deep sleep: no rapid eye movement (REM)

   b. lighter sleep: REM, limb movement

   c. drowsy alert: transitional

   d. quiet alert: awake, alert, and calm

   e. fussy: crying or agitated

   f. full agitation: crying and highly distressed

4. *Attention or interaction* is exemplified in the infant's ability to come to an alert, attentive state and to use this capacity to take in and process environmental information.

5. The *regulatory system* is behaviorally reflected in the infant's ability to integrate input from the various subsystems and to return to and maintain an appropriate state of balance and relaxation. Mastropaolo (1992) states that this system in the preterm infant may not be well managed until after the baby has left intensive care.

The initial response of an ill premature newborn to environmental stress is very different from that of a healthy newborn. This response is often manifested in physiological changes such as crying, gaze aversion, color change, or even vomiting (Catlett & Holditch-Davis, 1990). Moreover, these initial behavioral changes are frequently followed by rapid physiological deterioration and state disorganization, evidenced by sudden swings in state during which the infant may withdraw into a lower level of consciousness or "shut down" or stare fearfully or worriedly at his environment (Cole, 1985).

Catlett and Holditch-Davis (1990) have described their observations of a premature infant in a neonatal unit over a 2-hour period; the researchers documented 14 changes in state. At least one-half of these responses were prompted by noise and nursing or medical procedures. In view of the fact that newborns typically spend only a small percentage of time in waking states, frequent interruptions and interventions with preterm babies may result in deprivation of quiet sleep that is essential for the recovery of the acutely ill child.

Findings of other studies have pointed to correlations between compromised physiological responses and intrusive medical routines. Long, Lucey, and Philip (1980) used transcutaneous partial pressure of oxygen (Po_2) to study the effects of handling the premature infant. They recorded heart rate, respiratory rate, and Tc Po_2 in the first 5 days of life over a 20-hour period. Caregivers in the control group were unaware of the study; those in the experimental group were instructed in the operation of the monitors and told to use monitor feedback to modify procedures during "undesirable" time (when transcutaneous Po_2 was between 40 and 100 millimeters of mercury). The study results showed that control infants were handled more frequently and experienced more hypoxemia and that 75 percent of the hypoxic time was associated with handling. Moreover, the experimental group experienced only 6 minutes of "undesirable time," while control infants had an average of 40 minutes under stress. In a similar study, Norris, Campbell, and Brenkert (1982) looked at the effects of three routine nursing procedures (suctioning, repositioning, and performing a heel-stick) on blood oxygen levels, again using the transcutaneous oxygen monitor. Their study sample consisted of 25 infants with bronchopulmonary dysplasia who were observed over a 3-hour period. The authors reported that Tc Po_2, decreased significantly during suctioning with mechanical ventilation and during repositioning, but not during heel-stick. The greatest decline was seen after suctioning, with a gradual follow-up period of recovery. One can well speculate about the long-term consequences for the seriously ill infant with repeated prolonged decreases in oxygenation. Furthermore, diminished oxygenation frequently is accompanied by increased heart and respiratory rates, which concurrently increase oxygen consumption and caloric requirements (Catlett & Holditch-Davis, 1990)—two conditions that tend to delay growth and healing.

Given the compelling data, changes in best practice NICU intervention seem to be clearly indicated. No longer can professionals and families ask whether programing (intervention) is appropriate. The issue before us is *the nature* of neonatal intervention. Research focused on various types of environments and stimulation with high risk newborns is not new. Data collected over the past 20 to 25 years on intervention with premature, high risk, and developmentally delayed newborns in NICUs have been extensive. Unfortunately, however, although findings suggest that appropriate intervention improves outcome (Gorski, 1991; Schaefer, Hatcher, & Barlow, 1980), reviews on the effectiveness of programing leave many questions unanswered and consistently raise the need for refinement in methodology and design of such studies (Cole, 1985; Meisels, 1985; Oehler, 1985).

To move us beyond this point of controversy, research in the future will have to address many issues about the appropriateness and timing of interventions with varying degrees of prematurity. These issues include the nature of specific programing for purposes of protection as well as stimulation; sensitive measures of developmental change; the diversity of high risk populations; selection of the best individuals for program implementation; and the guidance that should be offered to parents in relation to earlier versus later stimulation. As demonstrated by prior research, in most instances it is not possible to enter in a study adequate numbers of infants within given categories at risk, define such classifications accurately, or impose control conditions in which babies are denied programing considered to be beneficial. Thus, future studies will need to be developed around these constraints. In addition, current researchers and practitioners now are advocating intervention for preterm infants that is individualized and adapted to abilities of the child to respond to various stimuli (Mastropaolo, 1992). Finally, with the present emphasis on family-focused involvement, programing for families will need to be tailored to individual priorities. Figure 16–1 illustrates the complexities of interactions and defines some of the processes critical to intervention with high risk infants and their families.

INTERVENTION WITH NEWBORNS

In a very real sense, interaction with newborns in the neonatal intensive care setting has come full circle. Prior to the 1960s, premature infants were considered too fragile to tolerate stimulation, and the philosophy that prevailed was one of minimal handling (Lester & Tronick, 1990). This thinking began to change with heightened concerns that the NICU environment and incubator, in particular, might be serving to deprive children of sensory stimulation (Lester & Tronick, 1990). Thus began a period of interventions, carried out with a variety of strategies focusing on three forms of stimulation: tactile-kinesthetic (Hasselmeyer, 1964; Korner, Kraemer, Haffner, & Cosper, 1975; Neal, 1968; Solkoff & Matuszak, 1975); auditory (Katz, 1971; Segal, 1972); and multimodal (Kramer & Pierpont, 1976; LaRossa & Brown, 1982; Leib, Benfield, & Guidubaldi, 1980). The decades of the 1980s and the 1990s have ushered in a period of contemporary research directed toward establishing a more compassionate, sensitive, and appropriate climate for both infants and families (O'Donnell, 1990).

Noise Protection and Auditory Stimulation

Noise levels in the NICU have been a major source of environmental stress for preterm infants (Catlett & Holditch-Davis, 1990). High risk newborns have a much higher incidence of moderate to profound hearing loss (2.5 to 5.0 percent) than infants in the general population (1 percent) (Schultz, 1987). Moreover, it is not uncommon for newborns admitted to the intensive care unit later in childhood to show evidence of high-frequency sensorineural losses, which are typically associated with excessive exposure to noise (Holmes, Reisk, & Pasternak, 1984). One study, conducted by Long, Lucey, and Philip in 1980, recorded sound levels in an NICU over an 8-hour period. Conclusions of the study were (1) that nursery

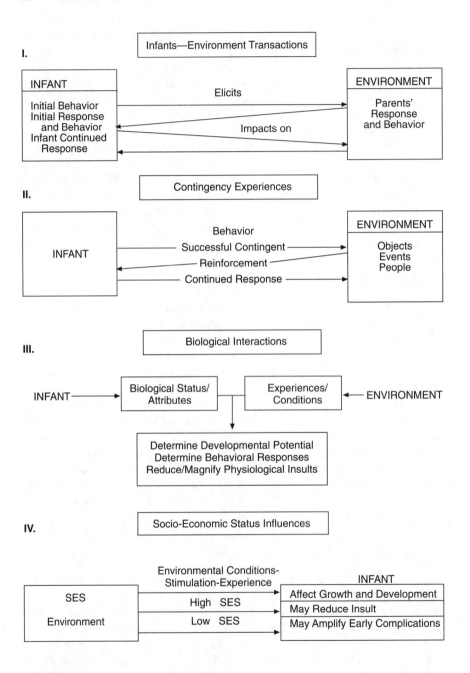

Figure 16–1 Some intervention considerations in the early environment of the high risk infant.

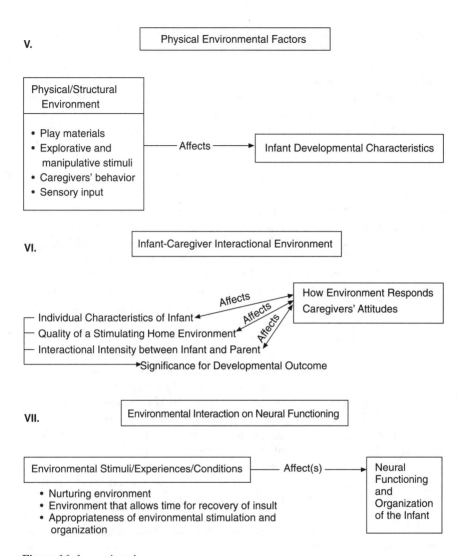

Figure 16–1   continued

staff were large contributors to noise levels, (2) that noise also may be an unrecognized cause of hypoxemia, and (3) that means for reducing noise levels in the nursery are readily available. Catlett and Holditch-Davis (1990) further reported that during 2-hour observations of each of five infants, 27 state changes occurred in response to loud noise, and more than 75 percent of the time, such noise caused physiological distress evident decreases in $Tc\ Po_2$ of more than 20 TORR, heart rate increases of more than 10 beats per minute, and one episode of bradycardia requiring mechanical ventilation. The authors cited the fact that noise levels of about 80 decibels, even for short deviations, have been shown to cause hearing loss in some adults. In 1974, the American Academy of Pediatrics expressed formal concern about noise pollution hearing loss attributable to high-intensity sounds and the interaction effects between these sounds and ototoxic medications (Gottfried, 1985). Although defining optimal noise levels for the premature infant is difficult, it is important for staff to have an awareness of noise levels and potential noise damage. Simple precautions may be the most effective and feasible (Mastropaolo, 1992). Such measures include protective strategies such as lowering voices, eliminating radios, limiting numbers of people, and using cloth diapers to drape incubators.

In addition to studies on auditory protection, research involving various types of intervention has been carried out. Study results indicate that quiet and intermittent auditory stimulation may be beneficial to preterm infants (Catlett & Holditch-Davis, 1990). It is important to note that such programing should be conducted only in NICUs where noise is maintained at a reduced level, when infants are physiologically stable, and when stimulation is individualized (Catlett & Holditch-Davis, 1990). Chaze and Ludington-Hoe (1984) suggested that the best auditory stimulus for a newborn is a parent's voice, which may be played for the child in the absence of the family. The authors recommended that parent voices be played for 2 to 3 minutes during alert inactivity, supplemented with classical music in 5-minute intervals as infants begin to show signs of positive responses to the music. Classical music has been utilized as well for periods up to 10 minutes in order to quiet agitated states and to promote deep sleep in premature infants (Barb & Lemons, 1989). In another study, Schmidt, Rose, and Bridger (1980) investigated responses of preterm infants to tape recorded heartbeats (72 beats per minute at 79 to 81 decibels). The sound was turned on immediately following sleep and continued while infant heart rate was monitored. The researchers found that the taped sounds did not lower heart rate but did have a substantial impact on sleep states, motility patterns, and cardiac responsiveness, bringing the preterm infant closer to the full-term newborn along those dimensions. If signs of stress such as crying, grimacing, yawning, changes in skin color, or hiccoughing appear, the auditory stimulation in any of these research contexts should be discontinued immediately (Catlett & Holditch-Davis, 1990).

Visual Protection and Stimulation

Until recently infants in NICUs typically have been exposed to high levels of fluorescent light, often on a 24-hour basis (Peabody & Lewis, 1985). In terms of lighting, American Academy of Pediatrics guidelines recommend 100-foot-candle intensity at the level of the infant at all times for adequate visualization (Peabody & Lewis, 1985). For years, it has been recognized that light has many effects on humans; light affects biological rhythms, endocrine glands, gonadal function, and vitamin D synthesis. Consequently, there is concern about the possible detrimental effects on infants exposed to high-intensity light. For example, Glass and colleagues (1985) compared the incidence of retinopathy of prematurity (ROP) among 74 infants in a standard bright nursery environment with the incidence among 154 infants of similar birthweight for whom light levels were reduced. They reported a 30 percent greater incidence of ROP in a subgroup of infants weighing less than 1,000 grams, and a higher likelihood for ROP to occur throughout the sample exposed to bright lights. In view of such data, modifications need to be made in what to date has been "standard" practice. Accommodating the imperatives of close observation, schedules should be flexible to allow periods of darkness or reduced lighting, especially for children in more stable condition. Diapers or blankets draped over incubators and individualized spotlights for dimming light during certain periods of the day and for simulation of day/night cycles can be used to offer periods of "time out" and protection from light exposure (Catlett & Holditch-Davis, 1990; Lott, 1989; Peabody & Lewis, 1985).

As infants are able to tolerate more interaction, visual stimuli may be presented—again with an eye to cues that signal overload. Gardner, Garland, Merenstein, and Merenstein (1989) have made several recommendations for appropriate presentation of visual information to accommodate an infant's needs. They suggest, for instance:

- holding the infant in a face-to-face position to feed, with gentle talking and rocking
- offering visual stimuli when the infant is in a quiet alert state
- placing mobiles and pictures at 8 to 12 inches from the infant's eyes, within the visual field
- alternating left and right sides for visual stimulation and changing the toys offered
- placing infants in positions such as lying on a side, which allows them to bring their hands together at midline, with oral exploration.

In conclusion, if by 34 weeks postconceptual age, a newborn is not responding to visual stimuli or not tracking moving objects to some extent, staff should recognize the possibility of visual impairment and the concurrent need for examination by an ophthalmologist (Schultz, 1992).

Tactile, Kinesthetic, and Vestibular Stimulation

Until recently, NICUs have been largely characterized by too much and inappropriate auditory and visual stimulation, and the amount of soothing tactile, kinesthetic, and vestibular intervention has been extremely limited. In fact, premature newborns in NICUs have had numerous experiences with touch and interaction, but these encounters have often been associated with pain and discomfort (Catlett

& Holditch-Davis, 1990; Colditz, 1991). In years past, the prevailing view was that pain is a learned response and that infants do not experience such sensations (Holmes, Reisk, & Pasternak, 1984). More recent research has offered strong evidence to the contrary, revealing a decline in oxygenation and increased heart rate in the presence of painful aversive touch procedures (Catlett & Holditch-Davis, 1990). Addressing the issue of painful stressors for the acutely ill newborn, Catlett & Holditch-Davis (1990) have recommended the following:

> The effects of procedural touch can be lessened by grouping care in short intervals and watching oxygen monitors so that procedures can be stopped whenever possible before hypoxemia occurs. For the sickest and smallest premature infants, long rest periods must be provided before and after periods of procedural touch to optimize oxygen levels and minimize prolonged stress.

> . . . Because acutely ill prematures are so sensitive to stimulation, interactional touch must be approached with great care and a good deal of expertise. If not, infants will respond as negatively to interactional touch as to procedural touch. Several studies have shown that, gentle, interactional touch during the neonatal period can decrease crying, increase weight gain, increase bowel motility, and improve developmental status at one year of age. (p. 24)

Several other researchers have noted the association between continuous handling of critically ill infants in neonatal settings and the potential for periventricular-intraventricular hemorrhage (Bada et al., 1990; Evans, 1991). Discussing the high incidence of hypoxemia associated with caregiving to preterm newborns, Evans (1991) has offered practical guidelines for implementation.

> Minimal handling policies and appropriate signs on incubators of infants at risk may reduce the incidence of multiple hypoxemia episodes. Setting aside specific rest periods so that others do not disturb infants who display wide physiological changes may help prevent intraventricular hemorrhage.

> Infants with limited energy reserves may need more time to recover between caregiving activities, or they may need caregiving spaced out over a longer time frame. Each infant must be evaluated for tolerance levels. Care plans can be individualized based on the infant's response to the stimulation and duration of caregiving activities. (p. 23)

Given that such precautions and specifications are now receiving endorsement from medical and developmental fields, NICU intervention programs focusing on tactile, kinesthetic, and vestibular stimulation are constituting an active area of research and inquiry. In 1986, Field and several colleagues published a study of the effects of tactile-kinesthetic stimulation on preterm neonates. These investigators studied a small sample of 40 premature newborns with a mean gestational age of 31 weeks and a mean birthweight of 1,280 grams. The research included a program of body stroking and passive movements of the limbs for three 15-minute periods per day for 10 days. Field and her colleagues found that, compared with the control group, the experimental group of infants averaged a 47 percent greater weight gain per day, were more active and alert during behavioral observations, showed more mature habituation, orientation, motor, and range of state behavior on *Brazelton's Neonatal Assessment Scale* (Brazelton, 1984), and had hospital stays that were shorter by 6 days. In a follow-up study (Scafidi et al., 1990), the findings were similar. The follow-up study included 40 preterm newborns with a mean gestational age of 30 weeks and a mean birth weight of 1,176 grams. The authors reported an average weight gain per day that was 21 percent greater, a hospital stay that was 5 days shorter, superior performance on habituation items of the *Brazelton Scale*, and greater activity during stimulation versus nonstimulation time. The program for intervention consisted of tactile-kinesthetic massage for three 15-minute periods during 3 consecutive hours per day for a 10-day period, once the infant's condition was stable. Despite the positive outcome, the authors did present several reservations regarding interpretation of the data.

> First, the reader must keep in mind that the infants in this study were healthy preterm infants. The intervention was administered only to medically stable infants in the intermediate care nurseries. Future studies should investigate the use of stimulation with smaller, sicker infants before adopting these programs universally. Second, routine handling of sick premature infants has been associated with hypoxemia (Long, et al. 1980; Speidel, 1978). The effect of tactile/kinesthetic stimulation on the oxygenation of the infant should always be examined by monitoring transcutaneous oxygen. Finally, it is unclear as to when in the infant's development tactile/kinesthetic stimulation would be most beneficial. Future studies should try to determine the most appropriate time for implementing stimulation programs. (pp. 185–186)

The method of kangaroo care, which involves parent-infant skin-to-skin contact, with the newborn wrapped into the parent's chest, is now being used in some form in modern NICUs in the United States. This type of tactile stimulation originated in Bogota, Colombia, in 1979 and has been associated with decreased hospital stays, shorter periods on ventilators, and increased alert states. In addition, some studies have explored mothers' reactions to kangaroo care, revealing a heightened sense of strength, self-esteem, and self-confidence in being able to monitor infant states and cues (Affonso, Wahlberg, & Persson, 1989).

Finally, there have been numerous studies of vestibular stimulation in preterm infants by actual rocking or through waterbed flotation. *Vestibular stimulation,*

which involves movement of the body in space, such as rocking, is closely associated with *kinesthetic stimulation,* which refers to the perception or sense of movement of a portion of the body in space.

Exemplifying research on vestibular stimulation, Korner and her colleagues
have carried out more than a decade of investigation on the use of oscillating
waterbeds. Specifically, these researchers intended to offer intervention that was
"compensating in nature," that would resemble intrauterine conditions, and that
would "supply gentle, passive movements designed to improve the infant's tonus"
(Korner, Kraemer, Haffner, & Cosper, 1975). The authors found that there were
no significant differences between the treatment group and control subjects in
terms of vital signs, weight, or frequency of emesis (vomiting). Yet, all infants
who were treated had significantly fewer apneic episodes than the control infants.
In a follow-up study to further test the reduction of apnea in preterm infants,
Korner, Guilleminault, Van den Hoed, and Baldwin (1978) investigated the effects of waterbed flotation on the sleep and respiratory pattern of eight preterm
infants with apnea. The subjects served as their own controls throughout the
course of intervention. Polygraphic recordings of sleep and respiratory patterns
were taken during a 24-hour period. The results confirmed those of the previous
study and demonstrated that apnea was reduced significantly while the infants
were on waterbeds. Moreover, the researchers found that the most extended apneic episodes and those associated with severe bradycardia showed the greatest
decline in frequency. Occurrences of shorter pauses in respiration and periodic
breathing were not decreased.

In a later study, Korner, Ruppel, and Rho (1982) focused on the influence of
waterbeds on the sleep behavior and motility of preterm infants treated with theophylline. Since sleep levels in theophylline-treated infants are often reduced, the
investigators were interested in determining whether waterbed flotation would
calm such newborns and increase levels of sleep. In a carefully designed study, 17
preterm infants were assessed on days 3 and 4 during treatment and control conditions. As in a prior study, infants served as their own controls. The researchers
reported that the infants displayed significantly more quiet and active sleep,
shorter length of time between periods of sleep, fewer state changes, less restless-
ness during sleep, less waking activity, and fewer jittery movements while on the
waterbed. The duration of theophylline therapy seemed to have a positive effect
on state changes and reductions in wakefulness while infants were on the
waterbeds. Perhaps most importantly, however, Korner and her colleagues found
that theophylline levels, which were considered to be low, did not affect state
changes. Specifically, they found that:

> ... flotation did not reduce residual apnea and bradycardia as it had
> done with two previous samples, composed of infants with uncompli-
> cated apnea of prematurity who were not treated with theophylline.
> Most of the infants in the recent study had protracted ventilator care and

had many more medical complications than the infants in the present study. The infants' failure to respond to waterbed flotation with apnea reduction confirms previous observation that suggests that waterbeds may not be effective in reducing apnea in this type of population. The infants' failure to respond may also have been due to the fact that the incidence of apnea and bradycardia in the theophylline-treated infants was so low that any effects of an additional intervention could not be discerned. (pp. 868–869)

With a somewhat different purpose, Korner, Schneider, and Forrest, in 1983, used a neurobehavioral assessment procedure to assess the impact of proprioceptive (kinesthetic) stimulation on premature neonates. Twenty infants were tested between 34 and 35 weeks post conceptual age. The authors reported that the treatment group demonstrated better skills in attending and pursuing animate and inanimate visual and auditory stimuli, performed with more maturity on spontaneous motor tasks, showed significantly fewer signs of irritability and hypertonicity, and were twice as likely to be in a visually alert, inactive state. Although the authors' conclusions were qualified, these results did support Neal's results (1968), which demonstrated that rocking preterm infants augmented their visual and auditory abilities. In closing, Korner, Schneider, and Forrest (1983) wrote:

We would like to stress that we consider the findings of this study as preliminary. The available sample was small and composed of infants who were critically ill when recruited and who, after selection, had many serious medical complications. Both the test-retest reliabilities and the suggestive evidence that compensatory vestibular-proprioceptive stimulation enhances the neurobehavioral development of preterm infants are therefore in need of replication with a larger and healthier sample of premature babies. (p. 175)

Stated in another way, further research is needed to determine at what point in the development of the high risk newborn various kinesthetic and vestibular interventions can be introduced effectively.

Calming Techniques

Calming techniques have been used in NICUs to minimize the many adverse environmental effects to which premature newborns are exposed daily. Three techniques in particular have been widely used to pacify infants and to promote sleep: positioning, swaddling, and nonnutritive sucking.

Positioning. The full-term infant normally comes into this world with well-developed flexor tone (physiological flexion) of all extremities (Barb & Lemons, 1989). On the other hand, the preterm infant, lacking this maturity, usually presents a pattern of generalized low muscle tone and is likely to assume extended positions of the limbs because of typically prolonged periods in the supine position (Barb & Lemons, 1989). Thus, positioning the infant should be aimed at promoting the development of flexor tone, which was not achieved in utero (Fay, 1988). Developmental specialists have often suggested that, among the options, prone positioning is beneficial for many infants in the NICU (Barb & Lemons, 1989; Fay, 1988). The infant can be positioned lying on one side instead of in a supine position, and rolls can be used to maintain this posture. In addition, placing a roll along the baby's abdominal surface helps to promote a flexion of the trunk and extremities (Mastropaolo, 1992) and offers the child boundaries that simulate the uterine environment. In the past, such issues have often been studied in healthier infants in more stable condition. Departing from this convention, Fox and Molesky (1990) studied partial pressure of arterial oxygen (PaO$_2$) in 25 premature babies with bronchopulmonary dysplasia, on ventilators, in prone and supine positions. The authors found that although no infant was hypoxic in the supine position, significantly higher PaO$_2$ readings were recorded and infants tended to calm more easily in the prone position.

Swaddling. It has been well documented that preterm infants often have a low threshold for stimulation and easily become irritable (Catlett & Holditch-Davis, 1990). Historically, swaddling is a technique found to be effective in promoting sleep and in calming and pacifying infants who are crying and colicky or fussy. Specific to the preterm neonate, specialists have reported benefits of swaddling for increasing oxygenation and decreasing heart rate (Mastropaolo, 1992). Observations in modern NICUs reinforce the continued utility of this simple but beneficial intervention.

Nonnutritive sucking. The third simple and growing technique for calming of the full-term and preterm infant is nonnutritive sucking. For years, mothers and fathers have confirmed the fact that babies who use their fingers, hands, or pacifiers early tend to soothe themselves more easily and quickly. With mounting knowledge and awareness of the impact of pain on the premature neonate, nonnutritive sucking has been adopted more and more in NICUs (Kling, 1989). Although questions remain, Kimble and Dempsey (1992) summarize the several positive effects that have been suggested in various studies.

> Nonnutritive sucking has been found to affect movement, sleep, state regulation and arousal, oxygenation, and nutrition and growth. Its quality is used as an indicator of central nervous system well-being. Speculations have been suggested about improved outcomes from respiratory distress syndrome, patent ductus arteriosus, and necrotizing enterocolitis. The possible effect of sucking movements on attachment between mother and infant has also been described. (p. 32)

As the reader easily can discern from this discussion of intervention strategies for the high risk newborn, there are no clear-cut answers relative to the optimal approach to offering developmental care. As Gorski (1991) has emphasized, "very early intervention programs during NICU hospitalization represent perhaps the boldest recent effort to actively consider and support infant and family development at the beginning of extrauterine life" (p. 1476). Unquestionably, problems of small sample size, short-term follow-up, insufficient descriptions of programing, and other methodological issues have limited the extent of our understanding of very complex issues with respect to the preterm and acutely ill infant, as well as our ability to generalize from findings of such studies. The challenge now lies in taking what we know to be most helpful and harmful and moving forward with further research to address questions, to protect children as individuals, and to enhance opportunities for their having a better start in the first year of life.

INTERVENTION WITH PARENTS

Research focused on the quality and nature of interactions between premature infants and their families has been fertile ground of inquiry over the past two decades (DiVitto & Goldberg, 1979; Field, 1979; Minde, Marton, Manning, & Hines, 1980; Parker, Zahr, Cole, & Brecht, 1992). Findings that parents may feel alienation, lack of control, poor attachment to their babies, sorrow, and tremendous stress should be no surprise. In recent years, however, researchers and developmental specialists have displayed an increasing appreciation of the individual priorities and needs of parents and a heightened sense of the important role that parents play following hospital discharge in guiding the developmental progress and physical well-being of their high risk newborns (Gorski, 1991). New questions about what parents need and feel when their babies are in intensive care are a natural extension of these trends (Bass, 1991; Hummel & Eastman, 1991; Kolotylo, Parker, & Chapman, 1990; McHaffie, 1992; Rogers et al., 1992). New intervention programs directed toward involving parents while infants are in the hospital, preparing for discharge, and assisting families with the transition to home are another result (Affleck, Tennen, Rowe, Roscher, & Walker, 1989; Boggs & LaPrade-Wolf, 1992; Brooten, Gennaro, Knapp, Brown, & York, 1989; Bruder & Walker, 1990; Gennaro, Brooten, & Bakewell-Sachs, 1991; Gennaro, Grisemer, & Musci, 1992; Hanline & Deppe, 1990; Jones, Struk, Hack, & Friedman, 1990; Martino & Pridham, 1992; Norr, Nacion, & Abramson, 1989; Rushton, 1990).

Although the specifics of planning with and for parents vary from model to model, there are common themes in research on intervention in the hospital and during the transition to home care. Five themes have emerged.

First, planning with and for parents toward discharge should start in the hospital and be organized around the individual needs and priorities of a continuum of families. How issues are dealt with in relation to parents of varying cultural backgrounds, the range of educated and less educated mothers and fathers, single caregiver families, and teen parents will require different kinds of support and information and different communication approaches.

Second, working with parents before and after discharge should incorporate teaching about meeting basic infant needs (such as feeding or care during oxygen therapy), as well as developmental concerns.

Third, careful follow-up is an essential component of the discharge process in order to build in continuity and support from hospital to home. In an attempt to augment traditional medical care and established approaches to monitoring infant development and teaching parenting skills, postdischarge services have been offered with a variety of follow-up services including traditional medical models, transitional units, technological assistance models, and public health and community health efforts (Gennaro, Brooten, & Bakewell-Sachs, 1991). With the implementation of Part H of Public Law 99–457 and designation of the health department as lead agency in many states, public health nurses undoubtedly will continue to play a significant role in the delivery of various postdischarge services. While the adoption of this approach is a natural extension of the hospital setting and is appropriate in light of the significant long-term medical and physical requirements of some infants, communities will need to exercise caution to individualize these support services, which must incorporate a strong developmental and educational component. These endeavors will call on the expertise of a variety of disciplines working in close collaboration. To address the complex needs of both infants and families, models will have to be eclectic and adaptable to changing situations.

Fourth, family-focused care during the transition from hospital to home ought to address changes in lifestyle commonly reported by parents of preterm and high risk infants. Among these very real problems are excessive fatigue, loss of sleep, lack of personal time, increased personal responsibilities, and concerns over out-of-control economic burdens. Some issues may be resolved by giving families information about local and state resources, while others will require offering services to support parents in carrying out their substantial commitments in a more personally compatible and self-fulfilling way.

Fifth, linking families to anticipated educational intervention programs prior to hospital discharge is increasingly recognized as best practice (Bruder & Walker, 1990) in building on the tenet of continuity of care.

In all of these aspects of intervention, active involvement of parents in the decision-making process, before and after discharge, is a critical dimension and goal in helping a family to finally gain control after the shock and upheaval of experiencing a premature delivery. There is, in fact, a fine line between offering genuinely needed support and gradually assisting and letting go of families to make the decisions that are rightfully theirs. Ultimately, these objectives will be most readily accomplished by emphasizing the strengths and capacities of families, as opposed to reinforcing their perceptions of what they cannot do. While there are many ways in which the preterm infant and family experiences differ from those associated with the full-term delivery, a basic sense of parents managing their own lives in the process is essential to the well-being and integrity of all concerned.

BIBLIOGRAPHY

Affleck, G., Tennen, A., Rowe, J., Roscher, B., & Walker, L. (1989). Effects of formal support on mothers' adaptation to the hospital-to-home transition of high-risk infants: The benefits and costs of helping. *Child Development, 60,* 488–501.

Affonso, D.D., Wahlberg, V., & Persson, B. (1989). Exploration of mothers' reactions to the kangaroo method of prematurity care. *Neonatal Network, 7*(6), 43–50.

Als, H. (1986). A synactive model of neonatal behavioral organization: Framework for the assessment of neurobehavioral development in the premature infant and for support of infants and parents in the neonatal intensive care environment. *Physical and Occupational Therapy in Pediatrics, 6,* 3–53.

Bada, H.S., Korones, S.B., Perry, E.H., Arheart, K.L., Pourcyrous, M., Runyan, J.W., Anderson, G.D., Magill, H.L., Fitch, C.W., & Somes, G.Wl. (1990). Frequent handling in the neonatal intensive care unit and intraventricular hemorrhage. *Journal of Pediatrics, 117*(1, pt. 1), 126–131.

Barb, S.A., & Lemons, P.K. (1989). The premature infant: Toward improving neurodevelopmental outcome. *Neonatal Network, 7*(6), 7–15.

Bass, L.S. (1991). What do parents need when their infant is a patient in the NICU? *Neonatal Network, 10*(4), 25–33.

Bellig, L.L. (1989). A window on the neonate's brain. *Neonatal Network, 7*(4), 13–20.

Boggs, K.U., & LaPrade-Wolf, P. (1992). Beyond survival: Strategies for establishing a follow-up program for infants treated with extracorporeal membrane oxygenation. *Neonatal Network, 11*(1), 7–13.

Brazelton, T.B. (1984). *The neonatal assessment scale* (2nd ed.). Philadelphia: Lippincott.

Brooten, D., Gennaro, S., Knapp, H., Brown, L., & York, R. (1989). Clinical specialist pre- and postdischarge teaching of parents of very low birth weight infants. *JOGNN, 18*(4), 316–322.

Brown, L. (1987). Physiologic responses to cutaneous pain in neonates. *Neonatal Network, 6,* 18–22.

Bruder, M.B., & Walker, L. (1990). Discharge planning: Hospital to home transitions for infants. *Topics in Early Childhood Special Education, 9*(4), 26–42.

Catlett, A.T., & Holditch-Davis, D. (1990). Environmental stimulation of the acutely ill premature infant: Physiological effects and nursing implications. *Neonatal Network, 8*(6), 19–26.

Chaze, B.A., & Ludington-Hoe, S. (1984). Sensory stimulation in the NICU. *American Journal of Nursing, 84,* 68–71.

Colditz, P.B. (1991). Review article: Management of pain in the newborn infant. *Journal of Paediatric Child Health, 27,* 11–15.

Cole, J.G. (1985). Infant stimulation reexamined: An environmental- and behavioral-based approach. *Neonatal Network, 3*(5), 24–31.

Cole, J.G., & Frappier, P.A. (1985). Infant stimulation reassessed: A new approach to providing care for the preterm infant. *JOGNN, 14,* 471–477.

DeVitto, B., & Goldberg, S. (1979). The effects of newborn medical status on early parent-infant interaction. In T.M. Field, A.M. Sostek, S. Goldberg, & H.H. Shuman (Eds.), *Infants born at risk: Behavior and development* (pp. 311–332). New York: SP Medical & Scientific Books.

Evans, J.C. (1991). Incidence of hypoxemia associated with caregiving in premature infants. *Neonatal Network, 10*(2), 17–24.

Fay, M.J. (1988). The positive effects of positioning. *Neonatal Network, 6*(5), 23–28.

Field, T.M. (1979). Interaction patterns of preterm and term infants. In T.M. Field, A.M. Sostek, S. Goldberg, & H.H. Shuman (Eds.), *Infants born at risk: Behavior and development* (pp. 333–361). New York: SP Medical & Scientific Books.

Field, T.M. (1990). Alleviating stress in newborn infants in the intensive care unit. *Clinics in Perinatology, 17*(1), 1–9.

Field, T.M., Schanberg, S.M., Scafidi, F., Bauer, C.R., Vega-Lahr, N., Garcia, R., Nystrom, J., & Kuhn, C.M. (1986). Tactile/kinesthetic stimulation effects on preterm neonates. *Pediatrics, 77*(5), 654–658.

Fox, M.G., & Molesky, M. (1990). The effects of prone and supine positioning on arterial oxygen pressure. *Neonatal Network, 8*(4), 25–29.

Gardner, S.L., Garland, K.R., Merenstein, S.L., & Merenstein, G.B. (1989). The neonate and the environment: Impact on development. In G.B. Merenstein & S.L. Gardner (Eds.), *Handbook of neonatal intensive care* (pp. 628–675). St. Louis: C.V. Mosby.

Gennaro, S., Brooten, D., & Bakewell-Sachs, S. (1991). Postdischarge services for low-birth-weight infants. *JOGNN, 20*(1), 29–36.

Gennaro, S., Grisemer, A., & Musci, R. (1992). Expected versus actual life-style changes in mothers of preterm low birth weight infants. *Neonatal Network, 11*(3), 39–45.

Glass, P., Avery, G.B., Subramanian, K.N.S., Keys, M.P., Sostek, A.M., & Friendly, D.S. (1985). Effect of bright light in the hospital on incidence of retinopathy of prematurity. *New England Journal of Medicine, 313,* 401–404.

Gorski, P.A. (1991). Developmental intervention during neonatal hospitalization: Critiquing the state of the science. *Pediatric Clinics of North America, 38*(6), 1469–1479.

Gottfried, A.W. (1985). Environment of newborn infants in special care units. In A.W. Gottfried & J.L. Gaiter (Eds.), *Infant stress under intensive care* (pp. 23–54). Baltimore, MD: University Park Press.

Gunderson, L.P., & Kenner, C. (1987). Neonatal stress: Physiologic adaptation and nursing implications. *Neonatal Network, 6*(1), 37–42.

Hanline, M.F., & Deppe, J. (1990). Discharging the premature infant: Family issues and implications for intervention. *Topics in Early Childhood Special Education, 9*(4), 15–25.

Harrison, L. (1985). Effects of early supplemental stimulation programs for premature infants: Review of the literature. *Maternal Child Nursing Journal, 14,* 69–90.

Harrison, L.L., & Woods, S. (1991). Early parental touch and preterm infants. *JOGNN, 20*(4), 299–306.

Hasselmeyer, E.C. (1964). The premature neonate's response to handling. *American Nursing Association, 1,* 15–24.

Holmes, D.L., Reisk, J.N., & Pasternak, J.F. (Eds.) (1984). Causes and correlates of high medical risk in the newborn. *The development of infants born at risk* (pp. 18–46). Hillsdale, NJ: Lawrence Erlbaum.

Hummel, P.A., & Eastman, D.L. (1991). Do parents of preterm infants suffer from chronic sorrow? *Neonatal Network, 10*(4), 59–65.

Jones, S., Struk, C., Hack, M., & Friedman, H. (1990). The premature infant home intervention program. *Caring,* December, 20–21.

Katz, V. (1971). Auditory stimulation and developmental behavior of the preterm infant. *Nursing Research, 20,* 196–201.

Kimble, C., & Dempsey, J. (1992). Nonnutritive sucking: Adaptation and health for the neonate. *Neonatal Network, 11*(2), 29–33.

Kling, P. (1989). Nursing interventions to decrease the risk of periventricular-intraventricular hemorrhage. *JOGNN, 18,* 457–464.

Kolotylo, C.J., Parker, N.I., & Chapman, J.S. (1990). Mother's perceptions of their neonates' in-hospital transfers from a neonatal intensive-care unit. *JOGNN, 20*(2), 146–153.

Korner, A.F., Guilleminault, C., Van den Hoed, M.D., & Baldwin, R.B. (1978). Reduction of sleep apnea and bradycardia in preterm infants on oscillating water beds: A controlled polygraphic study. *Pediatrics, 61,* 528–534.

Korner, A.F., Kraemer, H.C., Haffner, M.E., & Cosper, L.M. (1975). Effects of waterbed flotation on premature infants: A pilot study. *Pediatrics, 56,* 361–367.

Korner, A.F., Ruppel, E.M., & Rho, J.M. (1982). Effects of waterbeds on the sleep and motility of theophylline-treated preterm infants. *Pediatrics, 70,* 864–869.

Korner, A.F., Schneider, P., & Forrest, T. (1983). Effects of vestibular-proprioceptive stimulation on the neurobehavioral development of preterm infants: A pilot study. *Neuropediatrics, 14,* 170–175.

Kramer, L.I., & Pierpont, M.E. (1976). Rocking waterbeds and auditory stimuli to enhance growth of preterm infants. *Journal of Pediatrics, 88,* 297–299.

LaRossa, M.M., & Brown, J.V. (1982). Foster grandmothers in the premature nursery. *American Journal of Nursing, 82,* 1834–1835.

Leib, S.A., Benfield, D.G., & Guidubaldi, J. (1980). Effect of early intervention and stimulation of the preterm infant. *Pediatrics, 66,* 63–90.

Lester, B.M., & Tronick, E. (Eds.). (1990). Introduction: Guidelines for stimulation with preterm infants. *Clinics in Perinatology: Stimulation and the Preterm Infant, 17*(1), xiii–xvii.

Linn, P.L., Horowitz, F.D., & Fox, H.A. (1985). Stimulation in the NICU: Is more necessarily better? *Clinics in Perinatology, 12,* 407–422.

Long, J.G., Lucey, J.F., & Philip, A.G.S. (1980). Noise and hypoxemia in the intensive care nursery. *Pediatrics, 65,* 143–145.

Lott, J.W. (1989). Developmental care of the preterm infant. *Neonatal Network, 7*(4), 21–28.

Martino, R.J., & Pridham, K.F. (1992). Early experiences of parents feeding their infants with bronchopulmonary dysplasia. *Neonatal Network, 11*(3), 23–29.

Mastropaolo, A. (1992). The at risk infant: Medical insult and intervention. Unpublished lecture delivered in course at Syracuse University School of Education, Special Education Programs, Syracuse, NY.

McHaffie, H.E. (1992). Social support in the neonatal intensive care unit. *Journal of Advanced Nursing, 17,* 279–287.

Meisels, S.J. (1985). The efficacy of early intervention: Why are we still asking this question? *Topics in Early Childhood Special Education, 5,* 1–11.

Minde, K., Marton, P., Manning, D., & Hines, B. (1980). Some determinants of mother-infant interaction in the premature nursery. *Journal of the American Academy of Child Psychiatry, 19,* 1–21.

Neal, M. (1968). Vestibular stimulation and the development behavior of the small premature infant. *Nursing Research Reports, 3,* 2–5.

Norr, K.F., Nacion, K.W., & Abramson, R. (1989). Early discharge with home follow-up: Impacts on low-income mothers and infants. *JOGNN, 18*(2), 133–141.

Norris, S., Campbell, L.A., & Brenkert, S. (1982). Nursing procedures and alterations in transcutaneous oxygen tension in premature infants. *Nursing Research, 31*(6), 330–336.

O'Donnell, J. (1990). The development of a climate for caring: A historical review of premature care in the United States from 1900 to 1979. *Neonatal Network, 8*(6), 7–17.

Oehler, J.M. (1985). Examining the issue of tactile stimulation for preterm infants. *Neonatal Network, 4,* 25–32.

Parker, S.J., Zahr, L.K., Cole, J.G., & Brecht, M. (1992). Outcome after developmental intervention in the neonatal intensive care unit for mothers of preterm infants with low socioeconomic status. *Journal of Pediatrics, 120*(5), 780–785.

Peabody, J.L., & Lewis, K. (1985). Consequences of newborn intensive care. In A.W. Gottfried & J.L. Gaiter (Eds.), *Infant stress under intensive care* (pp. 199–226). Baltimore, MD: University Park Press.

Rogers, B.T., Booth, L.J., Duffy, L.C., Hasson, M.B., McCormick, P., Snitzer, J., & Zorn, W.A. (1992). Parents' developmental perceptions and expectations for their high risk infants. *Journal of Developmental and Behavioral Pediatrics, 13*(2), 102–107.

Rushton, C.H. (1990). Strategies for family-centered care in the critical care setting. *Pediatric Nursing, 16*(2), 195–199.

Scafidi, F.A., Field, T.M., Schanberg, S.M., Bauer, C.R., Tucci, K., Roberts, J., Morrow, C., & Kuhn, C.M. (1990). *Infant Behavior and Development, 13,* 167–188.

Shaefer, M., Hatcher, R.P., & Barlow, P.D. (1980). Prematurity and infant stimulation: A review of research. *Child Psychiatry and Human Development, 10,* 199–212.

Schmidt, K., Rose, S.A., & Bridger, W.H. (1980). The effect of heartbeat sound on the cardiac and behavioral responsiveness to tactile stimulation in sleeping premature. *Developmental Psychology, 16,* 175–184.

Schultz, M.C. (1992). Nursing roles: Optimizing premature infant outcomes. *Neonatal Network, 11*(3), 9–13.

Schultz, M.C. (1987). Hearing screening. In T.W. Taeusch & M. W. Yogman (Eds.), *Follow-up management of the high-risk infant* (pp. 109–114). Boston: Little, Brown.

Segal, M.V. (1972). Cardiac responsivity to auditory stimulation in preterm infants. *Nursing Research, 21,* 15–19.

Solkoff, N., & Matuszak, D. (1975). Tactile stimulation and behavioral development among low birthweight infants. *Child Psychiatry and Human Development, 6,* 33–39.

Spinelli, D.N. (1990). Plasticity triggering experiences, nature, and the dual genesis of brain structure and function. *Clinics in Perinatology: Stimulation and the Preterm Infant, 17*(1), 77–82.

Tichy, A.M., Braam, C.M., Meyer, T.A., & Rattan, N.S. (1988). Stressors in pediatric intensive care units. *Pediatric Nursing, 14*(1), 40–42.

Chapter 17

One Nursery: A Scenario of Change

Anne C. Mastropaolo, Larry Consenstein, and James J. Pergolizzi, III

PAIN

Imagine that you are an infant, born sick, frail, and 8 weeks premature. You have an abnormal white blood cell count, which raises suspicion of infection. Despite the fact that you have just been through the trauma of delivery, are chilled in a delivery room that has bright lights and noise, you are now subjected to one or more necessary but painful procedures. Often these experiences include needle punctures for blood drawing and the administration of intravenous fluid. In addition, you may be curled into a ball and have a needle placed between your vertebrae to obtain spinal fluid to complete your "sepsis work-up," or you are awake and alert as a tube is placed through your mouth and into your trachea. You cannot scream or cry, but you are conscious of every sound, every light, and each painful stimulus. The scenario goes on, on, and on . . . .

If you were an adult or even a small child, you would stand a better chance than most neonates of receiving analgesia to alleviate the pain and anesthesia to make the experience less stressful. The rationale for such situations is somewhat understandable but never defensible (see Figure 17–1).

Historically, our knowledge of the function of anesthesia and analgesia, as well as the technology for administration, has been limited for neonates. For those who were critically ill, hemodynamically unstable, or very tiny, it was thought that anesthesia and analgesia would jeopardize survival. *Anesthesia* is defined as a total loss of sensation, especially the sense of touch. General anesthesia for surgery results in loss of consciousness as well as sensation. Anesthetics, such as halothane, may cause hypotension and bradycardia in infants who are critically ill. *Analgesia* is defined as the loss of sensibility to pain. Analgesics, such as morphine, may induce respiratory depression and "withdrawal." Fear of these drug effects, even though they are rare, compounded by the myth that neonates cannot perceive pain, has delayed our ability to "do the right thing" (Rogers, 1992).

Berry and Gregory (1987) reviewed several published studies promulgating the concept that babies do not experience pain. He cited a study (McGraw, 1941) that suggested little or no response to a pin prick of the heel by full-term infants in the first week of life. The study results indicated further that infants developed increasingly appropriate responses, but not until the 3rd month of life. Gross and Gardner (1982) showed that twice as much electrical stimulation was needed to produce a given response in a 1-day-old newborn as in a 3-month-old infant. The findings of these studies and others suggested that neonates and older infants could not perceive pain. In recent years, however, these and similar studies have been found flawed as a result of poor controls, lack of stimulus standardization, and inappropriate definition of response to stimuli.

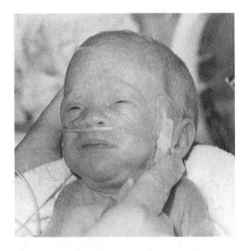

Change emerged in the early 1980s when researchers began to differentiate the cries of pain from the cries of hunger and discomfort (Levine & Gordan, 1982). For example, Williamson and Williamson (1983) used changes in physiological variables such as heart rate, respiratory rate, and blood oxygenation to define the pain response in

Figure 17–1 Infant in pain

infants undergoing circumcision with or without anesthesia. Anand and Hickey (1987), in the *New England Journal of Medicine*, reviewed over 200 published studies of pain and its effects on the human neonate and fetus. These authors summarized the physiological changes and behavioral responses associated with pain in the neonate. Their report helped to alter many unfounded beliefs regarding the newborn's *presumed* inadequate anatomical pathways for pain perception. In many of the 200 studies researchers suggested that nociceptive nerve endings or sensory receptors, which initiate the transmission of painful stimuli are decreased or absent from the skin in babies. Decreased myelination in a premature infant was proposed to support the argument that neonates could not perceive pain. To the contrary, it has now been shown that the synaptic connections all the way to the cortex, where the pain is perceived, are functional but not completely myelinated by midgestation. Anand and Hickey (1987) also reviewed articles demonstrating that neurochemical transmission of painful stimuli in neonates was probable, through high levels of substance P and substance P receptors. In addition, these investigators cited studies showing that beta-endorphin, which is known to modulate pain and to be produced in response to stress, is present in the blood of neonates at levels inadequate to produce analgesia (see Table 17–1).

In 1987, several articles in the medical literature demonstrated the relative safety of adequate neonatal anesthesia. For instance, Anand, Sippell, and Aynsley-Green (1987) demonstrated that there were, in fact, deleterious effects

---

Table 17–1 Development of Pain Perception*

Anatomic Development

Sensory Receptors	Neonates have as many as or more than are present in adults.
Myelination of Peripheral Nerve Fibers	Lack of myelination implies slower impulse conduction; however, slower transmission is offset by shorter distances to travel in neonates.
Spinal Cord Synapses	Development begins before 14 weeks gestation and is completed by 30 weeks gestation.
Myelination of Ascending Pathways	Myelination is completed in spinal cord, brainstem, and thalamus by 30 weeks gestation above thalamus to cortex and completed by 37 weeks gestation.
Cortex	Synaptic connection to afferent nerve axons established at 20 to 24 weeks gestation; cortical sensory evoked potentials elicited before 30 weeks gestation.

Development of Neurochemical Systems

Pain Transmission	Substance P appears early in fetal development (12 to 16 weeks gestation), and levels of substance P and receptors are higher in neonates than in adults.
Pain Modulation	Beta-endorphin is produced in response to stress in both fetus and neonate, but levels are much lower than those needed to produce analgesia.

* Based on information in Anand, K.J.S., & Hickey, P.R. (1987). Pain and its effects in the human neonate and fetus. *New England Journal of Medicine, 317,* 1321–1329. Reprinted with permission in Gordon (1990).

and a *worse outcome* for neonates not adequately anesthetized for surgery. Not only are neonates allowed to experience pain unnecessarily, but this experience is also potentially dangerous. Even today, the use of anesthetics and analgesics for painful procedures outside the operating room is not common practice.

In a recent survey of 35 neonatal intensive care units (NICUs), Bauchner, May, and Coates (1992) found that fewer than 10 percent used analgesia for invasive procedures such as intravenous cannulation, venipuncture, and lumbar puncture. Less than 27 percent cited the use of analgesia for even more stressful procedures such as paracentesis and arterial catheter insertion. In essence, little or no analgesia is being used in NICUs for many invasive procedures.

Bauchner and colleagues (1992) further describe the scenario of the critically ill newborn who was believed to be too "unstable" to tolerate anesthesia. As we have noted, anesthesia is used routinely in critically ill adults and children. Safe analgesics are available for infants with most medical conditions. However, many medical professionals who take care of neonates use explanations or excuses: "I can do the procedure more quickly without local anesthesia," or "Why stick the baby twice [first with lidocaine] when I can get the lumbar puncture on the first attempt without it?"

Babies are among the most vulnerable patients because of their inability to speak and act as advocates for themselves. Their cries of pain are often thought to be indistinguishable from their cries of hunger. At worst, their responses habituate into complete silence, as they withdraw or "shut down." Finally, their ability to complain is frequently impaired by medications (sedatives), which actually may accentuate their pain. The common excuse is well described in a quote from Rogers (1992) in the *New England Journal of Medicine* when he states: "It seems that we are better able to tolerate an infant's pain than to deal with our own discomfort and insecurity about the correct manner and dose of pain medication to give the infant" (pp. 55–56). These issues and others have been at the heart of the scenario of change at St. Joseph's Hospital (Syracuse, New York) over the past decade.

DEVELOPMENT OF THE NEONATAL INTENSIVE CARE UNIT (NICU)

History

St. Joseph's Hospital had a Level Two neonatal nursery, with the regional NICU center housed in a neighboring institution. The hospital administration always has had a commitment, which still remains, to the development of an improved NICU in St. Joseph's Hospital. During the course of several years, although the primary focus was improving the quality of the technical care provided, many new and valuable lessons have been learned from the staff, the parents, and the babies themselves. Our understanding of the baby as a part of a vital structure, the family unit, has grown and become the centerpiece of a new philosophy and blueprint for care in St. Joseph's NICU. We discuss here how this nursery has evolved toward having a more sensitive view of the needs of the newborn and his or her family and how this view has been incorporated into the structure and function of the present NICU nursery.

Environment

The first neonatal intensive care nurseries were designed to cluster specialized equipment in one area and to provide staff who had developed skills and experience necessary to use this equipment and understand the needs of the newborn patient. The model for these settings was the adult critical care unit, rather than the hospital nursery for normal newborns or the baby's nursery in the home. Areas were created to provide the greatest access to the patient and to ensure a clear view of the baby and the monitoring devices. These conditions resulted in brightly lit areas with flashing and beeping monitors surrounding each patient. Babies were placed in open beds, on their backs, with overhead warmers. Often, music played in the background, competing with the loud voices of the staff, and infants were reduced to depersonalized objects, whose physiological problems were monitored closely. The parents of these children frequently were viewed as being in the way, somehow interfering with the high energy flow of the unit, bringing a sometimes unwanted pathos into this surreal scene.

Nursing staff caring for ill newborns are a special group (see Figure 17–2). They frequently are drawn to this field by their concern for the infants or their need for an intense and challenging job experience. The potential exists for them to become mother surrogates, jealously guarding their patient from harm, because so much depends on their abilities to keep track of every detail of the child's care and to be sensitive to every change in condition.

To help cope with the death of an ill child and to deal with the suffering seen daily, medical professionals and parents develop defenses (Tyson & Speaks, 1987). Unfortunately, these defenses may serve to create a wall between the child and the natural parents. In their grief and worry, the natural caregivers may live as if in a fugue state. Thoughts may become ephemeral and feelings overwhelming. The invisible bond between parent and baby remain, but Mom is unable to access her baby, particularly in the beginning of the hospital course. The need to hold, to comfort, and to nurse is both overpowering and unobtainable. During the time the baby is hospitalized, which may extend for weeks or months, the parents may concede control and feel incapable of regaining it on their own. Later, there are other ramifications. Confident caregivers may try to re-establish control, which occasionally results in conflict with the nursing staff. Parents with less of a sense of self, those who are younger, or those without adequate social skills or emotional

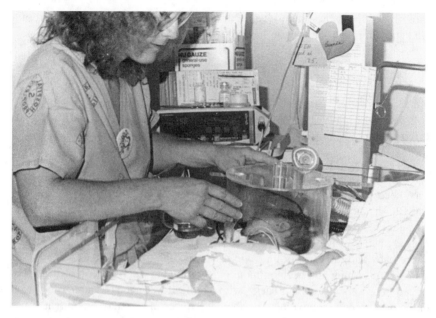

Figure 17–2 Nurse with infant at St. Joseph's NICU

support, may withdraw from the situation, becoming increasingly alienated from the child. In any case, the period when an infant is in the NICU is a difficult time.

Infection Control: Barriers to Visiting and Handling Newborns

In the early part of this century, physicians became aware of the significance of the spread of infection from person to person. Because the newborn has been long recognized as particularly vulnerable to disease, extensive precautions have been taken to prevent infection. Nurses and physicians have been draped with caps and long gowns and have used vigorous hand washing. Until very recently, other individuals have been prevented from entering the nursery, unless appropriately gowned. While a sensitivity to the risks of the spread of infection is important, this ritual has served also to further isolate the baby from the family and to set the NICU and its staff apart as a separate, exclusive world. More recent data have demonstrated that, if family members use careful hand washing, the greatest risk of infection comes from within the hospital, rather than from those dressed in street clothes (Umphenour, 1980). However, certain contagious infections such as human immunodeficiency virus (HIV) and hepatitis have necessitated that precautions be used. These measures follow a rigidly prescribed code of behavior, depending on the particular risk of exposure.

LESSONS LEARNED

Observation of patient care and suffering, family and staff interactions, as well as a new sensitivity to the needs of all, have led, in general, to a transformation in NICUs. Sporadically, articles in the medical literature have examined the effects of environmental factors on the development of the preterm infant (Als, 1982; Als et al., 1986; Cole, Begish-Duddy, Judas, & Jorgensen, 1990). Constantly juxtaposed to the stark reality of the NICU was the image of the fetus protected within the natural environment of the womb, floating in amniotic fluid and aware of light and dark and of sound muted by the natural insulation of the womb. Suspended, the baby moves and kicks against walls; sensation is modulated and temperature regulated. And then there is the sudden transition to the delivery room and then to the NICU—bright, loud, harsh, and painful.

The acquisition of a specialist in newborn development, in our case a physical therapist, was the key to changes in philosophy and in our treatment of newborns and families at St. Joseph's Hospital. At first, it was a difficult task to convince the hospital administrators about the importance of this position, since many of the services were not reimbursable. Through constant and gentle instruction, however, the NICU has become a different environment. The nursing staff for some time had been aware of the signals the babies were sending about their care. Even though infants are unable to speak, the furrowed brow, mottled skin, or high-pitched cry were recognized by experienced staff as signs of discomfort. For years, the staff had sublimated these observations, focusing on the necessities of caregiving techniques, viewing infant responses as inevitable outcomes.

Change required a sequence of steps. First, a consensus had to be reached among the nursing staff. Through a series of educational meetings with the neonatologists, nurse managers, the developmental specialist, and nurse practitioners, gradual acceptance was developed for the need to modify ways of caring for babies and their families. A stepwise plan was developed. It was recognized that the nursing staff needed to embrace these concepts through a deeper understanding of baby cues. Staff needed to understand behavioral states, the fragility of the nervous system, and the physiological ramifications of the disruption of the natural cycles of the child. With this knowledge, they would be both better able to communicate with their patients and would be more skilled in teaching parents about their unique children. Once this level of understanding was internalized after approximately 1 year, the next stage began.

Recognizing the significance of the various states the baby experiences (Brazelton, 1973) and dealing with the frequent disruptions the child endures (often more than 100 times within 24 hours), the medical staff initiated a policy of clustering care. At much less frequent intervals, the baby would have vital signs taken, blood drawn, and diapers and positions changed. After such a cluster of procedures, the infant would then be left alone again to return to sleep. A greater reliance was placed on technology. Instruments were used that allowed for minimal irritation in the monitoring of blood oxygen levels, heart and respiratory rates, blood pressure, and temperature. Like other NICUs across the country, routine care changed. Instead of inflating a blood pressure cuff, the nurse took the blood pressure reading from a transducer connected to the arterial line and, in especially unstable infants, the stethoscope was placed on the chest only when clinically necessary; heart and respiratory rates were read from the monitors. This sensitivity to the newborn's state continued during convalescence. It was a good experience for the staff, because they felt more in touch with the patient. Meanwhile, in the literature, more data (Als et al., 1986) which demonstrated the benefits of stage-appropriate stimulation were presented. Babies in the NICU grew faster, had fewer complications, and left the hospital sooner.

To make the environment more compatible with philosophical changes, physical modifications also were made. The radio went first, and there was no more loud background music in the NICU. Patient rounds were conducted either outside the unit or at some distance from the bedside, in consciously subdued conversation. Monitor alarms were linked to each other, the volume was decreased, and call lights were placed at each bedside to alert staff to problems. Bright fluorescent lights were all but eliminated and were replaced with incandescent lights controlled by dimmers at each bedside. Thus, a diurnal (day and night) cycle was established. Although there is little *hard* experimental evidence that establishment of a diurnal cycle is a direct benefit to babies, it seems teleological that such a pattern is part of their natural extrauterine cycle and, therefore, likely to be more appropriate. In addition, there is evidence that such environmental changes are helpful to a staff who work nights, allowing better adaptation and less stress (Thomas, 1989).

Protocol for Pain

In our continued efforts to manage neonatal pain, we have begun, by education and practice, to incorporate new principles into the structure and function of our NICU. Everyone involved in the care of the newborn—neonatologist, nurse, nurse practitioner, infant developmental specialist, house officer, and parent—is being educated formally and informally in the assessment of pain and appropriate interventions. The formal education component focuses on teaching behavioral cues and physiological and biochemical indicators of pain. Specific caregiving measures that include both pharmacological and nonpharmacological interventions are a critical part of the program (see Exhibit 17–1). Such measures are being achieved through in-service education, and have been incorporated into the standard orientation of all new staff. A nursing policy that addresses pain management has been developed. Informally, these principles are addressed daily during patient rounds and reinforced by role modeling. However, many challenges still remain before the treatment of neonates is elevated consistently to even the minimal level of adult patient care.

Exhibit 17–1 The NICU Protocol for Pain: St. Joseph's Hospital, Syracuse, New York

Goals of Pain Management

1. To minimize the intensity, duration, and physiological cost of the pain experience
2. To maximize the infant's ability to cope with and recover from the painful experience

Considerations in Pain Assessment

1. An infant's motor function is very immature and responses to stimuli such as pain are generalized and easily modified by environmental influences.
2. Absence of a response does not indicate lack of pain.
3. Response to painful stimuli may be delayed or cumulative. (The infant may appear to tolerate several procedures well and then exhibit signs of compromise and increased oxygen requirements in the absence of further stimuli.)
4. There may be no response to noxious stimuli in the very immature or very stressed infant. (The immature central nervous system has a limited ability to withstand stress—the absence of response may only indicate the depletion of response capability rather than the lack of perception.)

I. *Behavioral*
   A. Vocalization
      1. crying
      2. whimpering
   B. Facial expressions
      1. grimacing
      2. furrowing of brow
      3. quivering of chin
   C. Bodily movements
      1. limb withdrawal, thrashing
      2. clenching of fists
      3. rigidity versus flaccidity (in critically ill or very premature infant)
   D. State
      1. changes in sleep/wake cycles
      2. changes in activity level
      3. fussiness
      4. listlessness
II. *Physiological*
   a. increased heart rate
   b. increased blood pressure
   c. increased respiratory rate
   d. shallow respirations
   e. increased muscle tension
   f. pallor
   g. flushing
   h. diaphoresis
   i. palmar sweating
   j. decreased Tc PO_2 blood oxygen saturation
   k. dilated pupils
III. *Biochemical*
   a. hyperglycemia
   b. increased serum cortisol levels

continues

Exhibit 17–1 Continues

Nonpharmacological Measures to Reduce Pain

Goal: To arrange the environment so that the neonate can use internal and external resources to organize behavior and learn self-soothing techniques

Measures

1. Protect from light
   a. Shade infant's eyes with diaper or eyepatches.
   b. Cover isolette with blanket.
   c. Cover top of open crib with blanket.
2. Protect from noise
   a. Close incubator doors gently.
   b. Pad trash can lids.
   c. Minimize overall noise.
   d. Conduct rounds away from bedside.
3. Protect from overstimulation
   a. Cluster nursing care.
   b. Allow maximum downtime between care activities.
   c. Contain limbs during suctioning.
4. Provide boundaries
   a. Place in prone position or side lying.
   b. Swaddle, cover, or wrap the infant.
   c. Tuck blanket rolls around sides or back, and feet.
   d. Provide objects to suck or grasp.

Pain Management Guidelines

1. Analgesics are most effective when administered *before* pain reaches its peak. Waiting until there are recognizable pain cues results in
   a. undue suffering for the infant
   b. delay between onset of pain and relief
2. Barbiturates (phenobarbital) frequently produce hyperalgesia and increased reaction to painful stimuli; therefore, they are contraindicated for patients who have pain and also require sedation.
3. Neonates should *never* be treated for pain with sedatives or paralytic agents (e.g., Pavulon) unless an analgesic is administered concurrently.
4. Frequent and prolonged pain may have potentially harmful long-term consequences to the developing central nervous system.
5. Parents need to be reassured that their babies are not suffering unduly and that nurses and physicians are sensitive to the concept of pain. Parents should be encouraged to assist with nonpharmacological measures to reduce pain and discomfort.
6. Parents have a right to withhold consent for invasive procedures or surgery, contingent on the use of analgesic and/or anesthesic agents.

Note: TC P_{O_2} = transcutaneous partial pressure of oxygen.

FAMILY-CENTERED CARE AND DISCHARGE PLANNING

Clearly, having a sick newborn is extremely stressful. Parents experience grief, fear, anger, and loss of control, initially in the face of physical exhaustion and sorrow. Maintaining the natural bonds between the caregivers and the baby is part of the total care necessary for the newborn's best outcome. Many techniques to address this need should be incorporated into the daily routine.

Communication

For the family to feel part of the process of helping their child to recover, they should be fully informed of the patient's progress and problems (Perlman et al., 1991). (The "family" often includes extended family members and close friends.) Early in the process the family are often not knowledgeable about the medical issues and are stressed almost to the breaking point and physically put off by the hospital and the equipment itself. Thus, staff must begin slowly and simply. It is essential to first address the major issues: the risk of death or long-term morbidity. Information must be shared with the family even when the risks appear minimal. Presenting information with few scientific terms, in a realistically positive light, is important. For example, although a baby may be critically ill, the risk of death often is less than 10 percent. To counsel a family to be optimistic is not unrealistic, and they should be reassured that changes in their baby's course will be explained as they occur.

Maintaining a team approach to communication with the family is important. Since the physician cannot be present at all interactions with the family, it is essential that every member of the team be knowledgeable about the child's condition. Thus, instead of the family's being told by the nurse that they must wait to talk with a physician, the nurse may give up-to-date information about the hospital course. This kind of communication supplements ongoing teaching of the family about the basic medical issues. To accomplish this goal, daily physician rounds are attended by the bedside nurses, and this interaction results in a valuable exchange of information.

Visiting Policies

As we have noted, early theories of infection control prevented easy access to the NICU (Umphenour, 1980). Visiting policies precluded regular contact with the baby by the family, enhancing isolation and accentuating family stress. More recently, true risks have been identified. The importance of family involvement has been established philosophically (Lewis et al., 1991), and new NICU policies now allow almost unlimited visiting hours. Only the number of persons visiting at any one time is restricted, on the basis of space limitations. Provided that precautions are taken to minimize the risk of certain infections, siblings are now allowed to visit their baby brothers or sisters (Schwab, Tolbert, Bagnato, & Maisels, 1983). These practices may allay sibling fears and allow other children in the family to become part of the entire experience (Craft, Wyatt, & Sandell, 1985) (see Exhibit 17–2).

Exhibit 17-2 St. Joseph's Hospital-Health Center

General Policy for Visiting

1. Parents, grandparents, and siblings are allowed in the hallway of the Special Care Nursery.
2. Parent(s) may visit at any time.
3. With consent from the parents, grandparents may visit daily. Visits at the bedside may be limited to 15 minutes.
4. A primary support person for a single mother may visit at any time.
5. Only two visitors per baby are allowed in the nursery at one time because of limited space and in order to provide a quiet environment for the babies.
6. Parents are encouraged to hold their baby, providing he/she is not in critical, unstable condition. Otherwise, they are able to touch their baby on the warmer or through the portholes of the isolette.
7. The sibling visiting policy applies to brothers and sisters of the new baby. All siblings free of infection will be allowed to visit the nursery. Visitation at the bedside will be limited to 15 minutes.

Infection Control

1. All visitors must be free of any signs or symptoms of illness and/or infection.
2. Handwashing—All visitors are to wash hands thoroughly.
3. Gown—All visitors, prior to entering the nursery room, must put on a clean gown.
4. All siblings, before entering the nursery, must scrub and put on a gown, gloves, and mask.
5. Cameras are allowed in the nursery; hands must be washed between use and handling of the baby.

Policies on Holding the Newborn

Now that parents are viewed as a more significant part of their newborn's care, the importance of *holding* has emerged. Although there are times during the early and most critical stages of care that being held may be detrimental to the infant (Bada et al., 1990), this phase passes quickly.

If time out of the incubator is limited, and an infant's temperature is taken after a short duration, even tiny babies of less than 1,000 grams may be held briefly by their parents (see Exhibit 17–3). Close attention must be paid to temperature regulation in preterm infants. If babies are somewhat chilled, they burn extra calories to remain warm, which interferes with growth, and if they are allowed to get too cold, dangerous physiological changes may occur.

Holding is another step toward including caregivers in the process of caring for the newborn; it also enhances attachment and re-establishes the closeness experienced before birth—a clear benefit to the baby. Another important aspect of holding infants has been demonstrated by the practice known as *kangaroo care*, which

Exhibit 17–3 Policy for Parental Holding and Kangaroo Care of Infants Weighing 1,000 to 1,500 Grams

---

Conditions
1. Approval by attending physician
2. Temperature stable
3. Vital signs stable

Rationale
1. Increases parent-infant attachment
2. Addresses parent need to be involved in caregiving
3. Provides pleasant tactile stimulation
4. Enhances possibility of shortened hospital stay and improved weight gain, as indicated by some study results

Intervention
1. Discuss with parents; explain risks versus benefits.
2. Place baby blanket and hat inside incubator 30 minutes prior to holding.
3. Obtain vital signs, which must be within normal limits, with temperature between 36°C and 37°C.
4. Keep apnea/bradycardia monitor, temperature probe, and oximeter in place, as applicable.
5. Wrap in heated blanket with warm hat on or place on parent's chest and cover with blanket.
6. Place in parent's arms; encourage cuddling and holding close.
7. Observe infant throughout holding.
8. Limit maximum holding time to 10 minutes, 2 times a day. Holding time may be increased with improvement.
9. Return baby to isolette at any signs of distress.

Follow-up
1. Recheck temperature on return to isolette.
2. Call house officer or nurse practitioner for temperature less than 36°C.
3. Reinforce with parents how procedure was tolerated by their infant. Be sure to reinforce with parents whose child does not tolerate holding that the child's response is not a rejection of them and that holding will be tried again.
4. Record vital signs, especially temperature, after kangaroo care.

---

is discussed in Chapter 16 (see Figures 17–3 and 17–4). This intervention entails the daily holding of the infant in skin-to-skin contact with the parent. It has been shown that, during such periods, infant breathing becomes more regular and parents are able to maintain a perfect thermostat to regulate their baby's temperature. Newborns who experience this practice have been shown to grow better and to have shorter hospital stays (Affonso, Wahlberg, & Persson, 1989).

Discharge Planning

If the infant patient is viewed as part of a continuum that begins with the family and evolves through the hospital course to the start of life at home, several issues

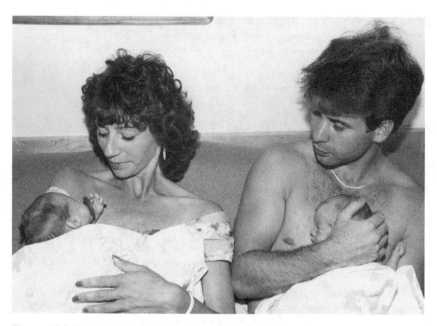

Figure 17-3 Mother and father doing kangaroo care with twins

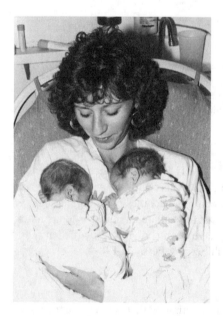

Figure 17-4 Mother with twins

relevant to discharge must be addressed during the hospitalization. These issues include temperature control, nutrition, stable medical conditions, and adequate home environment. Traditionally, it has been the purview of the nursing staff to teach parents various aspects of infant care prior to discharge. As hospital reimbursement practices have changed (Resnick et al., 1986), institutions have felt more pressure to discharge patients sooner, often requiring services that previously were offered only in the hospital to be provided in the home. If a child were to go home needing special equipment such as oxygen or apnea monitors, the specialized teaching required would often be the responsibility of the hospital nursing staff. Such training and preparation cost money, with hospital expenditures that are often hundreds of thousands of dollars (Phibbs, Phibbs, Pomerance, & Williams, 1986). It soon became clear at St. Joseph's Hospital that families were having difficulties in finding their way through the maze of agencies and funding sources in order to access the financial aid resources available to them.

The role of our discharge coordinator grew out of a need to link inputs from all relevant sources and to provide a liaison with the family so that their voice would become an essential part of the discharge process. The coordinator in the nursery thus serves as family advocate, offering experienced guidance throughout the hospitalization and during the discharge process. In our unit, a nurse has filled this role well, but a skilled parent who has been through the process could bring special qualities to such a position. Familiarity with nursing procedures and an ability to relate to parents are two essential skills. Another important aspect of this responsibility involves keeping abreast of changes in funding regulations and new program development and bringing information back to the nursery. Indeed, such an individual may become a force for change, with a sensitivity to the needs of the family and to the gaps in the system.

INFANT FOLLOW-UP PROGRAM

Infants who experience catastrophic illness or who are born prematurely are at risk for developmental delay. Perinatal risk factors such as intracranial hemorrhage or perinatal asphyxia are frequently compounded by social risk factors (e.g., low socioeconomic status or teenage pregnancy). At St. Joseph's Hospital, infants discharged from the nursery are assigned to one of four categories:

- Group A—no significant increased risk
- Group B—increased risk but no identifiable developmental or neuromotor abnormalities
- Group C—high risk, with subtle abnormalities
- Group D—abnormal with definite neuromotor abnormalities.

After discharge, babies in groups B, C, and D have follow-up in our Infant Follow-up Program. Group B has follow-up at 6 months, adjusted age, and group C at 2 to 4 months after discharge. Infants in Group D are referred directly into an early education program but are given the option of a follow-up appointment at 6 months, adjusted age. Routine follow-up occurs at 6, 12, and 24 months after the initial visit and at age 4 to 6 years. At the 6- and 12-month visits, babies are evaluated by the developmental specialist who saw the infant in the hospital, and one of several standardized developmental screening tests is administered. At 24 months, the *Bayley Scales of Infant Development* are used for evaluation; if further assessment is necessary, it is done by other members of the follow-up team, which includes speech and occupational therapists and a psychologist. A key aspect of the St. Joseph's program is that we emphasize s*ervice rather than developmental screening alone.* Parents of high risk newborns often harbor deep fears about the outcome for their children, and they struggle with perceptions of real or imagined problems. Developmental screening can easily be combined with support and encouragement to reinforce education and to give families important help for the future.

INFANTS AND FAMILIES: FURTHER IMPLICATIONS FOR INTERVENTION

In brief review, development is a complex process, and humans have a great capacity for plasticity. Although this ability may provide the advantage of greater adaptability, it also results in special vulnerabilities, which in the case of the preterm infant are particularly significant for optimal long-term development. Compared with full-term infants, preterm infants undergo a unique experience in development. During the first 40 weeks following conception, the fragile fetus is ideally situated within the womb. Developmentally, the womb serves a dual role: It provides safety from harmful forms of external stimuli, as well as affording a source of gentle, rhythmic stimuli. Extrauterine life is possible as early as 24 to 25 weeks following conception. During the time between a preterm birth and the natural 40-week gestation, the premature infant is exposed to stimuli that contrast sharply with those provided during uterine life. As we discussed earlier, preterm infants cared for in the NICU may be exposed to high levels of light and sound. Most of the touching experienced by the baby takes place during medical and nursing procedures, rather than being associated with parental bonding. Much of the infant's energy is used to maintain homeostasis (respiration, blood flow, and temperature regulation), which is affected directly by external stimuli.

We now know that information necessary to respond appropriately to infants is provided by their behavioral cues. Technology provides us with information about the autonomic nervous system function, which in turn gives us an even greater ability to "read" infant behavior.

Parents or parent surrogates are the most important stimuli that an infant can experience. This situation exists because infants are unique and they are totally dependent on their caregivers for sustenance, cleanliness, warmth, and social interaction. Once a preterm infant has left the hospital, support provided by nurses, physicians, therapists, social workers, and discharge planners disappears. Only the parents remain. Families of sick and preterm infants often are at significantly increased risk for various social and medical problems (Bernbaum & Hoffman-Williamson, 1986; Combs-Orme, Fishbein, Summerville, & Evans, 1988; Leventhal, Egerter, & Murphy, 1984). These problems include vulnerable child syndrome (children at risk for abuse and neglect), marital stress, and overdependence on medical services. From the initial stages of NICU admission, parents should be given a central role in their infant's care. This goal may be accomplished by involving parents in the provision of comfort care (see Figure 17–5) and by teaching infant cues and recognition of behavioral states, as described in Table 17–2.

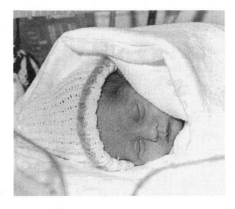

Figure 17–5 Swaddled infant in NICU

To minimize stress, comfort measures can be used when needed, at such times as during suctioning, chest physiotherapy, or drawing of blood. The sick preterm infant often displays disengagement cues such as gaze aversion, yawning, grimacing, eye closing, mottling, limpness, pallor, bradycardia, and apnea. If an infant's cues differ from parental expectation, caregivers may become discouraged and detached. Preterm infants generally have little energy for social interaction, providing few opportunities for eye-to-eye contact—a potent engagement cue. Parents must be taught to realize that the abilities of their infants to engage and socialize correlates largely with health and central nervous system maturation.

CONCLUSION

Many valuable lessons can be learned from our infant patients. First, by recognizing and responding to cues, it is possible to improve the quality of care provided, minimize stress, and maximize long-term development. If we teach these and other lessons to the families and recognize the critical importance of the relationship between the baby and the family, we can establish a collaboration between the health care provider and the family that may have profound and long-lasting benefits.

Second, we must come to grips with the enormous clinical significance of pain relief in the newborn. Not only can we learn to recognize the signs of pain, we can also treat it safely by using both pharmacological and nonpharmacological means. These practices will result in more effective and humane care for the most fragile of babies.

Table 17–2 Common Comfort Measures Parents Can Learn

Purpose	*Measure*
Containment	Hold the infant's arms and legs to the midline of the body.
Nonnutritive suck	Provide and facilitate use of a pacifier.
Infant grasp	Provide an object or parent's hand or finger.
Positioning	Position and support infant in prone position.

Finally, we are presently entering the next frontier in newborn care. Now that new technologies have allowed us to provide the physiological support necessary for survival, we must turn back to the infants themselves for direction on how to nurture and promote optimal long-term development.

BIBLIOGRAPHY

Affonso, D., Wahlberg, V., & Persson, B. (1989). Exploration of mothers' reactions to the kangaroo method of prematurity care. *Neonatal Network, 7*(6), 43–51.

Als, H. (1982). Towards a synactive therapy of development: Promise for the assessment of infant individuality. *Infant Mental Health, 3,* 229–243.

Als, H., Lawhon, G., Brown, E., Gibes, R., Duffy, F.H., McAnulty, G., & Blickman, J.G. (1986). Individualized behavioral and environmental care for the very low birth weight preterm infant at high risk for bronchopulmonary dysplasia: Neonatal intensive care unit and developmental outcome. *Pediatrics, 78*(6), 1123–1132.

Anand, K.J.S., & Hickey, P.R. (1987). Pain and its effect in the human neonate and fetus. *New England Journal of Medicine, 317,* 1321–1329.

Anand, K.J.S., Sippell, W.O., & Aynsley-Green, A. (1987). Randomized trial of fentanyl anesthesia in preterm babies undergoing surgery: Effects on the stress response. *Lancet, 1,* 243–247.

Bada, H.S., Korones, S.B., Perry, E.H., Arheart, K.L., Pourcyrous, M., Runyan, J.W., Anderson, G.D., Magill, H.L., Fitch, C.W., & Somes, G.W. (1990). Frequent handling in the neonatal intensive care unit and intraventricular hemorrhage. *Journal of Pediatrics, 117*(1), 126–131.

Bauchner, H., May, A., & Coates, E. (1992). Use of analgesic agents for invasive medical procedures in pediatric and neonatal intensive care units. *Journal of Pediatrics, 121,* 647–649.

Bernbaum, J., & Hoffman-Williamson, M. (1986). Following the NICU graduate. *Contemporary Pediatrics,* June, 22–37.

Berry, F.A., & Gregory, G.A. (1987). Do premature infants require anesthesia for surgery? *Anesthesiology, 67,* 291–293.

Brazelton, T.B. (1973). Neonatal behavioral assessment scale. *Clinics in Developmental Medicine, 50.* Philadelphia: J.B. Lippincott.

Cole, J.G., Begish-Duddy, A., Judas, M.L., & Jorgensen, K.M. (1990). Changing the NICU environment: The Boston City Hospital model. *Neonatal Network, 9*(2), 15–23.

Combs-Orme, T., Fishbein, J., Summerville, C., & Evans, M.G. (1988). Re-hospitalization of very low-birth weight infants. *American Journal of Diseases of Children, 142,* 1109–1113.

Craft, M.J., Wyatt, N., & Sandell, B. (1985). Behavior and feeling changes in siblings of hospitalized children. *Clinical Pediatrics, 24*(7), 374–378.

Fanaroff, A.A., & Martin, R.J. (1987). *Neonatal-perinatal medicine: Diseases of the fetus and infant* (4th ed.) (pp. 20–27). St. Louis: C.V. Mosby.

Gordon, P.C. (1990). Assessing and managing agitation in a critically ill infant. *MCN, 15,* 26–32.

Gross, S.C., & Gardner, G.G. (1982). Child pain: Treatment approaches. In W.L. Smith, E.L. Merskey, & S.C. Gross (Eds.), *Pain: Meaning and management* (pp. 127–142). New York: SP Medical and Scientific Books.

Leventhal, J.M., Egerter, S.A., & Murphy, J.M. (1984). Reassessment of the relationship of perinatal risk factors and child abuse. *American Journal of Diseases of Children, 138,* 1034–1039.

Levine, D., & Gordan, N.G. (1982). Pain in prelingual children and its evaluation by pain induced vocalization. *Pain, 14,* 85–93.

Lewis, M., Bendersky, M., Koons, A., Hegyi, T., Hiatt, M., Ostfeld, B., & Rosenfeld, D. (1991). Visitation to a neonatal intensive care unit. *Pediatrics, 88*(4), 795–800.

McGraw, M.B. (1941). Natural maturation as explained in the changing reaction of the infant to pin prick. *Child Development, 12,* 31–42.

Perlman, N.B., Freedman, J.L., Abramovitch, R., Whyte, H., Kirpalani, H., & Perlman, M. (1991). Information needs of parents of sick neonates. *Pediatrics, 88*(3), 512–518.

Phibbs, C.S., Phibbs, R.H., Pomerance, J.J., & Williams, R.L. (1986). Alternative to diagnosis-related groups for newborn intensive care. *Pediatrics, 78*(5), 829–836.

Resnick, M.B., Ariet, M., Carter, R.L., Fletcher, J.W., Evans, J.H., Furlough, R.R., Ausbon, W.W., & Curran, J.S. (1986). Prospective pricing system for tertiary neonatal intensive care. *Pediatrics, 78*(5), 820–828.

Rogers, M.C. (1992). Do the right thing (Pain relief in infants and children). *New England Journal of Medicine, 336,* 55–56.

St. Joseph's Hospital. (1993). Holding/handling policies for neonatal intensive care nursery. Unpublished information, Syracuse, New York.

St. Joseph's Hospital. (1993). Pain protocol for neonatal intensive care nursery. Unpublished information, Syracuse, New York.

Schwab, F., Tolbert, B., Bagnato, S., & Maisels, M.J. (1983). Sibling visiting in a neonatal intensive care unit. *Pediatrics, 71*(5), 835–838.

Thomas, K.A. (1989). How the NICU environment sounds to a preterm infant. *MCN, 14,* 249–251.

Tyson, J.E., & Speaks, S. (1987). Stress and the performance of neonatal intensive care unit staff. In A.A. Fanaroff & R.J. Martin (eds.), *Neonatal-perinatal medicine: Diseases of the fetus and infant* (4th ed.) (pp. 20–27). St. Louis: C.V. Mosby.

Umphenour, J.H. (1980). Bacterial colonization in neonates with sibling visitation. *JOGNN, 9*(2), 73–75.

Williamson, P.S., & Williamson, M.L. (1983). Physiologic stress reduction by a local anesthetic during newborn circumcision. *Pediatrics, 71,* 36–40.

Chapter 18

Families at Risk and Vulnerable Environments

For more than three decades now, professionals in child development, education, medicine, and other areas of human service delivery have sought to define preventive and remedial intervention for families at risk and with extraordinary needs. In particular, premature birth, unwed and/or teenage parents, severe poverty, unfinished educational agendas, and populations of children with exceptional needs have been cited again and again as contributors to vulnerability in children, heightened stress, and possible abuse within families. By the same token, attempts to accurately predict and then ameliorate circumstances that may eventually result in significant differences from the norm have met with scant success. The fact remains that newborns faced with cumulative detrimental insults do grow up to escape the ravages of deficit; other children, less traumatized yet less fortunate, early into their first and second years of life show signs of failure to thrive and departure from typical patterns of growth and development.

Current views of high risk families and of infants and young children with disabilities need to allow for less conventional expectations and more open-ended possibilities. A multitude of factors affect outcome. These factors include timing, the nature of medical insult, physical makeup and temperament of the child, resources and support available to parents, duration of hospitalization or separation, extent of poverty, evidence of substance abuse, parent state of health, the nature of any intervention, and the constellation of the family unit. As we have noted in other chapters, professionals need to be wary of excessive intrusion at inappropriate points. Our efforts often have led to misinterpretation and disillusionment. For example, educators and physicians frequently have shared concerns about the heightened probability of developmental delay in children of teenage parents. At times of referral, however, infants may not manifest any indicators of developmental or behavioral difficulty. Given current economic constraints, this dilemma is not easy to resolve.

With ever-increasing numbers of children and families in distress across this country, the question before us is undeniable: Politically, educationally, medically, and economically, when will the United States place a greater priority on prevention? Retrospective recognition of biosocial problems is helpful to a degree, but does not fully address prospective, preventive identification of and service to those families most in need of intervention. Underscoring our point of view, Jacobs and Davies (1991) have written:

> U.S. child and family policies are overwhelmingly treatment-oriented, with only those individuals and families already in difficulty being eligible; few preventive programs are broadly available. For example, families on the verge of having their children placed in foster care are eligible, in fact, are often required, to receive counseling; families in which problems are brewing but not extant usually cannot qualify for public services. This emphasis on treatment over prevention exemplifies what Grubb and Lazerson (1982) call a 'negative conception of *parens patriae*' ('the state as parent'). The reliance on treatment precludes helping families negotiate the normal stresses inherent in raising children, for example, by offering parent education, or by supporting reduced-hour work policies or parent leave for new parents. This latter type of assistance exemplifies the positive view of the 'state's role as parent' embraced by most industrial nations. But it is the negative conception of *parens patriae* that holds sway here: the state waits until parents fail and families become dysfunctional before assuming the obligation to protect children. *Parens patriae* applied in this fashion does, no doubt, protect some children from real and imminent danger; it also sacrifices the present and future integrity of many families in crisis. (p. 12)

CURRENT ISSUES

Families in Crisis: Common Themes

Research on families in crisis have followed many tracks, and issues continue to grow in complexity and volume; yet, familiar themes have been present since the earliest interest in parents, caregivers, and developmental environments. One recurrent area of study has focused on attachment and bonding (see Figure 18–1) and on the effects of events such as extended periods of separation, chronic illness, prematurity, multiple births, types and severity of disabilities, availability of day and respite care, and the support of extended family and friends. Of special importance have been (1) the long-term implications of interactions and relationships within families (among individual members and with the disabled child or infant at risk) and (2) the impact of these interactions and relationships on child development. Decidedly, there has been a shift away from the belief that, for child and caregivers, certain events are unalterably damaging.

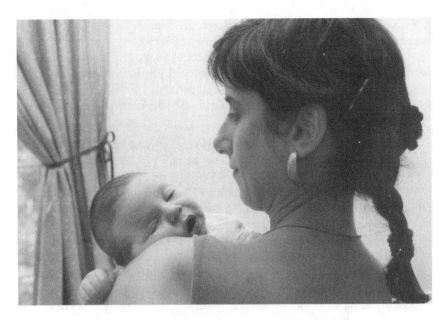

Figure 18–1 Mom and full-term baby, Matthew, 1 week after arriving home from hospital

In a second area of study, much of the work on prematurity and high risk deliveries has concentrated on analysis of the stages unique to families as they deal with the sorrow associated with acceptance of preterm and developmentally delayed infants. Again, contact with mothers, fathers, and siblings has taught us that, in contrast to prior assumptions, all families do not pass through universal stages. To some, for example, intensive care nurseries are understandably frightening; to others, they serve as a comfort and source of consolation. Also, we should not assume that, in the face of difficult circumstances, parents require uniform interventions. Support groups aid the healing process for some; for others, the desire to be alone needs to be respected. It is a well-established observation that families in the most serious need are often the most difficult to reach. For instance, while there is considerable documentation on middle to upper income caregivers and those who are the most stable, much less is known about the feelings and concerns of single, adoptive, or very young mothers and fathers and about meaningful and enduring solutions. In addition, what happens to families—their various stages of grief and their diversity of coping skills—may be largely a function of outside support. That process of interaction, though now given a great deal of credence, still remains open to question in terms of methods of enhancement and maintenance.

Abuse and violence—increasing at dramatic rates in our society among very young and elderly populations—is a third dominant issue. Reportedly, such events are more prevalent among poorer and less resourceful families and in situations in which premature, high risk, or developmentally disabled infants and young children live. Determining and precipitating factors include heightened stress, inadequate knowledge about young children, lack of behavior management skills, insufficient personal parent time, substance abuse, constrained financial resources, and caregiver histories of child abuse. Still, the unique combinations of circumstances that finally do precipitate abuse are difficult to document before the fact. Professionals in the field freely acknowledge our present paucity of data on middle income and upper income families, in which child abuse is more subtle and hidden. Perhaps the one variable but unifying key resides in the early study of parental interactions. The problem was well stated years ago by Solnit and Provence (1979):

> The weaknesses and intolerance of the infant often serve as a magnet and magnifier for environmental actions and reactions, for parental perceptions of and responses to the baby . . . . Included in this focus are vital past experiences that influence parental behavior and tend to utilize the newborn and young infant as a screen on which past feelings and attitudes, often inappropriate ones, are projected onto the baby and distort the current reality of infant and parent. Such adult behavior is not only inappropriate for the child but tends to promote the repetition and continuation of the adult's deviant behavior.
>
> What starts out for the child as a weakness or vulnerability may be magnified and elaborated by the parents' responses either because the parents lack resources or because the parents transfer inappropriate past attitudes or expectations onto the child. (p. 802)

The final issue, which is related to the other three concerns, is optimal developmental environments. Numerous studies have examined the relationships and dynamics between infants or young children and their primary caregivers. In the past, this kind of research has been limited largely to mother-infant dyads and associated patterns. Contemporary themes now recognize the centrality of the entire family unit and a family systems perspective (Barber, Turnbull, Behr, & Kerns, 1988). In the process of arriving at this realization, several fundamental questions have emerged; some have been answered but others are outstanding.

- How and why do interactions between preterm or developmentally disabled children and their caregivers vary from those between full-term or typical infants or preschoolers and their families?
- How do perceptions and attitudes of parents in regard to characteristics of the newborn affect the quality of relationships and developmental outcome?
- Which dimensions of interaction and of the developmental environment delay or facilitate cognitive, social, and emotional capacities and growth, and

are there stages when vulnerabilities and potentials are more likely to change?

- How do caregivers and siblings finally come to cope with having high risk and disabled children in the family and with the trauma of chronic sorrow throughout the early years and longer?
- Are there similarities between the lower income family that suffers from the damaging impact of their interactions and the middle or upper income parents who have lost faith that their children can change and learn?
- With the expanding regionalization of medical facilities and the associated difficulties of distance and separation, how can parents, siblings, and newborns achieve a better start and interact positively?

The issues and questions are unending and complex, and they demand multifaceted solutions. Just possibly, fruitful study of interactions may be found in some situations that defy the hardened stereotypes held by physicians and educators. Numerous infants of overburdened and overpopulated areas of the world such as Calcutta, India, are a case in point. Children are left on the streets, deprived of prenatal care, parenting, home, and country. The International Mission of Hope (IMH) is a registered agency in India and North America that is dedicated to "bringing hope to abandoned children."

Cherie Clark (1984), executive director of IMH, has eloquently stated the situation as follows:

> They come broken and defeated, and oftentimes premature and malnourished, ridden with disease that oftentimes makes the battle for their life a losing one. They come so late and so tired, often totally lacking the will to live. They struggle, unaware that there is more than pain involved in being. But the fact that within each tiny child lies the spark and the potential to grow gives our staff of doctors, nurses, and social workers the strength and the hope to struggle on for each and every new life, so that now far more tiny babies who come to us have lived than die.

> They come to us from the jails and streets, uneducated, unknowing, and unloved. What will they grow to be? How can they adjust? Watching them laugh and run and play and become children is our cause and our goal. To see them become educated, responsible, loving adolescents brings joy . . . . They come to us as survivors, who slowly wind their way through tons of paperwork and seals that must be affixed to documents before they are free. They make their way as photographs and papers through the courts, passport offices and immigration departments and all too often they die before the process can be completed.

The lucky ones go off as tiny ambassadors quietly and with complete trust into a world of love and acceptance. They travel across the ocean through the night to new food, new language and into the hearts and homes of a family who has waited and longed for their arrival. These children teach us that we are more alike than different and the right of each of us to love, family, and childhood is God given. (pp. 1-2)

This statement underscores the importance of quality parent-child interactions and their compelling influence on social, emotional, and intellectual development, irrespective of specific time periods, medical histories, and, in some instances, aberrant environmental experiences.

Parent-Infant Attachment and the High Risk Newborn

Many studies have documented the fact that preterm infants and newborns with other medical risks are less alert and less responsive to their immediate environments and more chronically irritable than full-term babies (Goldberg, 1978, 1982). These observations have set the stage for numerous investigations of the behavior of premature infants, parental attitudes and behaviors toward their offspring, and subsequent patterns of family interaction (Affonso et al., 1985; Lee, Penner, & Cox, 1991; Lowenthal, 1987; Miles, 1989; Miles, Funk, & Kasper, 1991). Historically, much of this research emerged from the work on parent-infant bonding by Klaus and Kennell (1976), which did prompt changes in hospital delivery and visiting practices for newborns and their families throughout the decade following their first publications. Their hard-line position of "sensitive period in the first minutes and hours of life during which it is necessary that the mother and father have close contact with their neonate for later development to be optimal" (1976, p. 14) has now been severely criticized and, some would say, discredited. Indeed, Klaus and Kennell themselves, in a work published shortly later (*Parent-Infant Bonding*, 1982), cautioned:

The human is highly adaptable, and there are many fail-safe routes to attachment. Sadly, some parents who missed the bonding experience have felt that all was lost for their future relationship. This was (and is) completely incorrect, but it was so upsetting that we have tried to speak more moderately about our convictions concerning the long-term significance of this early bonding experience . . . .

For some mothers one period may be more important than the other. If the health of the mother or infant makes this [early bonding] impossible, then discussion, support, and reassurance should help the parents appreciate that they can become as completely attached to their infant as if they had the usual bonding experience, although it may require more time and effort. (p. 56)

Other researchers have echoed concern about the stresses that caregivers initially experience with a stay in the neonatal intensive care nursery—in particular, feelings of isolation, uncertainty, and fear that their babies will not live and a sense of being out of control (Miles, Funk, & Kasper, 1991). At the same time, however, studies have indicated that, while differences for many parents of premature and other high risk infants may be evident at first (Affonso et al., 1985; Chess & Thomas, 1982; Cobiella, Mabe, & Forehand, 1990; Lee, Penner, & Cox, 1991; Lowenthal, 1987), families do not necessarily sustain long-term, adverse effects. As we have indicated in Chapters 16 and 17, many researchers and professionals in the field have suggested a need for early intervention that (1) focuses on helping parents to deal with their concerns and anxieties over having a premature or high risk infant, (2) responds to worries about future development, and (3) offers support during the first days, weeks, and possibly months of adjustment at home (Brooks-Gunn, Liaw, & Klebanov, 1992; Infant Health and Development Program, 1990; Klaus & Kennell, 1982; Pfander & Bradley-Johnson, 1990; Sigman, Cohen, Beckwith, & Parmelee, 1981).

Before Birth and Delivery

Our own experiences during the past 15 years in working with families of infants and young children at risk for or with identified developmental disabilities have confirmed many of the short-term observations cited in the literature. For many parents, the sense of concern arose even prior to delivery, yet no one seemed to listen; thus, there were feelings of isolation and loneliness for the duration of pregnancy. For instance, one mother we visited commented:

> From the day that I learned I was pregnant, I knew that there was something wrong with my baby. I told Bill constantly that something was not right and that something should be done. Everyone thought that it was just a feeling and that everything would be fine once I had the baby. Finally, when I was about 7 months along, I went to my doctor. He could not find a heartbeat and had not felt any life. I was hysterical. I told the doctor that he needed to find out if the baby inside me was dead or alive because I refused to deliver a dead baby. At that point, he did find the baby's heartbeat, which made me feel a little better. Yet, I still had a sense that something was not right. I could not get rid of that worry.

> Meanwhile, I started to feel life, very faint flutters and a faint kick now and then. That was all. A week before I delivered the baby, my obstetrician sent me for a second sonogram. The day before I had the baby I went in for the results, and the doctor told me that he was going to put off my delivery for another month. At that point, I knew that he was wrong because I was very sure about when I had gotten pregnant. The

doctor did not listen to me. Within 24 hours, I delivered Joey. [See Figure 18–2]

Nursery Experiences

Parents have reported to us equally traumatic experiences during and after delivery. They are fearful and naturally confused about the birth of a child 2 to 3 months early, and the initial perceptions of the crisis and of what is being said to them may differ between the mother and father. Despite the degree of prematurity, they may be worried, first, about whether the baby will live and, second, about whether the infant will have lasting problems. Frequently little is said in the delivery room because physicians themselves are uncertain about outcome. As our family accounts have shown, this period is commonly extremely difficult for parents to handle. Exemplifying these experiences, two parents shared these concerns:

> They showed me both babies (Figures 18–3 and 18–4) and informed me that Anna would need to go to the intensive care unit because she was so small. I worried some, but she looked good in color. I anxiously awaited the Apgar scores, knowing that they would give me an indication of the baby's condition. Margaret's scores were 8 and 9, and Anna's scores

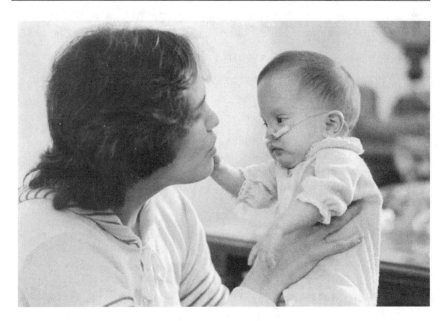

Figure 18–2 Mom and baby, Joey, born prematurely. For his first year of life, Joey suffered from severe pulmonary hypertension.

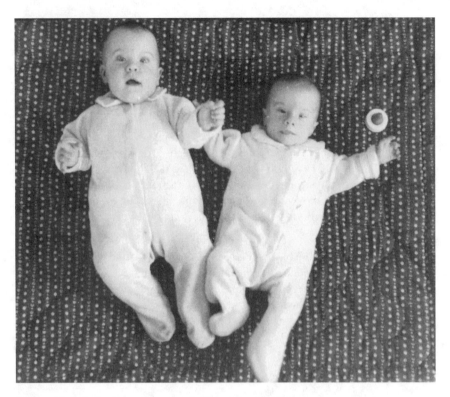

Figure 18–3 Twin sisters, Margaret (left) and Anna (right)

were 7 and 9. That information somewhat relieved me about Anna. Mike, my husband, brought Margaret to me in the recovery room. I had such afterbirth tremblings that I could not hold Margaret; I just touched her. My husband laid her next to me, but I was afraid that my shaking would unsettle her. Mike finally took Margaret to the nursery, and I slept.

The first hours were the worst. The special care nurses told me that Anna was doing well. I also knew that she would not be going home with me, and that knowledge was agony. I was trying the juggle my own recovery from the Caesarean section, breast-feeding with Margaret, and consulting with all the doctors and nurses. I got very little sleep, knowing the entire time that when I left that hospital I would be taking only one of my babies home. No one talked with me about my feelings and I felt very alone. Thank goodness, Margaret was learning to nurse well

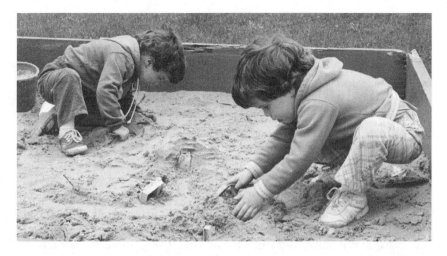

Figure 18–4 Twin sisters, Anna (left) and Margaret (right)

and gave me no problems. However, having at least one baby home was not the consolation that I thought it might be.

It was ironic that so many people came in to consult with me on breast-feeding, on caring for twins, on my physical care; but no one talked with me about those feelings that were the most painful. I needed someone at that time who had gone through the same kind of situation, who could comfort me and let me know that what I was feeling was not abnormal, that it was okay for me to cry for Anna.

In the words of another mother:

The next morning I was eager to see my baby. He nursed quite well for me in the morning, but as the day wore on he became disinterested and jumpy. I was slightly concerned that evening when one of my visitors asked why he was being kept at the back of the nursery. I decided to question the doctor about it in the morning. Early the next day, Brian's general practitioner told me that they were transferring our son to a neo-natal unit in a teaching hospital 120 miles away. He did not know what was wrong with the baby. He told me that Brian was rolling his eyes, twitching, and throwing his head back. I was stunned!

All of the problems recounted by these parents arose as a result of crisis circumstances and a rapid turn of events for which they were unprepared. Medical professionals always face the question of how such situations could be handled better in the future. First, it is important to recognize that parents remember selectively and that, in retrospect, they may believe that they have fully described symptoms during pregnancy when this really is not the case. Second, whenever mothers do have concerns, they should be sent and should refer themselves for second opinions so that their conditions can be monitored more closely. This practice ought to be followed especially when a mother has had previous complications with one or more pregnancies. Obstetrical services of regional perinatal centers have been designed specifically to manage such situations, which ordinarily cannot be handled by rural hospitals, for example. Routinely, mothers are now being transported before delivery to centers that offer newborn intensive care. In recent years, these changes have greatly improved both morbidity and mortality rates.

If problems are identified before birth, early contact can help caregivers in several ways. Medical technologies can possibly delay or avert premature delivery. Whatever the outcome, the counseling of parents at this stage by the attending neonatologist, who is familiar with the treatment of high risk infants and subsequently might be involved in the care of the newborn, can help to prepare families before they confront the reality of a premature delivery. Close collaboration between obstetricians and neonatologists prior to and during delivery is essential to the success of these kinds of services in the future.

Inevitably, the point of delivery is chaotic for physicians and parents alike. Families want to know about the immediate prognosis for their babies. In the majority of cases, it is impossible to give definitive information without a period of observation and the benefit of additional evaluation. Parents need to express all of their concerns and address these to one primary individual, namely, the attending physician. By their nature, teaching hospitals where neonatal intensive care units are located are staffed by large numbers of professionals at different levels of training. It is especially important in the beginning stages of communication with parents that information is provided consistently, simply, and soon after delivery. In addition, attending physicians are well aware that things said in the delivery room need to be repeated to both mother and father throughout the first days of intensive care because they often do not remember. Also, while time may be limited at delivery, parents need to be prepared by the attending neonatologist for the introduction to their newborn. The physical appearance of the baby and the collection of monitors and equipment are frightening to many families. Without exception, these initial communications come when mothers and fathers are emotionally in a state of shock and when the mothers themselves may require medical care.

From all of our parent accounts, it is clear that the first days and weeks of hospitalization, whatever the duration, were difficult to endure. Families were torn between home and their new babies. Frequently, they received conflicting information about the condition of the newborn from nurses, house officers, and rotating attending physicians. In addition, with the regionalization of neonatal intensive care facilities, many families are able to visit only on a weekly basis or sometimes less often. Thus, they are restricted to following the progress of their child primarily by phone. Because of the high costs, technology, and intense activity of such centers, most of the problems that families face are, unfortunately, difficult to resolve. Although these complications and issues alter forever the "typical" newborn period for families and babies, there are services that could help parents throughout these stressful transition periods. The recollections of families with whom we have worked speak to a few of these needs.

> The most frustrating part of Jennifer's nursery experience [Figure 18–5] was the fact that I could not see her enough. I could go into the unit 24 hours a day and stay, but I was not able to hold her as long as I wanted because she was on CPAP [constant positive airway pressure]. Also, with my 1-year old at home, I was limited in the time that I could spend at the hospital. At 10 o'clock at night, if I felt like going, I could go in and sit with her and talk to her. The nursing staff really made me feel that Jenny was my baby and that I was her mother, even though I knew they had total control over her. Whenever I was there and she needed to be changed or powdered, they always encouraged me to care for her. In that sense, I did not feel that I was left out totally during those 2½ months that she was in the hospital.

Another mother commented:

> As we left the hospital, the nurse handed us a booklet about the neonatal intensive care unit. Pictures prepared us for what we were soon to see.

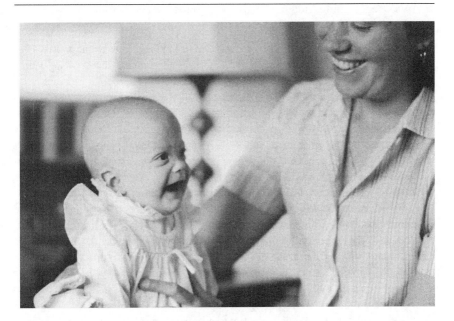

Figure 18–5 Mom and baby, Jennifer, born at 26 weeks gestation. Jennifer was hospitalized for approximately 2½ months in an NICU in Syracuse, New York.

However, there was little that helped us emotionally to deal with the stress of having our baby in an intensive care unit. Entering the hospital was like visiting a strange and frightening world.

Still another mother, who was a nurse, echoed similar thoughts:

The time that Rebecca was in the nursery was filled with many fears of her being handicapped. It was all such a delicate balance. She needed to have the right oxygen level; that was being monitored and measured. Too much oxygen could be harmful. She needed to have the right blood sugar level; in the beginning she could not regulate that very well. Again, that condition was being monitored. It was scary, relying on all these machines. Temperature was another problem. She was kept warm by a heating system, at first in an open crib and later in the isolette. This had to be checked. Exactly 2 weeks after the baby was born, Pat lost his job. I was still on leave of absence from my job. This situation added tremendously to our stress. For those who are familiar with the *Holmes Stress Scale*, we were getting pretty high in our score of traumatic life events.

Last, the words of another mother:

For those first 28 days, she was cared for totally—fed, changed, dressed, warmed, administered medication—by someone else. I went in to visit her, but she did not seem like my child.

Involving parents in the nurturing care of their babies to the extent possible has become routine in many intensive care nurseries over the past decade or so. While this participation does not resolve all of the irregularities and concerns that families face, it does help them to become a part of the healing process and to feel needed. Attachment to newborns who look so fragile and far removed from the condition of typical infants takes time for mothers, fathers, and siblings. The medical staff can attempt to enhance such relationships, but nurses and others need to let families work out their fears and feelings of distance. Following the progress of families through this period is beneficial in order to determine ways in which professionals can assist them prior to hospital discharge.

Communication of information is another continuing source of controversy and potential discontent in intensive care settings. Constant changes in staff are difficult because they rarely allow parents to establish lasting relationships with one physician. Obviously too, there are wide differences in personalities of attending physicians; some are much more family-oriented than others. Neonatal intensive care nurseries need better mechanisms to assist families with these transitions and to facilitate communication among professionals in the multitude of disciplines involved in such units. Regular meetings of nursery teams that include those professionals in primary decision-making roles can be a useful strategy to assist and communicate with families. In particular, such groups should draw on the expertise and feedback of the attending neonatologist; head nurse; social worker; pediatric physical or occupational therapists assigned to the nursery; developmental psychologist responsible for evaluation of babies in perinatal follow-up; early childhood special educators associated with child find or direction center services; the parents; and other specialists associated and familiar with intervention programs in a particular catchment area. For a given child, this team should have the capacity for sharing up-to-date medical and psychosocial information and for coordinating initial community-based, clinical, and educational services.

Physicians, nurses, social workers, and other professionals offer one kind of support for caregivers; yet, many families known to us over the years have suggested that they need something more. Nursery discussion groups that are directed by parents of babies discharged from the hospital and include mothers, fathers, and siblings of infants still receiving care can provide a critical outlet and source of emotional nurturing. Moreover, while every child follows a unique developmental course, the experiences of other families who have survived and resumed normal lives, with or without disabling conditions, can be a strength to those still in the midst of the unknown.

Discharge and Transition to Home

Finally, parents also have commented that the point of final discharge was especially traumatic despite their longing to have their babies home. When at last that day arrives, they can often hardly believe that the time has come. Understandably, they are fearful about a tiny infant who may weigh little more than 4 pounds and who still requires very special, continuing care. Consequently, families must cope with another in the long series of transitions—hospital to home. Public health nurses experienced in the care of high risk infants, who are assigned prior to discharge, offer a stabilizing resource for families. If the public health nurse makes the initial contact when the baby is still in the hospital, parents are better able to cope with the change and are not as likely to feel abandoned. Likewise, setting up perinatal center follow-up appointments and plans for intervention programing before discharge gives families support that is important to their well-being and to that of their babies in the first weeks at home.

Although many high risk infants may seem to approach typical development by 18 months to 2 years of age, professionals need to maintain a position of cautious optimism in the early weeks and months at home. The numerous worries and uncertainties parents carry from hospital to home are extremely difficult for them to manage and may impact adversely on family-child attachment. Recurrent hospitalizations serve to reinforce all of these concerns. In addition, an area of equal difficulty for many families with whom we have interacted and numerous families in research studies was that preterm and other high risk babies were often not easy to care for initially because of excessive irritability, sleeping problems, and lengthy feedings. These demands frequently were coupled with the realistic awareness of caregivers that they needed to isolate themselves and their other children from normal daily activities outside the home, at least temporarily, because of the risks of infection. Such pressures constitute a considerable burden—with little relief in sight for families during the first weeks and months at home.

The following are quotations from parents writing about their experiences shortly after hospital discharge.

> It was a hard time when Jennifer first came home. I could not sleep while she did because I had my 1-year old to take care of, too. Fortunately, I have a very supportive husband who was willing to get up with her at night to help out with the feedings. Nick would do anything for her. Meanwhile, it was very evident that she went through a transition period when she first came home. At first, she had to sleep with the light on all the time. She was comfortable only with people around and with constant noise. The staff at the hospital had warned us that she probably would have these kinds of problems.

> We still did not know if she was going to have any problems as far as her health or development. It was a wait-and-see time. That was hard and made us very tense. In fact, it was quite a while until we felt confident that she was going to be fine. We told ourselves and other people that she did not have problems, but inside we had a lot of doubts.

* * * *

> Wayne was growing, gaining weight, and everything seemed to be fine until one night when he was 2½ months old. He became very ill. We were giving him his bottle, and his father started to burp him. He began to spit up and choke. He stopped breathing and turned blue. Gary immediately called the ambulance, while I tried to get him breathing again. I had never had a course in CPR [cardiopulmonary resuscitation], but I had to try. He was in intensive care for 8 days in critical condition. We came very close to losing him.

* * * *

> When Brian was 9 weeks old, the public health nurse who had been visiting weekly and I noticed how stiff his muscles were becoming and how he was arching his head. Brian's general practitioner suggested that, again, we see a specialist 120 miles away. He did not warn us that Brian might be hospitalized. Therefore, we were totally unprepared for this event.

Every 3 weeks, we drove the 120 miles to see a specialist and physical therapist. We found dealing with the doctor a very frustrating experience. He was an extremely busy person and always pressed for time. Once, while Brian was in the hospital, we overheard him speaking to students about cerebral palsy in regard to Brian. It was 2 weeks before we could question him about that comment at our regularly scheduled appointment. Naturally, in those weeks we imagined the worst and worried incessantly.

* * * *

One of the most difficult pressures that I, as a new mother, had to cope with was an immediate return to work 2 weeks after Rebecca's discharge. I felt cheated, knowing that most people are home with their babies for at least 6 weeks. Indeed, it took me a great deal of time to work out these feelings of anger and resentment. I knew that it had to be, but I was not happy. I always had reminders at work. There were other people who were pregnant, and they made me recall that my pregnancy had terminated right at the time when I was enjoying being pregnant, and that it had not ended in a normal way. We had neither the typical nursery experiences nor a typical homecoming.

* * * *

After a while, we honestly felt as if we had entered "no man's land." We never got more than 4 hours of sleep. I remember getting up one day when Linda had gone to work, starting to get dressed, and putting on my suit to go to work. I had no job and had to take care of the baby, yet I almost went out the door. I remember hearing the baby and saying to myself, 'My God, what are you doing?' I was confused, disoriented, and did not even know what day it was.

* * * *

We could not go anywhere as a family unit without exposing Anna. It was bitterly cold during those days, and I could not take her out unless it was for a doctor's appointment or an urgent situation. After a while, the lengthy feedings caused me great agitation. At times, I simply wanted to say to Anna, 'Why can't you just be normal?'

While they cannot resolve all problems, primary care physicians interested in and knowledgeable about developmental issues and education can facilitate resolution of some problems and can give parents considerable guidance. They have the clear advantage of seeing families regularly, usually within 2 weeks of the return home. Furthermore, in terms of presenting consistent feedback to parents, pediatricians, educators, therapists, and staff of the perinatal center follow-up programs, primary care physicians need to take responsibility for sharing information and facilitating agreement on optimal courses of action for intervention, as they offer feedback to caregivers. In the short term and over the long term, parents need to be kept informed and realistically prepared. If concerns about disabling conditions must be discussed, physicians should give the family opportunities and time to raise questions and to talk about their fears. They should not be left to deal with these problems alone.

The Middle and End of the First Year at Home

For most parents, the middle months and end of the first year prove to be a turning point. Many marked delays begin to fade, and families see their babies looking and behaving in more typical ways. Visits to follow-up programs have been made and, with available resources, families have received information about their baby's developmental progress. Also, very importantly, the difficult periods of early adjustment are behind them, and they begin to feel more rested and comfortable with daily routines. If early intervention has been advised, caregivers have been able to proceed with those decisions. Such are the experiences of many families.

Unfortunately, however, another group of parents face continuing struggles that terminate sadly with serious disabling conditions or the loss of their child. These families obviously require a great deal of support.

Excerpts taken from the autobiographical stories written by eight sets of parents represent both sides of this continuum, with very different needs portrayed:

> This was the time when everything started to get better. Jenny did more, and we were less nervous. I think it was around the 8th month, which would have been her 5th month at home, when I finally felt confident that she was going to be all right. She started to sit up, she started to vocalize more, and she was more attentive. With Catherine's development, I remember this period as being a slow and gradual process. With Jenny, it was as if she did nothing one day, and the next day she did everything.

* * * *

> Things started to smooth out a bit during the middle months. My anger seemed to diminish, although at times it seemed ever present. I still had concerns about whether we were taking proper care of the baby. I felt as if I did not have enough time to do the reading that I wanted to do, take care of Rebecca, and continue my work. I remember the LaLeche coun-

selor saying that it is difficult for people with jobs because they feel that if they are doing their work successfully, they are not giving all they could to their children. If they are doing the most they can with mothering, they feel as if they are cheating their employer. It is difficult to come to a balance, and I was having trouble with that.

* * * *

In total, Anna did not look like a baby; she did not act nearly her age in comparison with Margaret. I was not able to nurse her, as I did Margaret and Peter. Finally, it came as a shock to me one day that I could not say to Anna very naturally, 'I love you.' This realization occurred some time in April, when I began to analyze some of my feelings. The recollection that kept coming back to me was an experience that I had as a child—watching a litter of pups, which had been born to our family dog. There appeared to be too many pups for the number of working nipples. I remember finding one little pup tucked under the mother's leg each time the puppies nursed. I recall being angry with the mother dog, questioning why she wasn't watching out for this little one, why she wasn't taking special care since it was so weak. Thinking back to this experience, it suddenly occurred to me that this was how I was feeling about Anna. In a sense, she was my 'runt of the litter.'

Despite this understanding, I still struggled with myself to feel love for Anna. She was scheduled for surgery in Boston on June 8 to correct three of her cardiac defects. It was not until 2 weeks before scheduled surgery that I allowed myself finally to admit that I did love her. Once I accepted that feeling, a myriad of other emotions surfaced. I took on a great burden and was almost consumed by it.

* * * *

The middle months were the very hardest—to sit back and watch Joey go from what we thought was healthy to what was just awful. At this point, he was about 6 or 7 months old. He weighed only 6 or 7 pounds. He was still wearing newborn baby clothes. Joey's being on oxygen was the most difficult part of these middle months. No matter where I took him, he had to have this portable oxygen tank. What hurt the most were the eyes of the other people who looked at him as if he were some sort of 'freak.' I could not imagine what they thought. In time, I was able to accept those looks because I knew that my little boy was a part of me and he was beautiful.

After Joey went on the oxygen [see Figure 18–6], he was a very hard child to care for at home. He was irritable most of the time. He never slept through the night and was awake most of the day. He still rarely ate more than 3 ounces at a feeding, and he refused cereal and fruit. Throughout this period, Joey stayed home possibly a week to 10 days at the most, then returned to the hospital for 1 or 2 weeks. He was never with us for more than 10 days at a stretch.

By this time, Joey was 9 months old, and things were not getting any easier. We took a trip to Rochester and spent the day with a pediatric pulmonary specialist. He examined Joey and looked at his X-rays. The doctors had not one bit of advice to offer, except to say that if Joey's pulmonary hypertension did not improve very soon, he would not live to see his second birthday. I was glad that they were so blunt. Again, all of the deep feelings that both my husband and I had since the day Joey arrived home came back. We knew deep down inside that somehow our son would never see his second birthday.

A few days prior to his birthday, I had talked to the doctors. They did not think that Joey could hold on much longer. It was a matter of a few days

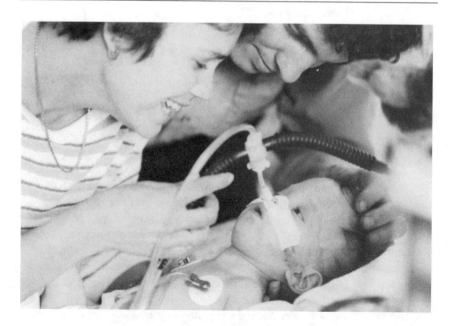

Figure 18–6 Joey, Mom, and Dad during his last days in the hospital. Joey died 1 week after his first birthday.

because his heart was getting so bad. It was just 7 days after his first birthday—exactly 1 week—that God took Joey to Heaven. As long as I had expected it, I could not accept what had happened. That was the hardest day of my life, saying 'good-bye' to my son forever.

Child Abuse and Neglect in Families

It is clear from the extensive chronicles in this chapter that these families were in severe distress—carrying burdens and responsibilities of little sleep, children who were difficult to care for at times, poor communication with professionals, concerns about the future, lack of employment at times, and frequent separation from their newly born infants. Clearly, these are conditions often cited in the literature and our daily newspapers that may lead to events of child abuse and neglect in families. Such was not the case with any of the eight families who worked with us; despite adversity, these parents were able to hang on and cope—and without exception, ultimately turn their problematic lives toward a positive outcome.

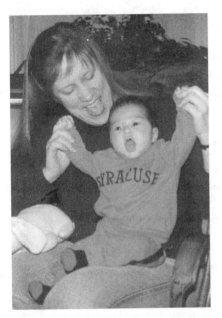

Figure 18–7 Olivia and Mom soon after her arrival from Taiwan

The question that continues to plague so many practitioners and researchers today is this: Why? Infants who are adopted do not join their adoptive families for the first several months of life (see Figure 18–7) and enjoy wonderfully meaningful relationships. What are those differences that make a difference, leading some caregivers to more severely troubled events with their children and others down another path toward healthier relationships?

Failure of infants to thrive, parental neglect, and physical and sexual abuse of children are extreme examples of violent and adverse relationships in families. Recently, such disturbances have received much attention as a result of the severity of the problems, their long-term consequences for children, and the dramatic rise in their occurrence in the United States (Kilpatrick, 1992; Ludwig & Kornberg, 1992; Report of the Twenty-Third Ross Roundtable on Critical Approaches to Common Pediatric Problems in Collaboration with the Ambulatory Pediatric Association, 1991). In a recent article published in the journal *Child Abuse and Neglect,* Ards and Harrell (1993) wrote:

Tremendous gains in public awareness of child abuse and neglect have been made in this country in the past 15 years, stimulated by the passage of mandatory reporting laws in every state. Since the Child Maltreatment and Prevention Act of 1974, the first national law regarding child maltreatment, the number of children reported to Child Protective Services (CPS) has steadily increased. Between 1980 and 1986, the number of children reported as maltreated in the United States rose from 1,154,000 to 2,086,000, representing an increase from 18.1 per 1,000 children to 32.8 per 1,000 children (U.S. Bureau of the Census, 1990). (p. 337)

Other authors (Trupin, Tarico, Low, Jemelka, & McClellan, 1993) cite similar statistics on reported incidence, indicating recent national figures of 2.2 million children referred to child protective services and an estimated 270,000 children nationwide placed in foster care as a result of some form of abuse or neglect.

The source of violence and abuse in families in the United States and the effective implementation of preventive and ameliorative programs have been a key focus of educational, medical, and other health care professionals for decades. Although we are now able to identify some of the causes before the events occur, this has not been the case in far too many instances. Both parties in broken relationships—caregiver and child—have been studied extensively in the past (Egeland & Vaughn, 1981; Jacobsen, 1986; Wolfe, 1987), but findings are varied. Moreover, there is a heightened sensitivity of researchers and practitioners to the fact that problems of abuse, neglect, and failure to thrive are not mutually exclusive. Given this observation, multiple factors have been linked to disturbed parent-child interactions that lead to abuse. As several authors have noted (Gelles & Lancaster, 1987; Wolfner & Gelles, 1993), these factors include past experiences of one or both parents, problems during pregnancy such as illness or the loss of significant relationships, complications during the perinatal period, marital problems, financial pressures, lower education levels, social isolation, and the use of alcohol and drugs. Specifically, in one national study in the United States, *A Profile of Violence toward Children,* Wolfner and Gelles (1993) reported the following:

A national probability sample of 6,002 households was surveyed by telephone in 1985, of which 3,232 households had at least one child under 28 years living at home. Minor violence, or physical punishment, was most common among mothers, caretakers 18 to 37 years old, fathers who were unemployed, caretakers with blue-collar occupations, households with two to four children at home, and among caretakers who used alcohol and other drugs, male children, and children 3 to 6 years old. The highest rates of abusive violence occurred in families located in the East, families whose annual income was below the poverty line, families where the father was unemployed, families where the caretakers held blue-collar jobs, families with four or more children, caretakers who used drugs at least once, male children, and children 3 to 6 years old. (p. 197)

Importantly, too, Wolfner and Gelles point out that despite this "profile" of families, abuse "crosses all social, racial, religious, educational, and financial boundaries" (1993, p. 209). Finally, these authors emphasize the critical role played by "socially learned" behaviors, in combination with stressful daily events.

In response to these widespread problems and the rising incidence of abuse and neglect, new models of intervention and support for children and families are being explored. Although the findings relative to outcome are still mixed, Intensive Family Preservation Services (IFPS) is one contemporary approach that is being implemented with a fair degree of success (Bath & Haapala, 1993). Specifically, the model involves provision of services:

. . . designed to prevent the unnecessary placement of children out of their homes while at the same time ensuring their safety. This is achieved through the provision of a mix of intensive therapeutic and support services tailored to the needs of families in crisis. (p. 213)

This approach is an outgrowth of the "HOMEBUILDERS program" of the Behavioral Sciences Institute (BSI) in Washington State, which was originated in 1974. Bath and Haapala (1993) indicate that the use of heterogeneous client samples may explain some of the equivocal findings of their research. Again, such findings and discrepancies should not be surprising in light of the complexity of the issues encountered by families who share some uniformity of precipitating events but also experience their own individual patterns of adversity and vulnerability.

FAMILY REACTIONS TO INFANTS AT RISK AND WITH DISABILITIES

Initial Feelings and Reactions

As we have indicated earlier in this chapter, families ultimately possess remarkable capacities of resiliency, which allow them to sustain enormous crises and, in a sense, to heal themselves. No one expects to have an infant with problems (see Figure 18–8). Newborn illness and impairment are traumatic and difficult to endure regardless of parental age, family composition, religion, or socioeconomic background. Some parents cope better than others; yet, all must inevitably confront feelings, attitudes, and anxieties. Initially, parents often experience a sense of shock and disbelief. As one father said in an account of family experiences with his daughter Becky, babies are not supposed to be born 3 months early, and babies are not supposed to have disabling conditions. Whether children are planned or come unexpectedly, parents anticipate that they will be healthy and beautiful. Mothers, in particular, sustain a sense of loss in not being able to carry their infants to full term, and, commonly, both parents feel guilty and blame themselves—often irrationally—for problems that have taken place. One family who worked with us actually attributed the premature birth of their baby daughter to the "strong coffee" they had made the morning of delivery. Parents frequently search for answers when there are none!

Coupled with the pain and shock over the birth of an acutely ill or disabled baby, families also must deal with the unfamiliar and overwhelming environment of intensive care nurseries. Even though they may be comforted by the excellence of care and technology of facilities, there is much they do not understand. This is a time of mixed emotions and constant change—joy over the survival of a baby, uncertainty about outcome, new learning about premature infants, new acquaintances with other families, and hope that perhaps things will be all right. The inevitable change and rotation of medical caretakers may be unsettling in already volatile circumstances. Not surprisingly, parents may feel starkly alone, yet, at the same time, strongly bonded to other families in a common state of insanity.

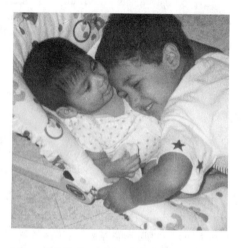

Figure 18–8 Stephen and sister, Helen. Helen experienced a number of medical problems when she first arrived in the United States from Guatemala. As a toddler, she is very active and she has the support of a loving and committed family.

If babies are extremely premature and/or suffer serious illness, the period of intensive care may be an emotional roller coaster. If their babies are "doing well," parents are ecstatic. If their children are not responding, family worlds fall apart. Some parents are able to involve siblings in the healing process, and that can be positive for the entire family in sharing thoughts and feelings. On the other hand, the questions that brothers and sisters may ask many times are difficult for mothers and fathers to answer, even for themselves (see Figures 18–9, 18–10, and 18–11). The larger world of family and friends also obviously plays a major part in caregiver adjustment and feelings of well-being. This is true with the birth of a typical newborn and possibly even more relevant when conditions are less than optimal.

Rarely is anyone prepared for the first glimpse of a baby born at 24 or 25 weeks gestation; the infant is barely visible amid the connections to monitors and other

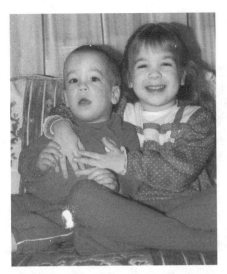

Figure 18–9 Steven and Michelle at home. Steven was born 10 weeks early and hospitalized for approximately 6 weeks. His older sister, Michelle, was a constant companion through many visits by home intervention teams.

equipment. All too frequently, parents have reported that neighbors fail to send cards or gifts or hesitate to acknowledge the birth of their new baby in any way, and relatives, attempting to cope with sorrow themselves, may refuse to return to the hospital after the initial visit. Such experiences tend to heighten the problems of dealing with the family crisis.

Understandably, parents feel angry. They ask themselves why this tragedy has befallen them. Friends and families who respond that it is "God's will" or that they can have other children offer little consolation. As one parent commented, "I ate the right foods, got plenty of rest, took care of myself and my baby before he was born. There was no reason for him to have been so sick or to have been in that unit." However well adjusted families are, living with the fear of developmental problems or even death exaggerates frustrations and feelings of helplessness. "How ridiculous," one parent explained, "to have to pick up the telephone each night to ask someone else how your baby is doing!" Parents naturally want to take care of their own children, and hospitals today are encouraging that participation as much as possible. When that care and contact are limited because of medical treatment in strange settings, the normal loving cycle of interaction is disrupted.

Resolutions

Eventually, after weeks, months, or perhaps years, order emerges from chaos, and most parents begin to take charge of their lives. For many, the pain and hard times bring strength, and families feel that they have grown

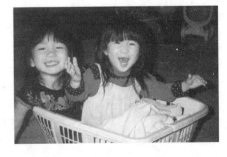

Figure 18–10 Korey and Kasey, two sisters adopted separately from Korea. They joined a family with three brothers.

from their experiences. The mother who lost her son Joey noted that never again would she take life and everyday events for granted. Having survived, many parents believe they are changed people. And indeed they are!

Resolutions come in different ways. Some parents need to work through their own attitudes and feelings alone before they can share with their partners and other members of the family. Others need to talk and confirm their thoughts from the beginning. It is difficult to hear all that is being said about one's baby; that too becomes a process, little by little letting in information. Situations become relative. Parents themselves sometimes are amazed

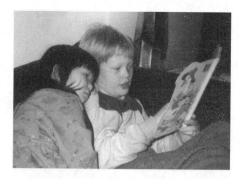

Figure 18–11 Korey and Patrick

that they can endure all that they do endure. Those who have grown through the experience discover within themselves that they are healthier human beings if they are able to dwell less on the negative and let go of their anger. Caregivers who have continued to harbor feelings of self-pity and who blame themselves and others for their misfortune run the risk of tarnishing the special joy of bearing and raising their children.

What brings parents to the point of acceptance is hard to define. Many eventually realize that, despite a persistent emphasis on perfection in this country, perfection is not reality for any child. We have been with families who have lost their babies during the first year of life and have known that that was inevitable soon after birth. Their faith and belief in the value of even a short life set an example for the rest of us who may take such gifts for granted. Again and again, our observations and interactions with families have confirmed that sick and developmentally delayed newborns may bring out the best qualities of love and unselfishness, which otherwise might not have risen to the surface. Parents have learned that they can love themselves and their children in spite of the terrible blow life appears to have dealt them. Much soul-searching, a trust in God, and supportive family and friends seem to be common strengths for many who have shared their feelings and experiences with us. Families begin to live their lives again, with a renewed optimism and hope, realistic expectations, and an ability to see the best, regardless of outcome.

One parent, Pam, who lost her son Joey 1 week after his first birthday exemplifies this strength in the following words:

> One of my greatest joys was watching what Joey did for other people and how he touched their lives. He gave so much love to everybody around him. It seemed almost impossible that this tiny baby could bring such happiness to so many people.

Most parents do well despite attempts of some professionals to help them. There is little that one can say to soften the pain and shock that families feel initially. One cannot remove doubt or cancel grief; time heals those hurts. The greatest injustice that professionals bring to families are promises that both know are unfounded.

Parents need to have essential medical information and our honest judgment about the current status of their child's development. They need to have resources of other parents and knowledge about intervention if they want it. They need to have sensitive, caring professionals who are not afraid to share the pain that families go through and who still can remain at a distance that allows them to offer sound guidance to the best of their abilities. Finally, families need to know that professionals—in medicine, education, social work, and other helping fields—do not have all the answers. They can provide support, but families themselves can and should make their own decisions about their children.

BIBLIOGRAPHY

Affonso, D.D., Hurst, I., Mayberry, L.J., Haller, L., Yost, K., & Lynch, M.E. (1985). Stressors reported by mothers of hospitalized premature infants. *Neonatal Network, 11*(6), 63–70.

Ards, S., & Harrell, A. (1993). Reporting of child maltreatment: A secondary analysis of the national incidence surveys. *Child Abuse & Neglect, 17,* 337–344.

Barber, P.A., Turnbull, A.P., Behr, S.K., & Kerns, G.M. (1988). A family systems perspective on early childhood special education. In S.L. Odom & M.B. Karnes (Eds.), *Early intervention for infants and children with handicaps: An empirical base* (pp. 179–198). Baltimore: Paul H. Brookes.

Bath, H.I., & Haapala, D.A. (1993). Intensive family preservation services with abused and neglected children: An examination of group differences. *Child Abuse and Neglect, 17,* 213–225.

Brooks-Gunn, J., Liaw, F.R., & Klebanov, P.K. (1992). Effects of early intervention on cognitive function of low birth weight preterm infants. *Journal of Pediatrics, 120*(3), 350–359.

Chess, S., & Thomas, A. (1982). Infant bonding: Mystique and reality. *American Journal of Orthopsychiatry, 52,* 213–222.

Clark, C. (1984). International Mission of Hope calendar introduction.

Cobiella, C.W., Mabe, P.A., & Forehand, R.L. (1990). A comparison of two stress-reduction treatments for mothers of neonates hospitalized in a neonatal intensive care unit. *Children's Health Care, 19*(2), 93–100.

Egeland, B., & Vaughn, B. (1981). Failure of "bond formation" as a cause of abuse, neglect, and maltreatment. *American Journal of Orthopsychiatry, 51,* 79–85.

Gelles, R.J., & Lancaster, J.B. (Eds.). (1987). *Child abuse and neglect: Biosocial dimensions.* New York: Aldine De Gruyter.

Goldberg, S. (1978). Prematurity: Effects on parent-infant interaction. *Journal of Psychiatric Psychology, 3,* 137–144.

Goldberg, S. (1982). Some biological aspects of early parent-infant interaction. *Reviews of research: The young child* (Vol. 3) (pp. 35–56). Washington, DC: National Association for the Education of Young Children.

Infant Health and Development Program. (1990). Enhancing the outcomes of low-birth-weight, premature infants. *JAMA, 263*(22), 3035–3042.

Jacobs, F.H., & Davies, M.W. (1991). Rhetoric or reality: Child and family policy in the United States. *Social Policy Report, Society for Research in Child Development, V*(4), 1–25.

Jacobsen, J.J. (1986). *Psychiatric sequelae of child abuse: Reconnaissance of child abuse and neglect, evaluation, prospects, recommendations.* Springfield, IL: Charles C. Thomas.

Kilpatrick, A.C. (1992). *Long-range effects of child and adolescent sexual experiences: Myths, mores, menaces.* Hillsdale, NJ: Lawrence Erlbaum.

Klaus, M.H., & Kennell, J.H. (1976). *Maternal-infant bonding.* St. Louis: C.V. Mosby.

Klaus, M.H., & Kennell, J.H. (1982). *Parent-infant bonding.* St. Louis: C.V. Mosby.

Lee, S.K., Penner, P.L., & Cox, M. (1991). Impact of very low birth weight infants on the family and its relationship to parental attitudes. *Pediatrics, 88,* 105–109.

Lowenthal, B. (1987). Stress factors and their alleviation in parents of high risk pre-term infants. *The Exceptional Child, 34*(1), 21–30.

Ludwig, S., & Kornberg, A.E. (Eds.). (1992). *Child abuse: A medical reference* (2nd ed.). New York: Churchill Livingstone.

Miles, M.S. (1989). Parents of critically ill premature infants: Sources of stress. *Critical Care Nursing Quarterly, 12*(3), 69–74.

Miles, M.S., Funk, S.G., & Kasper, M.A. (1991). The neonatal intensive care unit environment: Sources of stress for parents. *AACN Clinical Issues in Critical Care Nursing, 2*(2), 346–354.

Pfander, S., & Bradley-Johnson, S. (1990). Effects of an intervention program and its components on NICU infants. *Children's Health Care, 19*(3), 140–146.

Ross Laboratories. (1991). *Children and Violence.* Report of the Twenty-Third Ross Roundtable on Critical Approaches to Common Pediatric Problems in Collaboration with the Ambulatory Pediatric Association. Columbus, OH: Ross Laboratories.

Sigman, M., Cohen, S.E., Beckwith, L., & Parmelee, A.H. (1981). Social and familial influences on the development of preterm infants. *Journal of Pediatric Psychology, 6,* 1–13.

Solnit, A.J., & Provence, S. (1979). Vulnerability and risk in early childhood. In J.D. Osofsky (Ed.), *Handbook of infant development* (pp. 799–808). New York: John Wiley & Sons.

Trupin, E.W., Tarico, V.S., Low, B.P., Jemelka, R., & McClellan, J. (1993). Children on child protective service caseloads: Prevalence and nature of serious emotional disturbance. *Child Abuse & Neglect, 17,* 345–355.

Wolfe, D.A. (1987). Child abuse: Implications for child development and psychopathology. *Developmental Clinical Psychology and Psychiatry, 10.* Newbury Park, CA: Sage.

Wolfner, G.D., & Gelles, R.J. (1993). A profile of violence toward children: A national study. *Child Abuse & Neglect, 17,* 197–212.

Chapter 19

Sensory, Motor, and Regulatory Problems: Behavior and Early Intervention Strategies

Andrea M. DeSantis

Alex, born at 28 weeks gestation, exhibited mild developmental delays. He also had severe temper tantrums several times a day. Alex's parents approached a local developmental clinic for an evaluation to determine the origin of these tantrums so that intervention might be pursued. The clinic team was asked to determine whether this behavior was typical and, if not, what the causes might be. The following questions might be used in determining the cause(s) of Alex's behavior:

- Is Alex "merely" a temperamentally difficult 2-year-old?
- Are his temper tantrums provoked by mismanagement or limited parenting skills?
- Is Alex frustrated by being asked to perform above his developmental level?
- Does he exhibit a wide disparity between motor and cognitive development?
- Could it be that Alex's behavior is a result of sensory processing problems or poor self-regulation? (Self-regulation is the ability to maintain a balanced internal state in the presence of sensations and interactions from the external world [Greenspan, 1981].)
- Does he over-react or under-react to tactile, visual, auditory, or vestibular (gravity and movement) stimuli?
- What is the cumulative impact as Alex simultaneously processes these stimuli over time?
- If Alex has motor system impairments, is increased effort required to accomplish tasks that typically are automatic for a child of this age?
- Do frustration and fatigue affect his capacity to process sensory stimuli efficiently?

In this chapter, sensory aspects of the central nervous system will be discussed, along with the possible behavioral manifestations of inadequate sensory processing. Differentiating atypical sensorimotor development and its prevailing behavioral expressions from patterns that are truly age appropriate or "typical" is a complex task but one that is crucial for meaningful intervention (Brazelton & Yogman, 1986). Early identification of such atypical development is vital to family-focused strategies, so that secondary complications can be minimized. If sensory processing deficits are not identified in a child, the self-esteem of the child and that of his or her parents are in jeopardy. Unnecessary blame, power struggles, and a cycle of frustration are likely to follow. Parents may overlook sensorimotor influences on behavior. Furthermore, they may feel incompetent to manage their child's behavior, which often leads to feelings of resentment toward the child.

It is necessary to define three basic terms in order to understand sensorimotor problems in young children. *Regulation* is the body's adaptation to changing environmental conditions, which results in maintenance of normal sleep/wake cycles, feeding rhythms, and heart and respiratory rates (Greenspan, 1981). Researchers have postulated that *sensory processing* of visual, tactile, and vestibular sensations interfaces with the functions of regulatory systems (Greenspan, 1989). These two processes harmoniously coexist within a proficient nervous system. In this area of study, frequent reference is made to the *autonomic nervous system,* which keeps involuntary processes such as respiration, heart rate, and digestion in a state of equilibrium (Carlson, 1986; Kandel & Schwartz, 1985). A higher degree of neurological competence is recognized when a neonate achieves a state of alertness without autonomic stressors, such as respiratory pauses, spitting up, gagging, or motor stressors, such as flaccidity or hypertonicity (Als & Duffy, 1989).

In contrast to full-term infants, preterm babies typically reveal disorganized regulation of state and an inability to process visual, tactile, vestibular and auditory information simultaneously, which result in stress to the autonomic nervous system (Als, 1986). Furthermore, Als and Duffy (1989) have reported relationships between early neurobehavioral outcome and later behavioral manifestations in school-age children who were high risk, preterm infants. In follow-up studies, such children have frequently shown a range of disorganized autonomic and motor systems that are thought to be attributable to early neurological insult. Disorganized attention and disabilities in the areas of motor and spatial skills learning are also common (Als, 1985; Als & Duffy, 1889). Moreover, it has been hypothesized that later neurobehavioral inadequacies may take on more emotional and behavioral qualities, as demands become increasingly complex in the preschool and school years (Als & Duffy, 1989).

Early behavioral manifestations may elude the untrained observer. Knowledge of the nervous system and the principles of sensory integration is essential in detecting these subtle indicators. Many difficult behaviors exhibited by children are still misinterpreted as "stubbornness," "obstinance," or simply "bad" or "lazy" behavior. Reframing our understanding of these behaviors, hopefully, will permit more diverse insights and potential for programing.

SENSORY PROCESSING: PHILOSOPHIES, ASSESSMENT, AND INTERVENTION

Each of us has a unique set of sensory impulses that enters the brain for tuning, harmony, and interpretation. In addition, each person responds to environmental stimuli in a highly individual way. Some people dislike background noise when reading, while others require it to concentrate. Some are unable to attend to conversation in a busy shopping mall, appearing uninterested or rude; others can keep thoughts focused amidst utter chaos. Variations in the perception of touch and movement systems also cause individuals to behave in certain ways.

How do adults with intact, competent nervous systems respond to typical environmental stimuli? Frequently, people are able to self-regulate by removing themselves from a stimulating situation, decreasing environmental stimuli (e.g., turning off lights and music), or engaging in exercise. In today's demanding world, however, some individuals are ineffective in regulating their nervous systems, thus adding stress to the body. Reinforcing this notion, abundant research has revealed strong associations between emotional stress and physical illness in adults (Borysenko, 1987; Moyers, 1993). In young populations, self-regulatory and sensory processing problems may have a significant impact on overall development, personality, and interactional capabilities (Ayres, 1979; DeGangi, Craft, & Castellan, 1991; Greenspan, 1989).

In her pioneering theory of sensory integration, Ayres (1979) attempted to provide a framework for examining the relationship between brain and behavior. More recently, her early concept of the "organization of sensory input" has been elaborated to reflect the underlying premise that the central nervous system must take in sensations from one's own body and the environment and synthesize that information to allow for organized, goal-directed responses (Ayres, 1972, 1979; DeGangi, 1991; Fisher, Murray, & Bundy, 1991). In addition, a basic assumption of sensory integrative therapy is that higher level adaptive responses are elicited from the child as a result of stimuli specifically selected in the intervention situation and provided by the trained therapist. Likewise, it is anticipated that the child will achieve the optimal organization of these sensations within the brain by engaging in self-directed play (Ayres, 1972, 1979; Fisher, Murray, & Bundy, 1991).

Upon review of the sensory integration literature, one needs to differentiate the terminology and various authors' perspectives as to what constitutes sensory integration. For instance, researchers may attempt to delineate differences across approaches to sensory integration treatment, suggesting that, for example, only specifically designed suspended equipment combined with skillful administration of activities by a trained therapist genuinely qualifies as sensory integration (Murray & Anzalone, 1991). Other approaches entail less specific sensory stimulation involving the direct application of tactile, vestibular, olfactory, and/or visual input to elicit generalized behavioral responses such as calming or increased attention (Melnechuck, 1988; Wilbarger, 1984).

Commonly, sensory integration theory and intervention have been based on research with school-age children that was published in 1979 (Ayres). Interestingly, however, the first objective measure of sensory processing and reactivity in infants 4 to 18 months of age, the *Test of Sensory Function in Infants* (TSFI), was developed in 1989 by DeGangi and Greenspan. In conjunction with standardized tests of development, a sensory questionnaire, and clinical observations, the TSFI, with its potential to provide a valid and more precise measure of informal sensory functioning, is a valuable component in the process of identification and assessment of atypical sensorimotor development. Evidence exists that the entire instrument can be used reliably and validly for screening purposes, but more extensive research with groups of delayed and temperamentally difficult infants is needed (DeGangi, Berk, & Greenspan, 1988).

Sensory intervention that is applied within the context of a family-centered model to help the child who has sensory processing and regulatory problems should be integrated into the home environment and play arena. To achieve this integration, intervention must interface with both developmental and psychosocial parameters of the family-child and caregiver-child interactions. Both parent and child should be empowered to acquire self-awareness and self-directed strategies to develop more adaptive behaviors. Incorporating meaningful sensory information throughout play activities can heighten motivation for learning while, at the same time, providing experience with meaningful sensory opportunities essential to the child's overall development.

As described by Greenspan and Greenspan (1985), child-centered play ("floor time") can offer children multiple nonstressful play situations so that transitions can be modeled and, thus, more easily accepted. There are differences in the definition and implementation of this concept (DeGangi, Craft, & Castellan, 1991; Greenspan & Greenspan, 1985, 1989) as there are for all intervention strategies. Overall, constructs of child-centered play are similar in that they involve setting aside designated times each day for spontaneous play activities with the child. The Greenspan strategy, in particular, encourages the use of questions and themes for the child's play to facilitate a broad range of emotional expressions, communication, focused attention, and play schemes (Greenspan & Greenspan, 1985). A delicate balance of presenting ideas and allowing response time is determined by the child's individual temperament. As described by Greenspan and Greenspan (1989), floor time permits tuning into the child's motivations, communication, and emotions through gestural and pretend play; it offers the important benefits (1) of allowing the child to feel in control and (2) of facilitating an understanding of cause and effect within his or her immediate world.

Like Greenspan and Greenspan, DeGangi, Craft, and Castellan (1991) also describe the advantages of a child-centered play approach that includes sensory integration principles. Again, the parent learns to decipher child cues, behaviors, and emotions by allowing the youngster to take the lead in nonjudgmental playtime, while at the same time focusing on the preschooler's sensory, motor, and self-regulatory capabilities as parent and child interact. Accordingly, even though the child is perceived to be the leader in such play scenarios, specific props such as heavy toys and textured objects are chosen carefully to enhance sensory integration and offer an appropriate level of motor challenge and structure within a safe environment (DeGangi, Craft, & Castellan, 1991).

Intervention strategies using the principles of child-centered play described here represent a marked departure from traditional strategies of teaching and doing things "to" the child. In pediatric physical therapy, there are specific approaches that require hands-on, manipulative techniques such as stretching, weightbearing in all positions, and improving muscle tone and balance. Typically, therapists are trained to "give therapy," employing these hands-on strategies to improve function and foster independence.

Our best intentions are to help the child progress, but direct instruction may not be the most effective mode of learning at certain stages of development (Ames & Ilg, 1976a, 1976b; Armstrong, 1987). Alternatively, rather than hands-on intervention initially, the child first may be allowed to set the emotional tone and theme of the interaction. A delicate balance of turn-taking and more structured forms of intervention then may follow, depending on the child's needs. Always, a good learning environment addresses both physical and emotional needs, with the child ideally being an active, motivated participant. Unfortunately, much of our clinical and educational experiences for children have not held to this tenet. In his chapter on "dysteachia," for example, Armstrong (1987) describes a "mug jug" theory of learning, by which the teacher all too often "pours knowledge into the "child's mug." To the contrary, best clinical practice has taught us that children learn more efficiently in supportive environments that challenge existing concepts and use a wide array of methods. Recognition of the usefulness of alternative approaches is not easily attained, but support for such strategies is mounting.

Finally, as we indicated earlier, additional considerations of family intervention need to include an awareness of parent grief over "shattered dreams," which inevitably is fraught with feelings of inadequacy, hopelessness, and depression. Furthermore, issues relating to gender, cultural and religious beliefs and family of origin are also important considerations (Goldhor-Lerner, 1989; McGoldrick, Pearce, & Giordano, 1982). To ensure the success of a family-centered focus, professionals with a look to the future must make a commitment to expanding their knowledge, must be willing to release themselves from rigid discipline-specific roles, and must adopt methods of nonjudgmental, empathetic listening.

SENSORY, MOTOR, AND BEHAVIORAL PROBLEMS

Children with Regulatory Disorders

Many disabled children display difficulties with processing sensory and motor information. It is not uncommon for normal infants, during the first 4 to 6 months, to display transient sleep irregularities and/or colic that eventually resolve with maturity (DeGangi, 1991; Greenspan, 1991). If problems remain past 6 months, these "difficult" or "fussy" infants may, in fact, suffer from "regulatory disorders" (DeGangi, 1991; Greenspan, 1991). According to one recent longitudinal study (DeGangi, Porges, Sickel, & Greenspan, in press), persistence of such problems beyond the infant stage may be associated with a variety of later impairments in behavior, sensorimotor, and/or emotional development. Other studies (Als, 1985; DeGangi, 1991) have supported these findings.

The importance of early recognition of sensorimotor processing dysfunction—often referred to later as "sensory integration problems" (Ayres, 1972)—has been recognized by several researchers (Als & Duffy, 1989; DeGangi & Greenspan, 1988; Fisher, Murray, & Bundy, 1991; Greenspan, 1989). To date, longitudinal data have not been collected consistently within populations of preschool children at large; yet, early developmental histories of "nonlabeled" children who have come to the attention of professionals repeatedly have revealed patterns of later learning and behavioral difficulties (DeGangi, 1991). The manifestations of sensorimotor processing dysfunction are much like those described by parents of infants with regulatory disorders—difficulties with sleep/wake cycles; inconsolability and unexplained, undifferentiated persistent crying; colic; hypersensitivities to sensory stimuli; and/or an unwillingness to cuddle during infancy.

Not all early symptoms and characteristics of infants necessarily evolve into later developmental or behavioral problems (Turecki, 1989). Many children outgrow these difficulties by acquiring adequate neurological maturation within the first year, but others are not so fortunate (DeGangi, Porges, Sickel, & Greenspan, in press). In addition, a history of early sensorimotor problems has frequently been reported in populations of school-age children with emotional difficulties (Fish & Dixon, 1978; Walker & Emory, 1983). Given the complexities of human behavior and development, researchers have interpreted sensorimotor processing dysfunction from a variety of perspectives (Turecki, 1989). For instance, difficult temperament has often been cited as an explanation for "problem" children (Bates, 1980; Thomas & Chess, 1977), suggesting that such behaviors are inherent in a youngster's personality. The daily interaction of personality and environment inevitably shapes the behaviors of the developing child. Greenspan (1989) has viewed the behaviors of such children as "psychopathologic," while other investigators have focused on the characteristics of temperament that affect behavioral styles of children (Thomas & Chess, 1977; Turecki, 1989). To date, studies have not linked parent personality and the impact of home environment to evidence of difficult temperament (Daniels, Plomin, & Greenhalgh, 1984). Not to be discounted are specific infant characteristics with an etiology related to neurological maturation of homeostasis and sensory processing. All of these interpretations are viable considerations.

Children with Autism

Children with autism often have many sensory processing difficulties, ranging from little or no reaction to stimuli (e.g., avoiding eye contact or showing no response to verbal requests) to over-reaction to certain stimuli such as touch or movement (Ayres & Tickle, 1980; Greenspan, 1991). Ayres (1979) has described aspects of poor sensory processing in autistic children as an inability to register and modulate sensory input adequately, and many atypical behavioral manifestations have been noted as a consequence of this poor sensory processing ability (Ayres & Tickle, 1980). In particular, these behaviors may include motor planning deficits (Ayres, 1979), intolerance to touch, overactivity in response to movement, and hypersensitivity and/or hyposensitivity to visual and auditory stimuli (Greenspan, 1991). Attachment disorders, dysfunctional social interactions, and difficulties with language processing also have been documented in relation to autism (Greenspan, 1981, 1991). Grandin has discussed her personal challenges as an individual who has autism, expressing her belief that emotional reactions to certain stimuli may cause autistic children to retreat into a world of their own (Grandin & Scarino, 1986).

Autism is well recognized as a complex interaction of brain and behavior, and many speculations regarding its etiology have been made in the neuropsychological literature (Bauman & Kemper, 1985; Ritvo et al., 1986). In reality, several different etiologies probably account for these behavioral manifestations.

Children with Prenatal Exposure to Cocaine and Other Substance Abuse

In Chapter 13, we discussed the fact that it is almost impossible to identify the "pure" effects directly related to cocaine exposure in the fetus. While there is little argument that cocaine and alcohol do cause impairment in utero (Bingol, Fuchs, Diaz, Stone, & Gromisch, 1987; Chasnoff, Burns, Schnoll, & Burns, 1985; Chasnoff, Griffith, MacGregor, & Burns, 1989), many other factors also impact on the developing child. Genetic predisposition to disabilities, constitutional difficulties, poor nutrition, and little or no medical care all may be harmful to the developing fetus. In addition, as noted in Chapter 13, chaotic home environments and numerous transitions into foster care homes may intensify already existing negative prenatal effects of cocaine and alcohol use. Not surprisingly, self-regulatory difficulties, such as feeding and sleeping problems, in combination with inadequate processing of environmental stimuli, have often been noted in the young child exposed prenatally to cocaine (Dixon, Bresnahan, & Zuckerman, 1990). In addition, distractibility, poor interactive skills, limited facial expressions, language and motor coordination difficulties, and hypersensitivity to environmental stimuli have frequently been observed in later years (Chasnoff, 1992; Van Dyke & Fox, 1990). These findings are not unlike those related to learning difficulties due to other causes, but the association is perhaps more apparent because the disabilities occur in children of substance-abusing mothers.

Preterm Infants As Young Children

Als (1985) has described regulatory difficulties in preterm infants as young children as a mismatch between brain expectancy and adaptability to environmental stimuli. The child's inability to assimilate incoming stimuli often results in poor regulation of state behavior, overarousal, inadequate calming, and prolonged stress responses, all resulting from an incompetent autonomic nervous system. These findings mirror Ayres' (1972) concept of sensory integrative dysfunction and children with regulatory disorders (DeGangi, 1991). Als (1985) also has documented the persistence of disorganized neurobehavioral functioning into the school years in low birthweight populations. According to Als, despite the presence of "normal" intellectual capacity and an absence of documented brain injury, children born prematurely have frequently demonstrated greater autonomic reactivity, poor transition between tasks, articulation and language difficulties, and limited facial expression (1985).

As noted in our discussion of interventions in neonatal intensive care units (Chapters 16 and 17), differences in neurobehavioral organization in preterm infants require not only adapted, low stimulus environments in intensive care nurseries, but also predictable and structured intervention through the school years, in order to increase self-regulation and minimize stress responses. Such interventions may enhance both information processing and social interactions, minimizing later learning disorders and behavioral problems.

Children with General Developmental Delay

During the first year of life, infants with developmental delays have been found to exhibit sensorimotor dysfunctions such as tactile defensiveness, poor ocular-motor control, and vestibular problems (DeGangi & Greenspan, 1989). For the most part, these have been groups of young children without severe disabilities such as cerebral palsy, spina bifida, or other major orthopedic disabilities (DeGangi, Berk, & Greenspan, 1988; DeGangi & Greenspan, 1988).

In addition, sensory processing problems in the form of low muscle tone and poor tactile and vestibular modulation have frequently been observed later in life in more developmentally delayed school-aged children. While the causes of these characteristics may be related to known neurological insult, such children with more general delays, nonetheless, have been found to benefit from intervention using principles of the sensory integration theory and practice (Murray & Anzalone, 1991).

Children with Learning Disabilities

Although controversy over distinctions between youngsters with sensory integrative dysfunction and children with learning disabilities continues to exist, many similar behavioral patterns have been identified across these two groups. In both populations, there is a significant impact on behavior, temperament, and sensory thresholds during learning and social interaction. Descriptions of sensory integrative dysfunction in the learning disabled child (Ayres, 1979; Fisher, Murray,

& Bundy, 1991) parallel or mirror clinical manifestations of "nonverbal learning disabilities" (NLD) (Rourke, Young, & Leenaars, 1989). Moreover, in a 17-year longitudinal study, Rourke, Young, and Leenaars (1989) revealed evidence of maladaptive social and emotional development in this NLD population, placing such children at risk as they attempt to compensate for disability. Like sensory integration problems, long-term manifestations of NLD can jeopardize social and emotional stability into the school and adolescent years. A behavioral comparison of nonverbal learning disabilities and sensory integrative dysfunction is presented in Table 19–1.

In summary, specific labels or diagnoses related to children with sensory, motor, and behavioral difficulties possess some unique characteristics, but there are many similarities. In the field of pediatric intervention, professionals of all disciplines should recognize the overlap of regulatory and sensory processing difficulties within all populations of disabled children.

NEUROPHYSIOLOGICAL EVIDENCE OF REGULATORY DISORDERS

Many prominent researchers have found the nervous system to be the cause of "atypical" behavior. Porges (1983) attempted to understand children with regulatory disorders by studying patterns of response in the autonomic nervous system. Specifically, he hypothesized that cognitive development and behavior, theoretically, should be associated directly with central nervous system activity. Sophisticated technology now allows for measurement of such autonomic nervous system

Table 19–1 Comparison of Nonverbal Learning Disabilities and Sensory Integrative Dysfunction

Nonverbal Learning Disability	*Sensory Integrative Dysfunction*
Bilateral tactile-perceptual difficulties	Poor tactile discrimination
Bilateral psychomotor deficits	Bilateral integrative dysfunction (vestibular-bilateral disorder)
Visual-spatial organizational difficulties	Deficits in perceptual skills, especially in relation to body scheme, forms, and space
Tactile sensitivity	Tactile defensiveness
Psychomotor clumsiness	Developmental dyspraxia
Difficulty adapting to novel and complex conditions	
Delays in social judgment, perception, and interactions	

Source: (Data adapted from Ayres, 1979; Fisher, Murray, & Bundy, 1991; Rourke, Young, & Leenaars, 1989).

activity. Similarly, investigators have examined the psychophysiological effects of sensory and cognitive demands on normal infants and those with regulatory disorders (DeGangi, DiPietro, Greenspan, & Porges, 1991). In particular, baseline heart rate and vagal tone have been compared with heart rate and vagal tone during presentation of sensory and cognitive challenges. It is possible to use this method to determine neurobehavioral outcomes because heart rate variability (the change in the sequential beat to beat intervals over time) is influenced by the vagus nerve and neurotransmitters (Porges, 1983). Physiological factors such as posture, movement, and respiration affect heart rate variability.

In this research, while "normally functioning" infants were able to suppress heart rate variability and vagal tone in response to sensory and cognitive demands, babies with regulatory disorders were more apt to exhibit higher baseline vagal tone and inconsistencies in vagal reactivity. These findings suggest a close association of sensory reactivity and difficult behaviors with physiological components (DeGangi, DiPietro, Greenspan, & Porges, 1991).

Additional data linking behavior and neurophysiological factors have been presented in a study by Kagan, Reznick, and Snidman (1987). Specifically, these researchers found physiological differences between behaviorally inhibited (cautious and shy) and uninhibited (fearless and outgoing) children who were 2 to 6 years old. Concurrently, behaviorally inhibited children displayed lower thresholds to stimulation when presented with unfamiliar situations, as measured by special heart rate variability patterns noted among the groups. Elevated cortisol levels also were identified in this group. Cortisol, a stress hormone, was measured in this study through levels in saliva prior to and during specific activities. Furthermore, high levels of norepinephrine, a neurotransmitter in the autonomic nervous system, resulted in a greater "fight or flight" response in the behaviorally inhibited children of ages 4 and 5.

Overall, findings of these and other studies suggest, at least in part, a neurobiological foundation for behavior as manifested in the form of low frustration tolerance, hyperactivity to environmental stimuli, poor attention, sensory processing difficulties, motor incompetencies, atypical behaviors, and labile emotional state. Obviously, behaviors, in turn, impact on and are influenced by the immediate environment of the child.

SENSORIMOTOR INFLUENCES ON EMOTION AND BEHAVIOR

When a child with sensorimotor dysfunction exhibits challenging behavior, a common question from the parent or caregiver is: "How typical is this for the child's age?" As should be clear from our discussion, even a sound knowledge base of social, emotional, and sensorimotor development usually does not yield easy answers in terms of an accurate differentiation of the child's behavior. In this regard, Jean Ayres (1979) has cautioned that no individual displays *perfect* sensory integration of the numerous impulses bombarding the system. Nevertheless, contented, well-coordinated people, predictably, demonstrate a higher degree of nervous system integration than those who do not have these characteristics (Ayres, 1979). Emotional responses are a by-product of the nervous system's capabilities (Ayres, 1979). Nerve cells constitute the structural basis of the nervous system, modulated by an intricate blend of chemicals, metabolites, hormones, and electrical impulses. The brain organizes and integrates this myriad of impulses. Simply stated, the brain communicates to the body how it is to respond. The nervous system and all of its complexities are responsible for our thoughts, memories, perceptions, and feelings (Carlson, 1986). Feelings and emotions are just as crucial to consider during intervention as are problem-solving skills, movement, and language development.

Recent collaboration of neuroscientists, physiologists, and psychologists has moved us toward a realization that the ultimate outcome of nervous system function is behavior (Carlson, 1986). Moreover, the growing interest in psychoneuroimmunology is gaining increasing credibility (Melnechuck, 1988). (Psychoneuroimmunology is the study of how psychology and emotional states influence disease through the nervous, endocrine, and immune systems. Researchers have discovered areas of the brain abundant in chemicals that also control emotions and are receptor sites for the immune system. The interaction of mind and immunity offers important potential for understanding emotions (i.e., hopes and fears), which ultimately may influence the body's ability to defend itself (Melnechuck, 1988). For example, children with nervous system dysfunction have frequently been known to exhibit either suppressed or overactive immune systems, including a high incidence of allergies (McLoughlin, Nall, & Petrosko, 1985; Rapp, 1991). Thus, providing intervention in a nonstressful manner is paramount to any meaningful approach for maximizing a child's potential, while at the same time maintaining homeostasis of the nervous system.

MANIFESTATIONS OF SENSORIMOTOR PROBLEMS

Birth to 18 Months of Age

Although knowledge of social and functional milestones is useful in understanding behavior and sensorimotor problems, the interaction of parent styles, child characteristics, and environmental influences makes this process a substantial challenge. Let us consider the early building blocks that provide the foundation for more complex emotional capabilities. Greenspan's first emotional milestone is *homeostasis,* which is defined as the baby's ability to self-calm and modulate arousal in the presence of environmental stimuli and human interaction. Neurologically, homeostasis of the central nervous system refers to the ability of the body's internal, involuntary processes (e.g., heart rate and respiratory rate) to maintain a balanced state as the system receives external sensory stimuli (Greenspan & Greenspan, 1985).

If regulatory reactions and sensorimotor processing are inefficient, a baby's intense irritability will be expressed emotionally through muscle responses and the senses, thus compromising the child's early development of self and body schema (Greenspan & Greenspan, 1985). Parents often describe their child who lacks adequate regulation as being inconsolable and unable to acquire regular sleep patterns, self-calm through conventional methods, and/or modulate moods. As the child grows older, the precursors to the development of self-concept, trust, and predictability may suffer. If poor homeostasis persists, other stages of emotional development can be affected adversely (Greenspan & Greenspan, 1985). The following feeding scenario describes the intricate evolution of behavioral problems resulting from sensory, motor, and regulatory difficulties.

Sensory Hypersensitivities and Feeding

An infant who fails to thrive and who has tactile hypersensitivities learns early that arching away, rather than cuddling, during breast-feeding protects an overly sensitive tactile system. The nipple touching the infant's face and lips is perceived by the baby as uncomfortable. In addition, hypersensitivities may impact on the child's later ability to tolerate food textures. The baby's withdrawal during breast-feeding can be most devastating to the nursing mother since she may perceive this behavior as a personal rejection rather than the infant's inability to process tactile information. If the child also has low oral muscle tone, causing a poor suck and rapid fatigue during feedings, the mother may experience further frustration and even anger.

Complicating the situation, the parent's anxiety about inadequate caloric intake may become a dominant daily issue. Subsequent attempts to feed the baby may gradually result in an avoidance response, as the child learns to exert control by refusal. Also, the child may display limited eye contact, which may signify the baby's need to "tune out" other incoming stimuli as a result of tactile over-stimulation, reflecting general inability to simultaneously process sensory information efficiently. The dysfunctional interaction of forced feeding and rejection has been well documented in such parent-child relationships (Frank, Silva, & Needlman, 1993). A mother's apprehension about her child's weight loss generates intense anxiety because it challenges her self-image as a competent caregiver. In turn, the child's level of arousal and tactile discomfort with food textures, indeed, may impact on the ability to focus at mealtime.

A learned pattern of control occurs as the child approaches 12 months of age, when the baby can crawl away or can tightly close the mouth when food is introduced. The mother then begins to feed the child "on the run" to ensure adequate caloric intake, rather than moving through the ritual of food preparation, anticipation, sitting the child in the high chair, and engaging in face-to-face communication. The child may become even more disorganized by the rapid influx of environmental stimuli that occurs during feeding "on the run." The child is sensitive to earlier experiences of displeasure, by virtue of the mother's anxiety as she approaches and cajoles with a spoon full of food. What began as an early tactile rejection is compounded further by the development of emotional milestones of independence and autonomy. The child may reject cuddling because of the need for independence and the tactile hypersensitivity, thus making the parent feel more inadequate. If the child has a propensity toward hyperarousal, stressful feedings may perpetuate disorganized attention and power struggles in other areas of interaction. Thus, a ripple effect is likely to occur, creating conflict in daily activities such as play and sleep.

Sleep

Infants and toddlers with regulatory and sensory processing problems can also display sleep disturbances, which affect both the caregivers and child. The cycle of parent anxiety, lack of sleep, and frustration frequently leads to bringing the child into the parent's bed. Therefore, the child does not learn how to fall asleep independently. Many serious problems that are multifaceted and extensive may ensue (Ferber, 1986).

The following scenario exemplifies the complexities of parent-child interaction when a sleep disorder is present. A first-time mother of an active, irritable 9-month boy was concerned about her son's inability to settle in order to sleep and his frequent night awakenings. On evaluation, he exhibited difficulty in filtering out sights and sounds of his environment and demonstrated response to insignificant stimuli (e.g., noise and clutter), thus generating a cycle of overstimulation and hyperarousal. As a result, the baby required 3 hours of calming, using firm swaddling with a blanket and vertical bouncing, in order to sleep at night. Typically, he awakened six or seven times throughout the night and again required extensive calming measures to prevent uncontrollable crying. Because he was also unable to take a nap during the day, his behavior provided the mother with little time to recuperate or accomplish any self-nurturing activities.

Eventually, the mother's issues surfaced. She was often preoccupied with concerns about her inadequacies and thoughts that her son might be hyperactive, as his father was as a child. Given her child's high level of activity and irritability, the mother experienced guilt since she was not able to bond adequately with her baby in the way she had visualized prior to his birth. Furthermore, she believed that if she let her son cry without being present, he would experience mental and emotional harm. Allowing the child to sleep in his parent's bed provided a means for bonding and attachment. The mother needed to come to terms with the ways that her feelings and fears were contributing to her son's erratic sleep routine. Once she was able to confront her own fears, she was subsequently able to implement a bedtime routine, integrating a low-stimulus environment, sensory inhibition techniques, and repeated self-calming sleep techniques (Ferber, 1986). Only then did the parents learn to interpret appropriately the child's signals of overstimulation so that they could become skilled at adapting their strategies, with minimal guidance from the intervention professional.

Attention and Arousal

Infants who display tendencies toward hypoarousal or hyperarousal may lack expressions of joy, pleasure, and exploration. A hypoaroused infant often is referred to as "floppy" (hypotonic) and can appear apathetic and/or withdrawn (Greenspan, 1989). A less demanding, hypotonic infant may view the surroundings placidly, whereas a child with a tendency toward hyperarousal may disregard certain sensory stimuli, such as face-to-face imitation games, while focusing on irrelevant background sounds. In addition to attention modulation difficulties with visual and auditory stimuli, hand movement sensations may compound and intensify hyperarousal, resulting in diminished eye contact and limited interactive play.

By comparison, hyperarousal is often evidenced by a pronounced need for novelty and changing stimuli, which results in a poor attention span and play disorganization. Parents report that there is a constant need to keep their child occupied with toys and activities throughout the day. In such instances, it is likely that the child's ability to develop a toy preference and expand play schemes is severely limited (DeGangi, Craft, & Castellan, 1991). A cycle of overstimulation, mood lability, and irritability can easily develop. Hyperarousal can also be associated with sleep disturbances in both the infant and toddler stages.

The following vignette illustrates a familiar sequence of events in the life of a hyperaroused child. As a baby gains independent mobility, the frequency and amount of stimuli increase, causing the child to experience greater difficulty in playing with any one toy for an extended period. The hyperaroused child may seem "bright-eyed," appearing to need many toys to sustain interest and attention; however, this multisensory approach usually does not help the child to learn or focus. Instead, it may have the opposite effect of serving to perpetuate the hyperaroused state, creating disorganized play behaviors, limiting object manipulation, and restricting social interaction. In addition, such children may be unable to calm for sleep, despite the use of extensive sensory calming techniques.

Toddlers: 18 to 36 Months of Age

Toddlerhood is a period for achieving mastery of body-in-space concepts through skillful creeping, upright positions, and cause-effect relationships. The child's body now is more predictable. Acquisition of the ability to poke and manipulate small objects further teaches the toddler spatial relationships and problem-solving skills (Ames & Ilg, 1976b). The youngster experiences a range of affective expressions of pleasure and autonomy congruent with a newly kindled assertiveness and curiosity. These qualities eventually expand into symbolic representation through functional language and pretend play (Greenspan, 1989).

Toddlers continue to develop modes of communication and emotional contact, which began in infancy as "proximal modes" such as touch and holding. As the concepts of separation and individual identity emerge, "distal modes" evolve; these modes include the use of vision, vocalization, affective gestures, hearing for reassuring security, and reciprocal signaling (Greenspan, 1989). Greenspan (1989) suggests that distal modes are integral to the development of representational modalities and capabilities (ideation), which allow the youngster to label and integrate feelings through pretend play in addition to acting out themes. If a parent is overanxious or overprotective, the child with sensory processing limitations may have increased difficulty developing optimal use of these modes, particularly distal modes. For example, if visual-spatial organization is compromised, the child may have difficulty discriminating facial-gestural communication and rely primarily on proximal modes to obtain knowledge. Auditory processing difficulties may lead to restricted verbal decoding of commands. Challenging behaviors described by Greenspan (1989) at this stage, such as chronic temper tantrums, withdrawal, inability to exert self-control, sleep disturbances, chronic aggressive behavior, and lack of movement or emotional organization, may have their origins in sensory, motor, and regulatory difficulties.

The early sensory development of self in relation to objects (visual, tactile, olfactory, vestibular, and proprioceptive qualities) lays the foundation for multisensory cognitive representation. Consequently, sensory processing difficulties may also restrict the range and depth of social, emotional, and intellectual capabilities (Greenspan, 1989). This concept is reminiscent of Ayres' (1979) discussion of sensory integrative disturbances and Piaget's (1952) assumption that "sensorimotor" building blocks are essential for later preoperational skills, understanding, concrete operations, and representational capabilities.

Ames and Ilg (1976b) characterize emotional behavior of typical children at this stage during the toddler years as oscillating between equilibrium and disequilibrium, with no balance at the midrange. Months of calm, satisfied demeanor may be followed by periods of strong demands, as the child seeks to assert a new-found independence. The child also may experience frustration when desires are not met or when motor or language capacities do not match cognitive level. Often, for example, a 2-year-old requires fairly definite rituals in choice of clothing and food (Ames & Ilg, 1976b).

Because the behavior of typical toddlers is ritualistic and demonstrates disequilibrium, it is a challenge to identify behaviors that reflect sensory processing dysfunction in high risk toddler populations (Ames & Ilg, 1976b). However, a sound knowledge of child development and a perceptive sensitivity to parent-child interactions can help the astute teacher or clinician to accurately differentiate between typical and atypical behaviors. In particular, the child with regulatory and/or sensory disorders may be subject to periods of equilibrium that are short-lived and disrupted, as a result of stimuli that other children ordinarily can manage. Extremes of behavior such as severe temper tantrums may be identified readily, while more subtle nuances of behavior require careful analysis. Therefore, in conjunction with a developmental and/or psychological assessment, a thorough evaluation by a physical or occupational therapist with expertise in sensory integration may be required.

Play

A toddler with sensory hypersensitivities and motor difficulties may find changes threatening, since touch and movement opportunities are unexpected. In the scenario of "rough-housing," which is usually enjoyable for fathers and their toddlers, sensory and regulatory problems may cause misinterpretations. For example, a youngster may appear to enjoy this kind of play initially but quickly may become distressed or overly excited for "no apparent reason." Additional indicators of stress and overstimulation often reported by parents include increased motor activity, clumsiness, fleeting from toy to toy without purposeful play, aggressiveness, irritability, and pronounced temper tantrums. In turn, the caregiver may not understand the cause of the child's response, continue with the game, then become angry if the child becomes aggressive or withdraws from the play situation. Thus, a cycle of miscommunication is established, jeopardizing emotional stability and learning opportunities with people and objects and even limiting the types of activities that the child finds intrinsically motivating (Clifford & Bundy, 1989).

Alternatively, when parents are made aware of their child's tactile problems and behaviors, they can learn better to sort out priorities in setting limits and offering encouragement, because they understand that these problems are not under the child's voluntary control. Play interactions may require modification. For instance, many children with sensorimotor and regulatory problems demonstrate increased organization, attention, and age-appropriate play schemes with the benefit of short periods (10 to 15 minutes) of child-centered proprioceptive play— pushing and pulling heavy trucks, receiving firm pressure input down the back, and picking up couch pillows or pulling blankets. Firm proprioceptive input, it has been hypothesized, has an overall calming influence on the nervous system (DeGangi, Craft, & Castellan, 1991). Illustrating this intervention theory, an 18-month old "hyperalert" girl who mouthed toys excessively, despite normal cognition, received 15 minutes of proprioceptive play opportunities, along with the elimination of visual and auditory stimuli. Immediately following such intervention strategies, she discontinued mouthing behaviors and appropriately engaged in symbolic play; e.g., brushing a doll's hair.

Transition Difficulties

Many toddlers resist change to some extent, but most are able to transition with ample forewarning. Two-year-olds enjoy the consistency of sameness and routine, for instance, the repetition of reading the same stories or playing with the same cars, which may offer a sense of control and security (Ames & Ilg, 1976b). On the other hand, a child with regulatory and sensorimotor impairments may exhibit an excessive need for sameness and may persist in this rigid pattern well beyond the toddler years. The child may experience difficulty with translating play ideas into motor action. Such youngsters often are referred to as having "motor planning difficulties or developmental dyspraxia" (Ayres, 1979). A reportedly "stubborn" child may, in fact, be utilizing his or her only self-preserving, coping mechanism for protection against feelings of being "out of control." For example, the child may learn *one* method of getting on and off a riding toy but may lack the ability to make a motor adaptation if the riding toy happens to be stuck behind a chair. The child may become extremely frustrated in attempting to dislodge the toy. If change is then introduced, for instance, by saying, "Time to go to the store," the child may be unable to shift to a different motor routine, which may cause further anxiety.

Separation Anxiety

Although separation anxiety is often interpreted as a negative emotion, Greenspan and Greenspan (1989) believe that this milestone is an important growth process for both the parents and child. By 8 months of age, anxiety in response to strangers usually increases with the baby's heightened awareness of others in his or her surroundings. During the toddler months, these behaviors again evolve, as the now mobile youngster begins to develop a sense of autonomy and independence. In addition to discussing the emotional origins of separation anxiety, Greenspan and Greenspan (1989) also commented on the importance of visual-spatial components and the child's identification of body and space in relation to the caregiver. Various degrees of anxiety may emerge, depending on how the child perceives his or her world and communicates through proximal or distal modes. During developmentally less immature periods, additional assurance may be required for successful transition (Greenspan & Greenspan, 1989).

Many factors need to be considered with parents who, in a sense, have taken on the role of being the child's "sensor or antenna." In these instances, parents automatically may adapt to the child's sensory processing limitations by controlling the environmental stimuli (e.g., being overprotective or carrying the youngster more frequently). The parent may initially exert effective control against potential overstimulation inherent in a busy world of unexpected touch and noise, but such practices ultimately can impede the development of separation and autonomy, thus inhibiting the child's learning of how to deal with typical stimulation.

Unfortunately, if the source of a child's behavioral difficulties has not been identified when sensory and regulatory problems begin to arise, parents may experience years of anxiety and frustration. They may conclude that certain reactions are "normal" behavior for all children or believe that they possess inadequate parenting skills. The profound impact on the child's self-image can be equally devastating. For example, a child is likely to be disciplined regularly to "sit still" when, in reality, he or she may have little or no voluntary control over this behavior. The child may have low muscle tone, which requires constant movement in order to hold posture erect. Parents should be helped to understand that another possible cause of the child's behavior may be a reaction to environmental stimuli, that is, overstimulation resulting from an inability to process stimuli simultaneously. Then, discipline takes on a new dimension, with caregivers focusing on helping their child to learn appropriate strategies to minimize behavior problems and reserving disciplinary measures for more important issues such as safety.

In summary, rather than using age level alone as a basis for determining appropriate expectations and limit-setting strategies, professionals and parents should regard the child's sensory and motor capabilities as windows through which the integrity of emotional and behavioral maturity can be viewed. Learning to read early cues of sensory processing and/or regulatory difficulties can change the direction of behavior that is out of control and lead to establishment of more balanced, homeostatic levels for children struggling with such problems.

INTERVENTION PROCESS: ONE CHILD-FAMILY EXPERIENCE

History

Here, we share the experiences of a child with sensory, motor, and regulatory problems and how, through home and professional interventions, he and his family together began to learn how to cope with these difficulties.

Kevin was born at 38 weeks gestation with good Apgar scores and normal birthweight. Although he had jaundice at 3 days, no treatment was deemed necessary. In the first few days and weeks of life, Kevin began to manifest a variety of problems. He was slow to suck and had continuous swallowing problems. His extreme fussiness and colic initially were addressed through use of a special formula because of a history of milk intolerance in the family. Additional treatment with Levsin drops also was required. Nasal reflux began shortly after cereal was started at 4 months of age; projectile vomiting occurred up to 9 months of age and recurred at 21 through 24 months, when Kevin experienced severe separation anxiety.

Kevin's other developmental milestones were slow to emerge—rolling at 8 months, sitting at 10 months, pulling to stand at 15 months, and walking unsteadily by 16 months. Asymmetrical commando crawling, using primarily the right side, began at $10^1/_2$ months, while creeping on hands and knees developed at 14 months. Kevin especially disliked the prone position in his early months, and this displeasure likely was related to a tactile hypersensitivity. His acquisition of spoken words also was inconsistent.

Kevin received a comprehensive medical and developmental assessment from a local agency at 12 months as a result of his extreme inconsolability and developmental delays. Results of this evaluation indicated oral-motor problems, delay of $4^1/_2$ months in use of expressive language, inconsolability, a left asymmetry in the upper and lower extremities, mild motor delays, and slow development of object permanence and imitation concepts. These patterns of development, along with a family history of learning disabilities, placed Kevin at substantial risk for developmental problems.

Speech and language services were recommended, but Kevin did not qualify for other intervention services. Since his mother is a professional in early childhood education, Kevin's problems may have been attenuated by her ability to use educational techniques. Nonetheless, the family remained frustrated because professional assessment of developmental delay did not indicate the need for comprehensive intervention, despite Kevin's significant irritability and regulatory deficits. His parents felt trapped with expectations of "knowing how to deliver" intervention to their son, while at the same time desiring ongoing affirmation and the support from professionals necessary to address the full range of their child's behavior.

Evaluation

At 14 months of age, Kevin was brought by his parents for evaluation to determine whether physical or occupational therapy would be helpful; they had continued to seek guidance for their son's persistent regulatory difficulties. Specifically, they were interested in learning how Kevin's fussiness, speech and motor lags, and possible sensory dysfunction impacted his behavior, learning, sleep, and social interactions.

Kevin was a delightful, sociable child who readily engaged in appropriate interaction with adults and toys during the initial stages of the evaluation. At other times, he became frustrated when he was unsuccessful during play and was easily distressed with his lack of skilled motor control. His parents reported that Kevin frequently became irritable at home for no apparent reason and that this behavior quickly escalated to pronounced temper tantrums. This pattern had been manifested early in infancy, when Kevin's fussiness as a baby persisted despite numerous comforting strategies implemented by the family (e.g., swaddling with a warm blanket, use of a pacifier, and giving a warm bath). Attempts to employ Ferber's (1986) systematic approach to self-regulation of sleep was abandoned because the family lived in a one-bedroom apartment that was not soundproof. Thus, at the time of evaluation, a cycle of increasing frustration and hopelessness had added seemingly endless stressors to this family's life.

Kevin demonstrated severe hypersensitivities to tactile and vestibular stimulation on the TSFI. The TSFI, described earlier in this chapter, is a criterion-referenced measure that evaluates reactivity to tactile deep pressure, adaptive motor functions (motor planning), visual-tactile integration, ocular motor control, and reactivity to vestibular stimulation. During administration of the TSFI section on tactile items, Kevin became so distressed, with skin blanching and pronounced crying, that administration of the section on vestibular items could be performed only after a 20-minute calming period. Kevin's mother also reported that, at home, he needed to be fed in a vertical position and became distressed when he was tilted in space. While the use of a rocking chair had been somewhat successful to calm Kevin, other forms of movement caused him to become hyperaroused and agitated. The most successful mode to quiet this youngster was the presentation of visual information such as simple picture books or vertical bouncing, rather than rocking. Some of Kevin's distress signals were flushed and pale skin, hair twirling, increased flexion posturing of his left arm, and irritability. Additional tactile hypersensitivities were evidenced in Kevin's dislike of specific food consistencies, a lack of interest in textured toys, and failure to manipulate toys with the entire palm of his hand.

Attention

At times, Kevin's apparent decreased attention span impeded his interest in sustained interaction with adults or toys. He seemed to flee from toy to toy, without expanding play schemes with any specific item. Repeatedly, he interacted briefly with a toy and became quickly frustrated when he could not get his hands to manipulate the toy as desired. As is common in children experiencing sensory processing and regulatory problems, Kevin was beginning to manifest early signs of motor planning difficulties. At home, as this cycle progressed, Kevin required prolonged, external measures for calming throughout his day, since his autonomic nervous system was not capable of self-regulation. Even though his parents repeatedly attempted to anticipate this kind of cycle, they reported that they often "walked on eggshells," providing discipline inconsistently or avoiding interaction with Kevin to prevent such out-of-control behavior.

Transitions often were difficult for Kevin, who was keenly aware that he lacked the ability to calm himself. When routines changed, he was not able to adapt easily, even with adequate verbal preparation and visual cues. Ironically, although a calming approach was essential to help maintain a quiet state, Kevin seemed to process information more accurately when it was delivered with exaggerated facial and motor gestures. In reality, perhaps the supplemental information provided additional modes of input to assist with preparation for change. This statement does not imply that a multisensory approach is an advocated or effective technique for a child with significant sensory processing problems. In terms of early intervention, however, some children with learning problems do need to rely on repetition, facial expressions, and other strategies to determine the context of each new situation (Als, 1985; Smith, 1991).

Gross and Fine Motor Abilities

Kevin, who was large in stature and heavy, exhibited low muscle tone throughout his body, making it difficult for him to move. There was no evidence of high muscle tone or asymmetry on the left side of his body at rest, but Kevin's warning signs of early distress were often manifested in the form of increased muscle tone in his left arm and a subtle left arm neglect.

On the *Peabody Developmental Motor Scales* (Folio & Fewell, 1983), Kevin's performance was average for a 10-month-old child, even though his scores were compromised because he was not ambulating independently at the time. Because sensory organization is a necessary foundation for motor development and motor planning (Ayres, 1979), Kevin's opportunities for repetition of movements and mastery of body schema (i.e., interaction of his body with objects and people) were also jeopardized significantly.

Although Kevin's fine motor skills were age-appropriate at 14 months of age, his decreased shoulder stability and tactile hypersensitivity interfered with the quality of his motor performance. He used atypical posturing to manipulate toys, demonstrated exaggerated finger flaring when he released them, and lacked spontaneous use of his left hand.

In summary, Kevin was a child with major disparities between his cognitive and sensorimotor abilities. Sensory processing of tactile, vestibular, visual, and auditory information was disorganized, especially if two or more modalities were required.

Structured and Child-Centered Approaches

The degree to which environmental and parental facilitation was required to help Kevin regain an integrated balance of his regulatory and sensory systems was substantial, warranting extensive changes in parent-child and teacher-child interaction patterns. Conventional measures of comfort had been relatively ineffective for addressing all the aspects of Kevin's behavior. Initially, he required more child-centered opportunities to help focus his attention and to help him feel a sense of control. Evidence of more organized, focused periods of play were signals that Kevin could tolerate more structured sensory stimulation and hands-on techniques.

At home, adaptation of calming strategies was achieved because of new knowledge of Kevin's previously unrecognized tactile and vestibular hypersensitivities. For example, the home environment was altered to eliminate multiple toys and unneeded visual stimuli. A quiet corner behind the couch was established, since Kevin displayed a tendency to crawl behind it when overstimulated. In addition, modes of effective calming for Kevin were introduced regularly; these techniques included firm downward back stroking, swaddling in a blanket, and looking at simple books with him in his quiet corner.

Whenever Kevin became distressed by the introduction of tactile and movable toys, he typically withdrew and was inattentive. His parents accordingly adapted concepts of child-centered play, using heavy proprioceptive play at home to facilitate more advanced schemes. Kevin responded positively by playing with heavy, large trucks or repeating opportunities for lifting heavy pillows and stuffed animals in and out of boxes. Gradually, he expanded his area of exploration to tactile and symbolic play items. Eventually, Kevin tolerated brief forms of up-and-down bouncing, rocking in a head-to-toe fashion, while prone between two couch pillows, and side-to-side movement in supported sitting. He indicated his need for intermittent breaks from these vestibular activities by raising his head. Most importantly, Kevin needed to feel in control of the input at all times; otherwise, a stress response occurred. As a result of these measures, Kevin showed less distress and greater ease in making transitions to new activities.

Frequently, both at home and during therapy, it was difficult to discern Kevin's genuine anger and frustration from feelings that were prompted by overstimulation, inability to use body movements skillfully, or failure to communicate effectively. For example, one therapist first introduced a movable scooter with a doll riding it, so that Kevin could have a visual model of the activity. Given his vestibular dysfunction and the fact that he did not perceive movement as enjoyable, he resisted even pushing the scooter while on his knees, showing a fear response. Such a reaction could have been a symptom of gravitational insecurity, an irrational response to movement when the feet leave the ground (Ayres, 1979). During this same therapy session, a new activity was introduced using textured toys, which appeared to escalate his distress further. He began to hit the therapist, but his actions showed no malice; in fact they seemed to be guised as play. This common pattern, reported at home and in school, deserved careful analysis. It would have been easy for an untrained person not to see the prior cycle of overstimulation that resulted from his inability to regulate and integrate the tactile and vestibular stimuli presented. Kevin required firm boundaries; he had to be told, "We do not hit people." However, stern discipline was avoided. Such situations could easily have given rise to feelings of rejection, especially if discipline had been used repeatedly without astute recognition of the contributing factors.

At home, an increase in repetitive hammering, pounding, and violent crashing of large trucks often led to aggressive forms of play. Kevin may have been craving for more "whole body" forms of input to satisfy his sensory needs. Ultimately, however, these kinds of toys were replaced with safe play areas for whole body types of activities such as rolling, pushing, pulling, and jumping (Figure 19–1). Heavy bean bags to toss into a laundry basket provided added proprioceptive input. In the process, Kevin's aggressive behavior disappeared.

During the period from 21 to 24 months of age, Kevin experienced severe separation anxiety. Pronounced distress began when he awakened in the morning, on weekdays only. This distress seemed to be related to anticipation of his transition to school 3 days a week and to the babysitter's home 2 days a week. Kevin's parents needed to swaddle and gently bounce him to calm him when he awakened each morning. A security blanket, pictures of his parents and favorite toys, verbal reassurance prior to leaving home, and affirmation on separation at school did not improve the situation. After consultation with a psychologist and a therapist trained to treat sensory problems, a behavioral approach incorporating principles

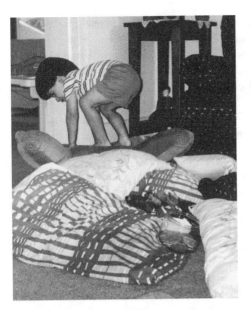

Figure 19–1 Nest of pillows offering safe area to acquire muscle and joint input. Modifying toys to match Kevin's sensory needs helped to supplement learning and interactional capacities.

of sensory integration was developed and implemented. Kevin's compromised visual-spatial body awareness was probably contributing to his anxiety of being "separate" from his parents. Careful analysis of the babysitter's home revealed an unstructured, busy environment with numerous active children. In retrospect, this situation was too unpredictable for Kevin's sensory and regulatory problems, particularly since his schedule for each day of the week involved numerous transitions. A switch to a less busy babysitter, continued verbal assurance, ample forewarning prior to each transition, and an increase in child-centered opportunities at home seemed to enhance his sense of security and control. Separation anxiety disappeared within 2 weeks of these changes.

At 24 months of age, Kevin's motor control was comparable to that of a 15- to 18-month-old child. These disabilities caused severe frustration, which often appeared to leave him in a state of "emotional disequilibrium" (Ames & Ilg, 1976b). With maturation and development, his problems began to resolve at about 30 months of age.

Intervention programing specifically focused on Kevin's motor problems was implemented finally by reframing traditional structured therapy sessions with a balance of child-centered activities. Kevin's need for a nonstressful play environment was paramount to his sense of security and control and, ultimately, to his ability to remain in a calm state. If too much movement or too many textures were introduced via a structured multisensory approach, Kevin tended to resist further activities and became distressed for the remainder of the day. Professional staff often expressed discomfort, feeling that by "backing off" from imposing necessary input, they were failing to provide Kevin with adequate intervention. In time, however, Kevin made tremendous progress by working in low stimulus rooms (Figure 19–2), and handling controlled amounts of sensory stimulation in an environment of predictable routines. The family and team were able to anticipate Kevin's pattern of distress in advance by discerning his signs of overstimulation.

Physical therapy provided multiple opportunities for weightbearing and heavy proprioceptive input, with these sessions being arranged at the beginning of each day. Periodic opportunities for such forms of input were incorporated into the classroom setting. Subsequently, Kevin began to initiate advanced motor sequences, using body symmetry while demonstrating improved balance reactions. A greater range of joy in his facial expressions began to emerge, as he gained a sense of mastery over his body in space. Speech, language, and occupational therapies were combined to avoid multiple transitions, as well as to provide a means for integrating activities and sensory components. For example, pictures fastened to a rug with velcro promoted opportunities for weightbearing through crawling, and additional proprioceptive shoulder input was provided when Kevin pulled the pictures off the rug. He also seemed to be better focused when these proprioceptive activities fortified language-based tasks.

Kevin's classroom was set up with props to facilitate sensory, motor, and social development. The kitchen area was carpeted to muffle sound and lined with bookshelves, which limited distraction from other areas, affording a low stimulus environment (see Figure 19–2). Velcro strips were used to stick plastic play food to a surface, which provided more resistance, offered proprioceptive input, and minimized the frequency of frustration due to objects rolling off the table. Empty grocery boxes and plastic grocery carts were weighted with beans and sand (Figure 19–3). Eventually, stair steps and opportunities to climb and reach for groceries were introduced to challenge Kevin's balance and ability to functionally integrate his adverse responses to gravity and movement in a play scenario. Frequently, child-centered play was incorporated into Kevin's classroom routine, followed by structured sensorimotor activities, as directed by the physical and occupational therapists.

Kevin required repeated introduction of new sensory play materials such as Play-Doh or cornmeal, dictated on his terms. Prior to exposure to new textures, the therapists provided whole body tactile and proprioceptive desensitization activities such as firm massage and rolling and jumping into a crash area made with pillows. These experiences served to prepare his body to accept touch to selected areas such as finger, hands, and face. A low table, about 12 inches high, allowed him to have multiple opportunities for upper body weightbearing while he kneeled (Figure 19–4). This input offered a steady routine for desensitization as Kevin manipulated various tactile media.

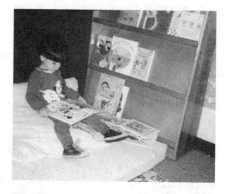

Figure 19–2 Enclosed, low stimulus classroom environment

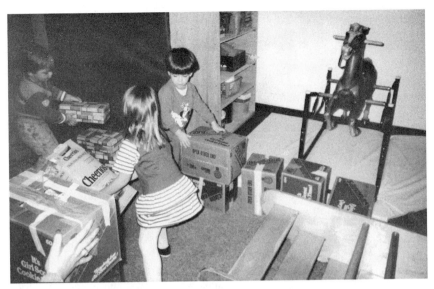

Figure 19–3 Play area showing large weighted boxes used during block building and grocery shopping play to provide additional muscle and joint input

In a "quiet corner," Kevin was able to engage in dress-up play and social interaction, which often involved unexpected touching from other children. These experiences were enhanced further by using soft clothing or heavy cloaks or by placing weights in jacket pockets, which provided firm pressure input.

In conclusion, heightened awareness in reading Kevin's signals greatly assisted caregivers, teachers, and therapists to determine a needed balance of daily child-centered versus structured activities. Kevin is now 32 months old with age-appropriate cognitive and language skills. Asymmetry has diminished, and balance has improved dramatically. Although motor planning and motor execution continue to be a challenge, he is showing more motivation and focused attention to practice both gross and fine motor skills. He is learning to identify his own early signs of distress and to initiate self-calming strategies such as taking deep breaths when the environmental demands become overwhelming. Ongoing reassessment and adaptations to determine the most advantageous intervention principles and strategies will continue as Kevin faces new challenges and milestones in the future.

CONCLUSION

Children with sensory processing problems are a diverse group, with high risk for later behavioral and learning difficulties. To address the complex, unique needs of each child with a strategy that will achieve reliable behavioral differentiation in approaches to intervention, professionals need to consider multiple variables relating to neurophysiology, behavioral psychology, genetics, sensorimotor factors, parent-child interactions, cultural expectations, and environmental influences.

In addition to clinical expertise, teachers and developmental specialists must be able to elicit support from and foster rapport with families as equal colleagues in problem solving. Moreover, in this area of expertise, professionals are increasingly challenged to set aside their traditional desires to "fix" the child or the family's problems. Intervention must evolve as a natural process of open, nonjudgmental partnerships.

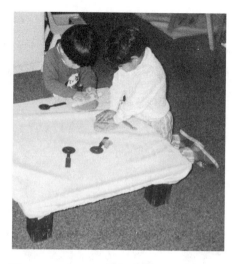

Figure 19–4 Table with shortened legs, allowing exaggerated upper and lower body weightbearing (note that table edges are padded for safety)

BIBLIOGRAPHY

Als, H. (1985). Patterns of infant behavior: Analogues of later organizational difficulties. In F.H. Duffy & N. Geschwind (Eds.), *Dyslexia: A neuroscientific approach to clinical evaluation* (pp. 67–92). Boston: Little, Brown.

Als, H. (1986). A synactive model of neonatal behavioral organization: Framework for the assessment of the premature infant and for support of infants and parents in the neonatal intensive care environment. *Physical and Occupational Therapy in Pediatrics, 6,* 3–53.

Als, H., & Duffy, F.H. (1989). Neurobehavioral assessment in the newborn period: Opportunity for early detection of later learning disabilities and for early intervention. *Research in Infant Assessment, 25*(6), 127–152.

Ames, L.B., & Ilg, F.L. (1976a). *Your one year old.* New York: Dell.

Ames, L.B., & Ilg, F.L. (1976b). *Your two year old.* New York: Dell.

Armstrong, T. (1987). *In their own way.* New York: St. Martin's Press.

Ayres, A.J. (1972). *Sensory integration and learning disorders.* Los Angeles: Western Psychological Services.

Ayres, A.J. (1979). *Sensory integration and the child.* Los Angeles: Western Psychological Services.

Ayres, A.J. (1989). *Sensory integration and praxis tests.* Los Angeles: Western Psychological Services.

Ayres, A.J., & Tickle, L.S. (1980). Hyper-responsivity to touch and vestibular stimuli as a predictor of response to sensory integration procedures by autistic children. *American Journal of Occupational Therapy, 34*(6), 374–381.

Bates, J.E. (1980). The concept of difficult temperament. *Merrill-Palmer Quarterly, 26,* 299–319.

Bauman, M, & Kemper, T.L. (1985). Histoanatomic observations of the brain in early infantile autism. *Neurology, 35,* 866–874.

Bingol, N., Fuchs, M, Diaz, V., Stone, R.K., & Gromisch, D.S. (1987). Teratogenicity of cocaine in humans. *Journal of Pediatrics, 110,* 93–96.

Borysenko, J. (1987). *Minding the body, mending the mind.* Toronto: Bantam.

Brazelton, T.B., & Yogman, M.W. (1986). *Affective development in infancy.* Norwood, NJ: Ablex.

Carlson, N.R. (1986). *Physiology of behavior.* Boston: Allyn & Bacon.

Chasnoff, I.J. (1992). Cocaine, pregnancy, and the growing child. *Current Problems in Pediatrics, 22*(7), 302–321.

Chasnoff, I.J., Burns, W.J., Schnoll, S.H., & Burns, K.A. (1985). Cocaine use in pregnancy. *New England Journal of Medicine, 313,* 666–669.

Chasnoff, I.J., Griffith, D.R., MacGregor, S., & Dirkesk Burns, K.A. (1989). Temporal patterns of cocaine use in pregnancy. *JAMA, 261,* 1741–1744.

Clifford, J.J., & Bundy, A.C. (1989). Play preference and play performance in normal boys and boys with sensory integrative dysfunction. *Occupational Therapy Journal of Research, 9,* 202–217.

Daniels, D., Plomin, R., & Greenhalgh, J. (1984). Correlates of difficult temperament in infancy. *Child Development, 55,* 1184–1194.

DeGangi, G.A. (1991). Assessment of sensory, emotional, and attentional problems in regulatory disordered infants: Part 1. *Infants and Young Children, 3*(3), 1–8.

DeGangi, G.A., Berk, R., & Greenspan, S.I. (1988). The clinical measurement of sensory functioning in infants: A preliminary study. *Physical and Occupational Therapy in Pediatrics, 8*(2–3), 1–23.

DeGangi, G.A., Craft, P., & Castellan, J. (1991). Treatment of sensory, emotional, and attentional problems in regulatory disordered infants: Part 2. *Infants and Young Children, 3*(3), 9–19.

DeGangi, G.A., DiPietro, J.A., Greenspan, S.I., & Porges, S.W. (1991). Psychophysiological characteristics of the regulatory disordered infant. *Infant Behavior and Development, 14,* 37–50.

DeGangi, G.A., & Greenspan, S.I. (1988). The development of sensory function in infants. *Physical and Occupational Therapy in Pediatrics, 8*(4), 21–33.

DeGangi, G.A., & Greenspan, S.I. (1989). *Test of sensory function in infants.* Los Angeles: Western Psychological Services.

DeGangi, G.A., Porges, S.W., Sickel, R.Z., & Greenspan, S.I. (in press). Four year follow-up of a sample of regulatory disordered infants. *Infant Mental Health Journal.*

DeGangi, G.A., Wietlisbach, M., Goodin, M., & Scheiner, N. (1993). A comparison of structured sensorimotor therapy and child-centered activity in the treatment of preschool children with sensorimotor problems. *American Journal of Occupational Therapy, 47*(9), 777–786.

Dixon, S.D, Bresnahan, K., & Zuckerman, B. (1990). Cocaine babies: Meeting the challenge of management. *Contemporary Pediatrics, 6,* 70–92.

Ferber, R. (1986). *Solve your child's sleep problems.* New York: Simon & Schuster.

Fish, B., & Dixon, W.J. (1978). Vestibular hyporeactivity in infants at risk for schizophrenia. *Archives of General Psychiatry, 35,* 963–971.

Fisher, A.G., Murray, E.A., & Bundy, A.C. (1991). *Sensory integration: Theory and practice.* Philadelphia: F.A. Davis.

Folio, M.R., & Fewell, R.F. (1983). *Peabody developmental motor scales.* Chicago: Riverside.

Frank, D.A., Silva, M.A., & Needlman, R. (1993). Failure to thrive: Mystery, myth, and method. *Contemporary Pediatrics,* February, 114–123.

Goldhor-Lerner, H. (1989). *The dance of intimacy.* New York: Harper & Row.

Grandin, T., & Scarino, M. (1986). *Emergence: Labeled autistic.* Navato, CA: Arena.

Greenspan, S.I. (1981). *Psychopathology and adaptation in infancy and early childhood: Principles of clinical diagnosis and preventive intervention.* Madison, WI: International Universities Press.

Greenspan, S.I. (1989). The development of the ego: Insights from clinical work with infants and young children. In S.I. Greenspan & G.H. Pollock (Eds.), *The course of life: Infancy* (Vol. 1, pp. 85–164). Madison, WI: International Universities Press.

Greenspan, S.I. (1991). Regulatory disorders: I. Clinical perspectives. *NIDA Research Monograph, V*(114), 165–172.

Greenspan, S.I., & Greenspan, N.T. (1985). *First feelings: Milestones in the emotional development of your baby and child.* New York: Viking.

Greenspan, S.I., & Greenspan, N.T. (1989). *The essential partnership.* New York: Penguin.

Kagan, J., Reznick, S., & Snidman, N. (1987). The physiology and psychology of behavioral inhibition in children. *Child Development, 58,* 1459–1473.

Kandel, E.R., & Schwartz, J.H. (1985). *Principles of neural sciences* (2nd ed.). New York: Elsevier.

McGoldrick, M., Pearce, J.K., & Giordano, J. (1982). *Ethnicity and family therapy.* New York: Guilford Press.

McLoughlin, J.A., Nall, M., & Petrosko, J. (1985). Allergies and learning disabilities. *Learning Disability Quarterly, 8,* 255–260.

Melnechuck, T. (1988). Emotions, brain, immunity, and health: A review. In M. Clynes & L. Panksepp (Eds.), *Emotions and psychopathology* (pp. 181–247). New York: Plenum.

Moyers, B.D. (1993). *Healing and the mind.* New York: Doubleday.

Murray, E.A., & Anzalone, M.E. (1991). In A.G. Fisher, E.A. Murray, & A.C. Bundy, (Eds.), *Sensory integration: Theory and practice.* Philadelphia: E.A. Davis.

Piaget, J. (1952). *The origins of intelligence.* New York: International Universities Press.

Porges, S.W. (1983). Heart rate patterns in neonates: A potential diagnostic window to the brain. In T. Field & A. Sostek (Eds.), *Infants born at risk: Physiological, perceptual, and cognitive processes* (pp. 3–19). New York: Grune & Stratton.

Rapp, D. (1991). *Is this your child?* New York: William Morrow.

Ritvo, E.R.l, Freeman, B.J., Scheibel, A.B., Duong, R., Robinson, H., Guthrie, D., & Ritvo, A. (1986). Lower Purkinje cell counts in the cerebella of four autistic subjects: Initial findings of the UCLA-NSAC autopsy research report. *American Journal of Psychiatry, 143*(7), 862–866.

Rourke, B.P., Young, G.C., & Leernaars, A.A. (1989). A childhood learning disability that predisposes those afflicted to adolescent and adult depression and suicide risk. *Journal of Learning Disabilities, 22*(3), 169–175.

Smith, C.R. (1991). *Learning disabilities: The interaction of learner, task, and setting* (2nd ed.). Boston: Allyn & Bacon.

Thomas, A., & Chess, S. (1977). *Temperament and development.* New York: Brunner/Mazel.

Turecki, S. (1989). *The difficult child.* New York: Bantam.

Van Dyke, D.C, & Fox, A.A. (1990). Fetal drug exposure and its possible implications for learning in the preschool and school age population. *Journal of Learning Disabilities, 23*(3), 160–163.

Walker, E., & Emory, E. (1983). Infants at risk for psychopathology: Offspring of schizophrenic parents. *Child Development, 54,* 1269–1285.

Wilbarger, P. (1984, September). Planning an adequate sensory diet—Application of sensory processing theory during the first year of life. *Zero to Three: Bulletin of the National Center for Clinical Infant Programs,* pp. 7–12.

Chapter 20

Early Intervention: New Themes, Programing, and Research

Gail L. Ensher, Mary Elizabeth Redmond, Margaret P. Ninno,
and Helen Harrison

HISTORICAL PERSPECTIVE

Throughout history, one of the primary goals of many cultures has been the care and education of the young. In most Western countries, the family traditionally has assumed this responsibility, and when the family could not perform this function, society has found other ways to care for children—in orphanages, in foster homes, and, as a last resort, in institutional settings. The outcome for children cared for by society has, more often than not, been negative. In the 1940s, with the publication of studies on early development by Goldfarb (1943) and by Spitz (1945) and research on individualized care for infants with disabilities by Skeels and Dye (1939), society and educators in particular began to understand the seriously detrimental effects of various environmental settings.

During the 1950s, the programs of kindergartens and nursery schools were affected by such educators as Froebel, Montessori, and Dewey, as well as by the theoretical approaches of Piaget, Gesell, and Erickson. Preschools afforded better child care and a supportive environment to middle class childhood in the United States on a fee-paying basis. Subsequently, important social, economic, and political changes, together with new attitudes about child development, began to exert a direct influence on American early childhood education and intervention. The role of women in the United States changed, and a career outside the home became a major consideration for many mothers. During the 1960s, more than one-third of the women with children below school age had jobs; by 1970, that proportion had risen to about one-half. In addition, the traditional nuclear family also began to change, and a dramatic increase in single-parent households made early education programs an absolute necessity.

Subsequently, the highly charged political climate of the 1960s gave birth to several movements, the most important of which engendered a heightened sensitivity to civil rights. Throughout this decade, there was a major effort to address issues of socioeconomic "class" differences, which was perhaps most clearly reflected in Lyndon Johnson's "War on Poverty." One noteworthy outgrowth of these changes was the initiation of Head Start, the preschool intervention program implemented "in the hope of providing young children with a sort of inoculation against the ill effects of poverty" (Zigler & Berman, 1983, p. 895). Meanwhile, increasing numbers of researchers and child development specialists (Frost, 1973; Gordon, 1969) added new empirical evidence to substantiate the association between poverty and poor school performance. Concern was expressed that infants and young children living in low socioeconomic circumstances were particularly vulnerable.

In addition to potent social and political changes, new theories of childrearing and caregiving surfaced during the 1960s and 1970s. Bloom (1964) and Hunt (1961) were two early scholars who provided educators with an ideological framework for preschool intervention programs (see Figure 20–1). Coinciding with these positions, Piaget's writing on genetic epistemology (1963) focused on the child as an active participant in the learning process, a view that was reinforced by Bruner (1973) in his groundbreaking studies on learning and thinking. Armed with these theoretical foundations, early educators thus emphasized structured learning experiences and appropriate stimulation, both inside and outside the home. With this position, a new trend emerged in the field of early intervention.

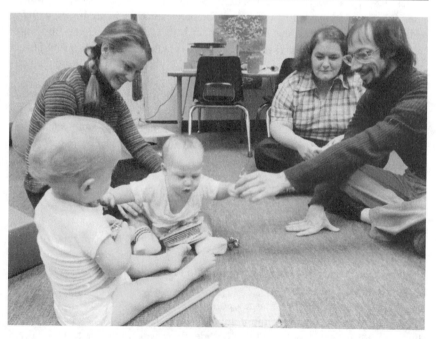

Figure 20–1 Center-based early intervention program with parents and children

The majority of early childhood programs that were designed and subsequently implemented during the 1960s focused on low income and minority children. Most were compensatory in nature and were patterned after a learning-deficit model. In contrast, programs in the 1970s placed a greater emphasis on prevention, and the passage of Public Law (PL) 94–142 (the Education for All Handicapped Children Act) in 1975 added a new dimension to the provision of services for persons with disabilities. Public Law 99–457, which amended PL 94–142, specifically mandated free and appropriate educational intervention and programing for all children with special needs and, as we have noted in earlier chapters, offered strong incentives for states to make services available to infants and toddlers. Finally, in 1990, a full spectrum of programing was reauthorized at the federal level with the passage of PL 102–119 and Part H, which explicitly address the needs of infants and toddlers from birth to 3 years of age. With the implementation of these new pieces of legislation, early childhood education has achieved a genuine integrity of its own, reinforcing and extending the rationale that "behavior and developmental potential are neither fixed in early life by genetic factors nor impossible to change after a supposed sensitive period" (Meisels, 1989, p. 452).

PUBLIC LAW 99–457: A NEW PHILOSOPHICAL BASE

Since 1986, virtually hundreds of articles and books have speculated about and defined the implications of PL 99–457, in particular Part H, for the field of early childhood special education, research, and training. One of the most insightful of these publications was written by Odom and Warren. Published in 1988, the article took a close look at the "internal" and "external" factors that would be most likely to shape the nature of early childhood special education by the year 2000 (p. 263). As we now approach the middle 1990s, many of these predictions have already become reality. They are explicitly related to a new philosophical base offered by PL 99–457, largely characterized by seven considerations (Odom & Warren, 1988, pp. 264–268):

1. serving children in least restrictive inclusive settings
2. collaborating toward optimal programing
3. focusing on caregivers
4. focusing on research in organizational and ecological contexts
5. serving new populations
6. coordinating statewide systems of service
7. training new personnel.

Serving Children in Least Restrictive Inclusive Settings. Public school systems throughout the United States are still in the formative stages of implementing PL

99–457 and its companion amendment PL 102–119. One of the foremost requirements of the legislation is to serve children in least restrictive inclusive settings (Peck, Odom, & Bricker, 1993). Across the board, this mandate has presented and will continue to raise challenges to every aspect of our educational and service delivery system. Critical components of the system include the physical locations where programs are administered, the curricula and methods used, personnel required to carry out such services, costs, the new roles of professionals, and the training procedures that will be utilized in higher education teacher preparation programs. Emphasis on *integration* of developmentally delayed children into the learning activities of typical children is not a newcomer to the field of special education. For years, it has been a focal point of much research designed with varying degrees and types of disabilities. As Peck, Odom, and Bricker (1993) state, the question has been greatly complicated by the myriad of factors that affect outcome. Clearly, however, quality programing in inclusive settings offers a superior model of intervention for all children and families, with the "implicit recognition that the segregation of a child with disabilities is in itself a powerful social act that may negatively affect the child's social and educational future" (Peck, Odom, & Bricker, 1993, p. 3).

Collaborating toward Optimal Programing. As we indicated in our discussion of assessment, the terms *interdisciplinary, crossdisciplinary,* and *transdisciplinary* describe various ways in which professionals have collaborated in the past across diverse disciplines. The concept of cooperative service delivery systems is the second essential component of the new early childhood legislation, which has given this concept new meaning. Such cooperation in delivery of services is now recognized as a defining quality of future professional-parent relationships. Issues of turf, which historically have served as barriers to effective cooperative efforts, are being challenged as never before. Moreover, consultative and collaborative approaches are fundamentally tied to the implementation of best practice inclusive programing. Implied in these contemporary efforts are cooperation across agencies and disciplines and between professionals and caregivers, shared "ownership" in the decision-making process, shared resources, and a need for new and different training endeavors (Hanson & Widerstrom, 1993, pp. 164–165). This hallmark of PL 99–457 and PL 102–119 is one of the most difficult efforts to legislate. Implementation will require close monitoring and evaluation, as well as carefully designed research studies to determine optimal strategies for facilitating and maintaining collaborative and cooperative interactions and working relationships.

Focusing on Caregivers. Caregiver-centered intervention is a third landmark of the new early childhood legislation and future models of intervention (Brown, Thurman, & Pearl, 1993). Families are to be explicitly included as part of the decision-making process of intervention, and their priorities for their children are to be recognized as a central focus of the Individual Family Service Plan (IFSP).

Describing the legislative context for early intervention services, Safer and Hamilton (1993) have written:

> Thus, Part H reflects not only a respect for families and what they know, but also an assumption that the family plays the key role in the development of the young child, and that the responsibility of the service system is to support that role. The needs of the family are as much a focus of Part H as are the needs of the child, and the family is given the authority to determine which services it will accept and which it will not. (p. 5)

Translated into operation, strategies for recognizing the caregiver role in the process of intervention should include the following practices, at a minimum:

- involving families as *active* participants in the team process
- meeting parents and families at their current level
- soliciting and answering all questions
- giving all known information
- putting information into a perspective that facilitates understanding
- encouraging parent-to-parent support
- keeping families in a position of control
- empowering families to be observers of their child
- giving credibility to parental reports. (Songer, 1993)

Focusing on Research in Organizational and Ecological Contexts. As the total context for intervention moves toward implementation in natural, least restrictive environments, it will be critical to perform new research on factors affecting the outcome of such efforts, the initiation and maintenance of inclusive programs, process and organizational variables, and the influence of training (Peck, Furman, & Helmstetter, 1993). Likewise, best strategies for interfacing family-program impact for the child will need to be examined closely. Finally, in contrast with studies of the 1960s, 1970s, and 1980s, which centered almost exclusively on the efficacy of early intervention, research of the 1990s will address new questions of best matches between curricular interventions and children, best timing for intervention, peer modeling for the development of social interaction and competence, strategies for transitioning from home to school, facilitation of play strategies for learning, and the impact of cultural diversity on the implementation of programing.

Serving New Populations. Without question, the heightened national interest in infants and young children spawned by enactment of PL 99–457 and PL 102–119 has increased the need for serving larger populations. Facing policymakers and professionals across the United States is the stark reality that at least one of four preschool children is growing up in this country in poverty (Odom & Warren, 1988, p. 267). In addition, the potential pool of youngsters to be served has been enlarged by implementation of new eligibility criteria for entry in intervention programs for high risk infants, along with changes in the limits for viability and survival of preterm infants. Finally, the escalating number of young children who prenatally have become the victims of HIV/AIDS has greatly affected the incidence of disabilities. In conclusion, Odom and Warren (1988) speculate that "we should assume that far more personnel and programs will be needed in the year 2000 and beyond" (p. 267).

Coordinating Statewide Systems of Service. Safer and Hamilton (1993) have indicated that the response of states to the mandates of PL 99–457 and PL 102–119 has varied tremendously in the degree of coordination across systems of service delivery and in the assignment of primary responsibility to lead agencies of Health and Education Departments. Also networking across local service providers, in many instances, has been problematic, and thus the need for new alliances to facilitate effective programing and efficient utilization of resources has become evident. Because there had been little precedence for the systematic provision of services prior to the new legislation, models for optimal coordination and organizational activities have been in short supply, and it has been necessary to institute new plans and processes for implementation. Since the passage of these new pieces of legislation, many states have already made changes in the designation of the agencies responsible for implementation of Part H (Safer & Hamilton, 1993, p. 11). These changes have been needed to create greater coherence between existing and newly developed structures. Increased economic constraints on financial resources at state and national levels have further complicated implementation of this legislation.

Training New Personnel. Finally, the passage of PL 99–457 and PL 102–119 has called on faculty of undergraduate and graduate programs to re-examine both the goals and processes of training. Over the past 6 years, more than four-fifths of the states involved in a national survey have indicated shortages of adequately trained personnel in early childhood intervention programs, and all have reported needs for qualified therapists (Safer & Hamilton, 1993, p. 11). Teachers and professionals in clinical disciplines (e.g., speech and language therapists, psychologists, social workers, and physical and occupational therapists) in the future will be required to demonstrate competency in many new areas of expertise, with respect to their own specific domains of study as well as those of their professional colleagues.

LEARNING FROM RESEARCH: WHAT DO WE KNOW ABOUT EARLY INTERVENTION?

Traditional education dies hard. Historically, curricular emphasis was placed primarily on preparing the child for performance as an adult, with less attention paid to the activities of childhood. However, as attitudes toward children have evolved and changed over the years, children have increasingly been recognized in their own right. Thus, more appropriately, curricular and programatic goals have shifted from preparing for adulthood to strengthening competence. Moreover, Sandall (1993) has addressed some of the specific dimensions of "exemplary programs" as follows:

> Exemplary early intervention curricula include a number of necessary components: a philosophical framework, a scope and sequence, sound instructional methods, a variety of activities and experiences, methods of promoting generalization, strategies for the use of the physical environment, systems for adapting to unique needs, and methods for data collection and use. (p. 134)

By extension, important instructional components minimally should include:

- enrichment—a provision of a stimulus-rich environment that sets the stage for growth, learning, and development (see Figure 20–2)

- direct instruction—attainment of critical goals and objectives of curricula through sequential learning steps

- incidental teaching—use of child-directed, child-selected situations and events to pursue instructional goals

- activity play-based intervention—facilitation of active participation in the natural events and situations of intervention (Fox & Hanline, 1993)

- focus on primary developmental areas—use of appropriate methods to develop key skills, including social competence, language, neuromotor abilities, sensory and perceptual skills, cognitive skills, adaptive behavior, and emotional development

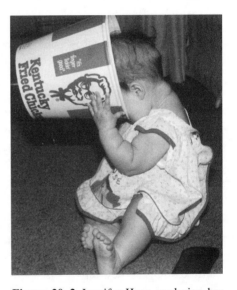

Figure 20–2 Jennifer Hope exploring her environment

- focus on engagement, mastery, and skills of independence—goals to be utilized in a variety of natural settings and with a range of peers and adults

- use of a culturally relevant environment for all children

- emphasis on caregiver priorities for the child—incorporation of these priorities as a major consideration and target for programing

- individualization to meet the needs of the child in terms of setting (e.g., home, center, or the combination of both).

Overall, even though much remains to be learned about the effectiveness of early intervention, researchers and practitioners now know a great deal more about the dimensions of optimal programing and the questions that need to be addressed. Global issues raised in the past have become almost irrelevant and indeed are viewed by many experts as inappropriate in light of the diversity of populations served, the variability of family circumstances, and the distinctive histories and additional legitimate demands that such groups bring to the intervention process. Guralnick (1988) has stated the complexity of evaluating the effectiveness of intervention:

> Within this framework, it is not surprising that existing efforts to review and evaluate the effectiveness of early intervention programs have taken more global approaches. The absence of sufficiently specific descriptions in the early studies and the lack of systematic evaluations of important program variables have yielded conclusions that tend to be based on outcomes aggregated across many different disability groups, intervention approaches, outcome measures, and numerous other subject, program, and goal characteristics. Compounding this situation, methodological problems characteristic of reviews in this area have been an additional challenge to the validity of many of their conclusions. (p. 77)

Presently, researchers examining the effectiveness of early intervention programing are focusing on questions of the optimum benefit of specific types of strategies for specific "populations" under specific conditions of service delivery, carried out in cooperation with various family supports and constellations, and applied in various natural settings. Obviously, the issues are multidimensional and outcome will be integrally connected to a number of changing, interdependent factors. Furthermore, the lockstep, universal approach to educational services, clearly, is no longer a viable or defensible model, despite the press of economic realities and constraints for community-based programs. Thus among several key considerations in developing "best practice" interventions are the following guidelines:

- Children living in fragile home situations may require additional day care or respite services (Deiner & Whitehead, 1988; Ramey, Bryant, Sparling, & Wasik, 1985; Wasik, Ramey, Bryant, & Sparling, 1990).
- Children at risk for later academic delay or failure will benefit from a literacy-rich, language-based early intervention experience.
- Infants and young children with complex medical and psychosocial problems such as the human immunodeficiency virus (HIV) infection may ben-

efit from foster care in private homes or nurturing "boarding" home programs (Cohen & Durham, 1993; Rendon, Gurdin, Bassi, & Weston, 1989).

- Some children will require intervention programing specifically designed for and congruent with "the behavior and expectations of the members of a particular culture" (Hanson, Lynch, & Wayman, 1990).
- Some children, given the nature of their disabilities, will benefit most from continuous programing from birth and throughout their preschool and school-age years; e.g., youngsters born with Down syndrome (Guralnick, 1988).
- Children with extensive medical needs may require extended periods in a supportive, family-centered medical care facility with supportive transition services to home (Long, Artis, & Dobbins, 1993).
- Some children will require special hospital-to-home discharge planning and transitioning supports (Affleck et al., 1989; Bruder & Walker, 1990).

These guidelines underscore conclusions of two researchers who commented recently on the status of early intervention efficacy studies—Shonkoff (1992) and Meisels (1992). Shonkoff (1992) reported on experiences of the Early Intervention Collaborative Study, a 7-year longitudinal study of 190 children and their families enrolled in 29 early intervention programs in Massachusetts and New Hampshire:

> One of our most important findings about the experience of an early intervention program raises significant questions about the interpretation of previous research on service efficacy, and has considerable implications for further investigation. Specifically, we learned that the children and families in our study received such a wide range of services, in such different settings, and with such varying frequency that it is meaningless to talk about an "average" or "typical" early intervention experience. Early intervention programs are complex, and many families are involved in multiple service systems. Sometimes formal intervention has a major influence on the life of a young child and family; sometimes it may be relatively inconsequential and overwhelmed by other forces. As practitioners, we continue to appreciate the importance of an individualized service approach for each child and each family. As researchers, we have learned about the importance of looking closely at the actual services received by different subgroups of children and families. (p. 7)

> . . . A central challenge for the 1990s is the need to reframe the questions that are addressed by researchers and policymakers. We should be asking not "How do children with developmental delays change as they grow older?" but "Why do some children and families do better than

others?" We need to ask not "What is the best early intervention model?" but "What is the best approach to use for a particular child and his or her family to achieve a specified outcome?" (p. 9)

Similarly in an article entitled *Early Intervention: A Matter of Context,* Meisels (1992) wrote:

> . . . for almost 20 years we have continued to stumble over the issue of "efficacy," which I call the "Big Question" of early intervention. Many of my colleagues concur that this is actually a pseudo-question. It was not a poorly formed question . . . . But it is now, because "Early Intervention" has changed and evolved and so has our understanding. Early intervention does not refer to something singular, but to a complex, multifaceted, and dynamic set of phenomena. (p. 2)

> . . . As we review the efforts of the past, and as we anticipate the needs of the future, we can see a distinct need for a better match between the child and family's lived context and the context of early intervention, with particular attention paid to the manner in which services are delivered. It is essential that we shift the way that systems and structures are organized so that they work more effectively for families. No longer can we consider the child as isolated from his or her family. No longer should we attend to the needs of parents without also recognizing that they must know how to respond to the changing needs of their children. No longer is it appropriate to follow the dictates of a theoretical view of intervention without questions of its relevance to a particular child and family's social and community situation. Rather, we must foster highly individualized programs of intervention that consider the needs of children in tandem, and that seek to address these needs through theoretically driven and empirically substantiated models that are consistent with the family's world. (p. 6)

Always, a really top-flight early education program must proceed from a strong theoretical base. Far from being a mere written statement in a brochure, this philosophical foundation should infuse every phase of the program, guiding practitioners as they translate theory into practice. By extension, an early education practitioner working with the population from birth to 3 years of age and their families has a difficult job, calling for a wide array of skills, considerable energy, and emotional resilience. In addition, a meaningful level of administrative and peer support is a prerequisite to the success of the staff in their everyday work. Time must be set aside in order to make helpful support translate into reality.

Preserving and enhancing a child's predisposition to learn, whatever the level of impairment or disability, is a primary task of early education and a central part of the curriculum. Nothing is more valuable than a child's enthusiasm and active engagement in learning in all of its various forms and formats. Protecting and nurturing this innate desire is a constant in best practice.

In terms of prevailing controversies about "structured" versus "unstructured" experiences for young children, extreme positions have been taken. In reality, the nature of activities and events for infants, toddlers, and preschoolers is rarely this dichotomous. Adult rules and expectations can and should be conveyed unobtrusively, and this "structure" is indeed necessary for optimal development of all children, not just those with special needs. Within a framework provided by the adult, children benefit from having a wide array of choices and opportunities to influence within their own environments and thus feel a sense of mastery in the completion of activities of their choosing. From this perspective, structured and child-directed learning, rather than being mutually exclusive, are complementary aspects of best practice.

Paralleling these decisions, the "responsive environment" is another important concept for the early years. It was Piaget who definitively described the essence of a baby's first attempts to affect his or her environment throughout the six sensorimotor stages of development (1963), and, clearly, teachers and other educational specialists need to convey strongly to the infant and the young child a sense that "What you do really matters." Again, in practice, implementing a responsive environment means different things to different children, at different stages and ages of development. For the 6-month-old, it may mean helping a mother to understand that her baby's sneezing or yawning says "I have had enough." For the 18-month-old toddler, on the other hand, it may mean putting away attractive and beckoning figurines. For the 3-year-old, at still another stage, it may involve having a broom and dustpan available so that the child may assist with clean-up. Basically, best practice in early intervention suggests that teachers and parents are always alert to the "teachable moment" in creating a responsive environment.

Flexibility is more important than ever in the wake of PL 99–457 and PL 102–119. Without resilience, incorporating the parent's or caregiver's agenda will be extremely difficult, if not impossible. Every home visit requires that the practitioner be ready to demonstrate an active ability to change in response to the unique situation of a given home on a particular day, whether the event is an emotional crisis or the celebration of a newly achieved milestone for a family member. A willingness to adapt is an educator's best ally in facilitating change and beneficial outcome for all involved in the intervention process.

"Decentering"—another fundamental quality of best practice—has at least two meanings relevant to the context of early educational programing. It first refers to an early developmental watershed whereby a child comes to a realization that others have feelings and different perspectives. In another sense, for the professional and the parent it means a lifelong process of education whereby a thoughtful person evolves into a greater awareness of the multiplicity of factors affecting his or her world and that of the children entrusted to his or her teaching. Decentering encompasses cultural issues and political realities, as well as considerations relative to race and class. The sensitive practitioner struggles constantly to try to avoid making inappropriate and incorrect assumptions from his or her corner of the world. By taking another point of view, hopefully, he or she may be more effective at bringing about a better outcome for young children and families of all cultural and ethnic backgrounds.

Finally, as most recent research and literature have noted at great length, preparing for transitions is another crucial dimension of best practice. Current studies of family systems have stressed the important role played by "typical" or "normal" life transitions and have underscored the frequent difficulties involved in such transitions, no matter how commonplace. These transitions include events such as adding a new family member and beginning school, which present changes for families and, almost without exception, precipitate periods of instability and vulnerability (Becvar & Becvar, 1993). Best practice needs to include strategies for offering ways to help families through these predictable transitions.

In summary, the new early childhood legislation presents vast challenges for the helping and educational professions. If these challenges are met successfully, there are numerous opportunities to create a shining example of enlightened public policy as we proceed into the next century.

CONTEMPORARY MODELS FOR COLLABORATION IN COMMUNITY SETTINGS

As we have discussed, many program components and dimensions must interface to reflect optimal educational opportunities for infants, young children, and their families. Two nationally recognized programs, although different from each other, have incorporated many facets of contemporary thinking about best practice in early childhood intervention: the Jowonio School and the Main Street Early Education Program.

The Jowonio School: A Setting for All Children and Families

Philosophy

Along with the inclusive preschool center-based setting available at the Jowonio School, a home-based program strives to offer families a model that meets their needs. The home-based program originally was developed as a natural extension of the inclusive philosophy and child-centered practices of the school in Syracuse, New York, which has been a nationally recognized leader in the field of integration since 1969. With the belief that families who have children with special needs should have the same options for the care and education of their children as do families with typical children, an assortment of choices for intervention have been made available.

For practical reasons, the youngest children enrolled in Jowonio were selected for home-based services. With early diagnosis, infants and toddlers are being referred for these services, for several reasons. First, many parents want to keep their babies and young children home, if possible. Second, parents can continue to be the primary caregivers, and many children can benefit from the intimate and familiar home setting. Third, a variety of medical problems, including fragile immune systems or dependence on medical equipment, make it important that some children have the option to remain at home. Fourth, there are few center-based programs in rural areas. Home-based services thus allow rural children and their families to receive support. Fifth, the Jowonio staff provide teacher and therapy services in a family-based (center-based) day care center and in community nursery programs in order to meet the various needs of families and children. (See Figures 20–3 and 20–4.)

Beliefs about parent-program partnerships are the basis of the principles that guide much of the service offered at Jowonio. In particular, staff seek to:

- provide an "enabling approach" that allows families to use their abilities and to acquire new skills to meet their needs and those of their children
- "empower" caregivers by helping them to maintain or acquire a sense of control over their families and develop the confidence to negotiate the human service system on behalf of their children

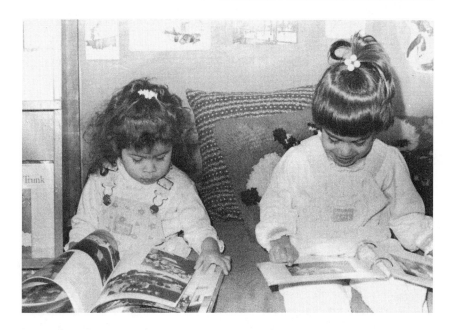

Figure 20–3 Ali and Lindsey at the center-based program of the Jowonio School

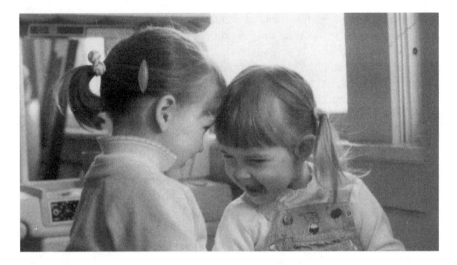

Figure 20–4 Alison and Dani playing in kitchen area

- respect and accept each family's values, beliefs, and lifestyle
- be sensitive to individual differences and acknowledge that there are strengths and resources present in all families
- involve key family members and other family support systems in all aspects of the program
- offer services in the least intrusive and most natural setting
- provide services to families on the basis of their priorities and choices for their children and themselves.

Program Activities

Jowonio's home-based program staff consists of special education teachers, occupational therapists, physical therapists, speech therapists, a social worker, psychologists, and a coordinator. Each professional has specific skills and strengths, but all have the ability to remain flexible and understanding, therefore offering their services in a manner that has the potential to match the individual needs of each family.

In addition to functioning as a strong transdisciplinary team, the home-based program staff also interacts cooperatively with community agencies that may already be involved with families. In many cases, referrals to these community agencies are made when families are in need of and ask for additional support. The support offered to families includes such services as facilitating social security income applications; participating in protective and preventive services teams;

providing aid in finding housing, clothing, and food; and helping caregivers to gain access to medical professionals with sensitivity to disability issues.

In accordance with the principles and guidelines for enabling and empowering families outlined by Dunst, Trivette, and Deal (1988), members of the home-based program at Jowonio view the child as a member of a family system. For productive intervention to occur, a broad-based approach that takes into account any given family's concerns, aspirations, and strengths is critical. The programs specifically strive to:

- tailor parent involvement activities to the responsibilities, interests, and time availability of caregivers
- provide education information relevant to particular families
- offer opportunities for parents to learn assertiveness and advocacy skills
- help caregivers to strengthen existing support networks and to develop new ones
- assist parents in identifying their priorities and in developing strategies for action on these priorities
- support children in a variety of settings including home, day care, baby-sitter's home, and nursery school
- model appropriate activities and expectations to meet child needs.

Jowonio's program remains in a state of constant reassessment. In the 5 years that the home-based portion of the school program has been in existence, significant changes have taken place. These changes have been based on feedback from families involved, changes in state and federal regulations, and interactions and meetings with other early intervention service providers. The home-based program began with service to four families and currently serves 30 families annually. With these experiences at hand, the initial enrollment procedures, assessment processes, and implementation of the Individualized Family Service Plan all have been redesigned. At this time, as a result of the enactment of the early care legislation PL 99–457 and PL 102–119, transitions and changes are again taking place. In the midst of such constant flux, efforts are being made to assure that these changes are driven primarily by what is best practice for children and their families, rather than solely by fiscal considerations, which are always a prevailing constraint.

Program Process

Services at Jowonio presently begin with a referral from parents, physicians, public health nurses, or other professionals to an Early Childhood Direction Center, a clearinghouse for early education programs. Some families choose to have a County Health Department service coordinator help them through the referral process. After explaining the various philosophies and services offered by the different programs, the service coordinator or the Early Childhood Direction Center staff makes a referral for an assessment to the program chosen by the family. If a referral is made to Jowonio's home-based program, the coordinator schedules an evaluation.

For each family, the assessment procedure is different. A process is designed to meet the needs of the child being evaluated and the family's schedules. Families may be offered an assessment in their home or in their day care setting. Sometimes, two members of the assessment team work together, some families prefer that evaluations be performed by one person at a time. An arena type evaluation, during which one professional interacts with the parent/caregiver and the child, while all other team members observe and record, is also available. Some standardized tests are used, along with functional observations of play and interaction. The home-based program staff then prepare a written report of background and medical history, parental and caregiver concerns, observations, and results of the assessment, with recommendations. This report is provided to the family and, with their permission, to the family doctor or primary care pediatrician. A copy of this evaluation with recommendations also is given to the County Health Department, so that the responsible individuals can approve services for funding purposes.

The next step in the process, which is related to programing, is the development of the Individualized Family Service Plan (IFSP) by the service coordinator, members of the home-based program, and the family. The development of the IFSP, like the assessment procedure, differs for each family. Some families may be ready to identify needs and areas for attention immediately after the evaluation. Other families may need some time to adjust in order to understand their options and to decide on how they would like their priorities and those of their children to be met. There are some basic underlying factors that remain the same in each IFSP. The most important of these considerations is that the family is the constant in the child's life and that, consequently, service systems and personnel must support, respect, encourage, and enhance the strength and competence of the individual family unit. The extent to which caregivers want to be involved is determined by the family. Moreover, the IFSP should promote independence of child and caregiver alike.

The delivery of services is also determined by family choice. The number of visits per week and the times of visits are planned to fit into the family's existing schedule. Often, teachers and therapists pair their visits to facilitate carry-over of goals and strategies. Evening visits, too, may be needed to enhance clear communication with the many parents who work and are not available during the day.

Weekly, the entire home-based team meets to support each other and to plan and coordinate the short-term and long-range goals of the IFSP, which are the responsibility of Jowonio staff. On a monthly basis, each child's IFSP is updated, with notations of progress and new activities. This coordination and planning is the process that allows the team to offer services in a unified and effective manner.

Much thought and discussion with family and team members occur regarding a child's transition to a new setting. Families are offered home-based programing for children from birth to 5 years of age; however, at any point they may want and request a change. Often, families want their children to have other children to play with, or they come to believe that their children are ready to spend time in different surroundings with different routines. In addition, family members may reach a point when they need time for themselves, for work, for other children, or for various other reasons. Caregivers and parents are encouraged to visit and explore different programs and centers in order to learn about different philosophies, expectations, rules, and routines. Some families undertake this responsibility by themselves; on the other hand, members of the home-based program often visit other programs with parents. The needs of any given family and child are always paramount in selection of the most appropriate setting, and time of transition is planned for both child and caregivers. Visits are made to the program of choice to see the site and to meet teachers and therapists, if possible. Along with parents, the home-based team meets with the new team to discuss effective strategies and long-range goals and concerns. This transition for some children and families happens quickly and smoothly; for others, a slower process is necessary.

Main Street Early Education Program: A Public School-Based, Collaborative Model

Located within a public school district in North Syracuse, New York, the Main Street Early Education Program (EEP) was opened in 1980 as a pioneer effort in the development of community-based services for young children. The Early Education Program provides special education and related services to children from birth to 5 years of age and their families, including 42 infants, 36 toddlers, and 90 preschoolers with identified special needs, as well as a population of typical peers. The program is fully integrated, offering opportunities for children with disabilities to participate in a child-centered and socially stimulating environment with preschool children of more normal development. Family education and support services are an integral part of the program.

Preschool Intervention

Center-based programing is provided for children between the ages of 2 and 5 years of age. Both full- and half-day programs are available to youngsters on the basis of educational and therapeutic needs and parent/caregiver preference. Special education teachers and therapists, in addition, support children in community preschool programs.

As defined in Part 200.1 of the Regulations of the Commissioner of New York State, children identified as having developmental delays may be eligible for special education services. Specific classifications, as described in the regulations, include autistic, emotionally disturbed, learning disabled, mentally retarded, deaf, hard of hearing, speech impaired, visually impaired, orthopedically impaired, other health impaired, and multiply handicapped.

Daily classroom programing at Main Street emphasizes learning and social development through play, art, music, and language activities. Adapted physical education, monthly family participation events, and periodic field trips are additions to the educational program. (See Figures 20–5 and 20–6.)

Each classroom is developed heterogeneously, with the intent to educate in the "least restrictive environment." Children participate in learning activities within an inclusive setting of preschool age-appropriate peers. Youngsters in each classroom demonstrate a wide range of abilities and interests, which offers an excellent opportunity for cooperative learning. The integrated environment promotes awareness, understanding, sharing, problem solving, and collaboration among all children and their families. Main Street serves children throughout a large three-county area, encompassing urban, rural, and suburban communities.

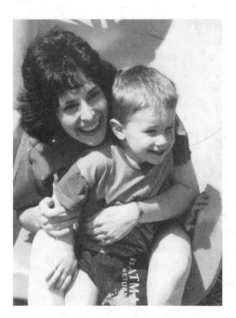

Figure 20–5 Sliding on the Main Street School playground

The guidelines of the National Association for the Education of Young Children (NAEYC) serve as the base for the curriculum, a growing trend in special education (Bredekamp, 1993). Sequential lessons and exposure to a variety of cognitive, social-emotional, language, and neuromotor tasks of an age-appropriate and individually appropriate level constitute the focus of programing. Classroom materials and organization combine with learning and teaching styles to create an educationally rich curriculum that meets child needs and extends learning and growth. Infants, toddlers, and preschoolers are challenged with activities of interest at appropriate stages for their learning, behavioral, and developmental growth.

The education and therapy needs of each child determine the specific nature of the Individual Education Plan (IEP). The classroom team and related service therapists jointly assess each child for current levels of performance and develop transdisciplinary annual goals, with short-term learning objectives. The comprehensive classroom program is supported by ongoing team evaluation. The transdisciplinary approach sets the stage for the regular staff meetings, where each child's program and Individual Education Plan are reviewed thoroughly. Teaching strategies and evaluation techniques appropriate for each child's rate of progress and learning style are monitored through this process.

Intervention with Infants, Toddlers, and Families

The Main Street Early Education Program of the North Syracuse School System also serves children from birth to 2 years of age. A multidisciplinary team provides an evaluation of the infant or toddler in the home setting. The first step in this assessment is carried out by the school psychologist, who takes a social, developmental, and medical history. At a second session, the child's skills in all areas of behavior and development are assessed by a team consisting of a speech therapist, a psychologist, an infant-toddler special education teacher, and, as appropriate, by physical and occupational therapists and a teacher of the visually impaired. Children who qualify for the program are then offered the services needed to facilitate their learning and growth.

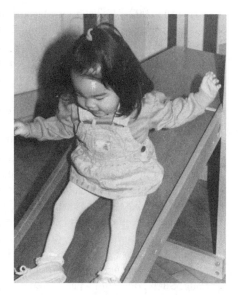

Following the evaluation, caregivers who opt to utilize a county service coordinator work with the coordinator and the evaluation team to develop an IFSP for the family. (This process is similar to processes followed by staff of the Jowonio School.) The IFSP is then implemented by the early intervention team and the family and reviewed twice a year.

The focus of the home-based infant and toddler program is to work with families and primary caregivers to stimulate growth in key areas of development. Parents are viewed as

Figure 20–6 Sliding in the "Zoom Room" at the Main Street School

the child's "real" teachers and play an essential role in the provision of a comprehensive educational program. Teachers and therapists interact directly with the infant or toddler, make suggestions to family members, and, on home visits, provide activities and adaptive devices for the child to use. They assess the child's functional activities in the home setting and address parental concerns. Feeding, bathing, positioning, and mobility are frequently targeted by families and professionals as areas of concern.

In addition, interaction skills are modeled and guided by the transdisciplinary team. They also focus on techniques of teaching turn-taking and imitation in order to develop the social and language skills of the young child. Older infants and toddlers whose expressive language is severely delayed are provided with alternative communication strategies such as sign language and facilitated communication.

Offering support to families of young disabled children is another target area of the home-based team. Families frequently require emotional support as they go through the grieving process when they discover that their child has a disability. Often, the family experiences much stress, too, as a result of the frequent medical appointments, hospitalizations, and financial difficulties. At these times, teachers and therapists provide nurturing and give help by making referrals to appropriate agencies that deal with respite, counseling, or financial entitlements. Also, the program offers support groups that provide child care for families who choose this service.

During the 1992–1993 school year, the home-based team added a new component to their program. Weekly parent-child play groups were established for children who are 18 months to 3 years old. These groups afford an opportunity for small groups of toddlers and their parents to come together for a more social learning experience. Teachers and therapists facilitate play and provide music and snack activities that incorporate specific individual child goals and objectives. Parents and caregivers enjoy social opportunities of being with other families and of playing with their children.

In recent years, the home-based team has seen many more medically fragile young children. Infants, toddlers, and preschoolers who are ventilator-dependent, have tracheostomies, gastrostomy tubes, and round-the-clock nursing care also are seen by the home-based teachers and therapists. These children present with a variety of new, different, and challenging problems. Often alternative communication is crucial to the development of these children. Frequently, they have not eaten orally and, consequently, oral-motor treatment is a prime concern. In addition, since they have experienced limited typical activities, the development of normalizing experiences is paramount through the course of intervention programing. Such populations have strengthened not only the transdisciplinary concept within the Main Street Early Education Program itself, but also working relationships with other professionals across communities and counties in New York State.

In conclusion, both the Jowonio School and the Main Street Early Education Program have been integrally involved in the training of undergraduate and graduate students in the School of Education at Syracuse University. Staff actively participate in classes, and both settings offer best practice experiences for practica and student teaching, as well as important opportunities for regular observation across disciplines.

Finally, reflecting the newest thinking in the field of intervention with infants and young children, numerous models have been conceptualized and implemented across the United States in recent years. Some of these programs have originated as a result of funding by the Office of Special Education Programs (OSEP), the Division for Innovation and Development (DID), and the Early Education Program for Children with Disabilities (EEPCD) (Decker, 1992). Other programs have developed in association with hospital and medical centers or universities, in order to meet service delivery needs of children, in addition to the need for preparing future professionals in teaching and related clinical disciplines.

There are many early childhood and/or special education programs that represent unique perspectives on common themes. The following programs have attracted national recognition because they exemplify contemporary trends in service delivery to infants and young populations:

- the School for Constructive Play at the University of Massachusetts, Amherst, Massachusetts (Forman, 1993)
- the Portage Project, which had its beginning in Portage, Wisconsin, and is now located at the Civitan International Research Center of the University of Alabama, Birmingham, Alabama (Shearer, 1993)
- the Family Center of Nova University, Princeton, New Jersey (Segal, 1993)
- the High/Scope Curriculum for Early Childhood Care and Education located at the High/Scope Educational Research Foundation of Ypsilanti, Michigan (Weikart & Schweinhart, 1993)
- the Discharge Planning Project for Hospital to Home Transitions, University of Connecticut, Storrs, Connecticut (Bruder & Walker, 1990)
- Niños Especiales Outreach Project, New York Medical College, Valhalla, New York (Bruder, 1992)
- the Family Enablement Project, Western Carolina Center Foundation, Morgantown, West Virginia (Dunst & Deal, 1992)
- the early education program located at the Pennsylvania State University, University Park, Pennsylvania (Neisworth & Buggey, 1993)
- the Early Intervention Collaborative Study of the Division of Developmental and Behavioral Pediatrics located at the University of Massachusetts Medical School, Amherst, Massachusetts (1992).

This list of programs is not exhaustive. Each of these projects, however, is indicative of a new "agenda" for early childhood special intervention in the 1990s. Shonkoff (1992) has characterized this new agenda as follows:

> The marriage of advocacy and science in early childhood intervention is long overdue. With the proper balance between faith and skepticism, we will be ready to address the meaningful yet difficult questions that remain unanswered. (p. 9)

BIBLIOGRAPHY

Affleck, G., Tennen, H., Rowe, J., Roscher, B., & Walker, L. (1989). Effects of formal support on mother's adaptation to the hospital-to-home transition of high-risk infants: The benefits and costs of helping. *Child Development, 60,* 488–500.

Becvar, D.S., & Becvar, R.J. (1993). *Family therapy: A systematic integration.* Needham Heights, MA: Allyn & Bacon.

Bloom, B.S. (1964). *Stability and change in human characteristics.* New York: John Wiley & Sons.

Bredekamp, S. (1993). The relationship between early childhood education and early childhood special education: Healthy marriage or family feud? *Topics in Early Childhood Special Education, 13*(3), 258–273.

Brown, W., Thurman, S.K., & Pearl, L.F. (1993). *Family-centered early intervention with infants and toddlers: Innovative cross-disciplinary approaches.* Baltimore: Paul H. Brookes.

Bruder, M.B. (1992). Niños Especiales outreach project. In M.J. Decker (Ed.), *1991–1992 Directory of selected early childhood programs.* Chapel Hill, NC: The University of North Carolina, NEC*TAS, Frank Porter Graham Child Development Center.

Bruder, M.B. (1993). The provision of early intervention and early childhood special education within community early childhood programs: Characteristics of effective service delivery. *Topics in Early Childhood Special Education, 13*(1), 19–37.

Bruder, M.B., & Walker, L. (1990). Discharge planning: Hospital to home transitions for infants. *Topics in Early Childhood Special Education, 9*(4), 26–42.

Bruner, J.S. (1973). *Beyond the information given: Studies in the psychology of knowing.* New York: W.W. Norton.

Cohen, F.L., & Durham, J.D. (Eds.) (1993). *Women, children, and HIV/AIDS.* New York: Springer.

Decker, M.J. (Ed.). (1992). *1991–1992 Directory of selected early childhood programs.* Chapel Hill, NC: The University of North Carolina, NEC*TAS, Frank Porter Graham Child Development Center.

Deiner, P.L., & Whitehead, L.C. (1988). Levels of respite care as a family support system. *Topics in Early Childhood Special Education, 8*(2), 51–61.

Dunst, C., & Deal, A. (1992). Family enablement project. In M.J. Decker (Ed.), *1991–1992 Directory of selected early childhood programs.* Chapel Hill, NC: The University of North Carolina, NEC*TAS, Frank Porter Graham Child Development Center.

Dunst, C., Trivette, C., & Deal, A. (1988). *Enabling and empowering families.* Cambridge, MA: Brookline Books.

Forman, G. (1993). The constructivist perspective to early education. In J.L. Roopnarine & J.E. Johnson (Eds.), *Approaches to early childhood education* (2nd ed.) (pp. 137–155). New York: Merrill.

Fox, L., & Hanline, M.F. (1993). Preliminary evaluation of learning within developmentally appropriate early childhood settings. *Topics in Early Childhood Special Education, 13*(3), 308–327.

Frost, J.L. (1973). *Revisiting early childhood education.* New York: Holt, Rinehart & Winston.

Goldfarb, W. (1943). The effects of early institutional care on adolescent personality. *Journal of Experimental Education, 12,* 106–129.

Gordon, I.J. (1969). *Early child stimulation through parent education: Final report to Children's Bureau, Department of Health, Education, and Welfare.* Gainsville, FL: University of Florida, Institute for Development of Human Resources.

Guralnick, M.J. (1988). Efficacy research in early childhood intervention programs. In S.L. Odom & M.B. Karnes (Eds.), *Early intervention for infants and children with handicaps: An empirical base* (pp. 75–88). Baltimore: Paul H. Brookes.

Hanson, M.J., Lynch, E.W., & Wayman, K.I. (1990). Honoring the cultural diversity of families when gathering data. *Topics in Early Childhood Special Education, 10*(1), 12–131.

Hanson, M.J., & Widerstrom, A.H. (1993). Consultation and collaboration: Essentials of integration efforts for young children. In C.A. Peck, S.L. Odom, & D.D. Bricker (Eds.), *Integrating young children with disabilities into community programs: Ecological perspectives on research and implementation* (pp. 149–168). Baltimore: Paul H. Brookes.

Hunt, J.M. (1961). *Intelligence and experience.* New York: Ronald Press.

Long, C.E., Artis, N.E., & Dobbins, N.J. (1993). The Hospital: An important site for family centered early intervention. *Topics in Early Childhood Special Education, 13*(1) 106–119.

Meisels, S.J. (1989). Meeting the mandate of Public Law 99–457: Early childhood intervention in the nineties. *American Journal of Orthopsychiatry, 59*(3), 451–460.

Meisels, S.J. (1992). Early intervention: A matter of context. *Zero to Three: Bulletin of the National Center for Clinical Infant Programs, XII*(3), 1–6.

Neisworth, J.T., & Buggey, T. (1993). Behavior analysis and principles in early childhood education. In J.L. Roopnarine & J.E. Johnson (Eds.), *Approaches to early childhood education* (2nd ed.) (pp. 113–135). Baltimore: Paul H. Brookes.

Odom, S.L., & Warren, S.F. (1988). Early childhood special education in the year 2000. *Journal of the Division for Early Childhood, 12*(3), 263–273.

Peck, C.A., Furman, G.C., & Helmstetter, E. (1993). Integrated early childhood programs: Research on the implementation of change in organizational contexts. In C.A. Peck, S.L. Odom, & D.D. Bricker (Eds.), *Integrating young children with disabilities into community programs: Ecological perspectives on research and implementation* (pp. 187–205). Baltimore: Paul H. Brookes.

Peck, C.A., Odom, S.L., & Bricker, D.D. (Eds.). (1993). *Integrating young children with disabilities into community programs: Ecological perspectives on research and implementation.* Baltimore: Paul H. Brookes.

Piaget, J. (1963). *The origins of intelligence.* New York: W.W. Norton.

Ramey, C.T., Bryant, D.M., Sparling, J.J., & Wasik, B.H. (1985). Project CARE: A comparison of two early intervention strategies to prevent retarded development. *Topics in Early Childhood Special Education, 5,* 12–25.

Rendon, M., Gurdin, P., Bassi, J., & Weston, M. (1989). Foster care for children with AIDS: A psychosocial perspective. *Child Psychiatry and Human Development, 19*(4), 256–269.

Safer, N.D., & Hamilton, J.L. (1993). Legislative context for early intervention services. In W. Brown, S.K. Thurman, & L.F. Pearl (Eds.), *Family-centered early intervention with infants and toddlers: Innovative cross-disciplinary approaches* (pp. 1–19). Baltimore: Paul H. Brookes.

Sandall, S.R. (1993). Curricula for early intervention. In W. Brown, S.K. Thurman, & L.F. Pearl (Eds.), *Family-centered early intervention with infants and toddlers: Innovative cross-disciplinary approaches* (pp. 129–151). Baltimore: Paul H. Brookes.

Segal, M.M. (1993). Classes for parents and young children: The family center model. In J.L. Roopnarine & J.E. Johnson (Eds.), *Approaches to early childhood education* (2nd ed.) (pp. 33–45). New York: Merrill.

Shearer, D.E. (1993). The Portage Project: An international home approach to early intervention of young children and their families. In J.L. Roopnarine & J.E. Johnson (Eds.), *Approaches to early childhood education* (2nd ed.) (pp. 97–111). Baltimore: Paul H. Brookes.

Shonkoff, J.P. (1992). Early intervention research: Asking and answering meaningful questions. *Zero to Three: Bulletin of the National Center for Clinical Infant Programs, XII,* 7–9.

Skeels, H.H., & Dye, H.B. (1939). A study of the effects of differential stimulation in mentally retarded children. *Proceedings and Addresses of the American Association on Mental Deficiency, 44,* 114–136.

Songer, N.S. (1993). Unpublished communication on parent-professional collaboration. Syracuse, NY: Early Childhood Direction Center.

Spitz, R.A. (1945). Hospitalism: An inquiry into the genesis of psychiatric conditions in early childhood. *Psychoanalytic Study of the Child, 1,* 53–74.

Wasik, B.H., Ramey, C.T., Bryant, D.M., & Sparling, J.J. (1990). A longitudinal study of two early intervention strategies: Project CARE. *Child Development, 61,* 1682–1696.

Weikart, D.P., & Schweinhart, L. (1993). The High/Scope curriculum for early childhood care and education. In J.L. Roopnarine & J.E. Johnson (Eds.), *Approaches to early childhood education* (2nd ed.) (pp. 195–208). Baltimore: Paul H. Brookes.

Zigler, E., & Berman, W. (1983). Discerning the future of early childhood intervention. *American Psychologist, 38,* 894–906.

Chapter 21

New Collaborations: Professional-Family Partnerships

Dianne S. Apter and Nan S. Songer

Valuing collaborations means valuing empowerment, growth, and diversity. It means moving from programmatic to systemic thinking, from short- to long-term visions. It means understanding that equity and access are conditions of quality, not factors ancillary to it. It means being realistic about what collaborations can accomplish within the context of deeply entrenched American institutions and deeply rooted American values. Above all, valuing collaboration means believing in and bringing out the best in all of America's children, families, and institutions. (Kagan, 1991, p. 93)

During the last decade, there have been some dramatic shifts in the ways that early intervention services have been conceptualized and delivered. Early intervention has come to encompass much more than specific activity with a specific child to ameliorate or rehabilitate specific deficits. In current best practice, there is a fit between *family-prioritized* needs and the services delivered. Numerous labels have been applied to name this service delivery approach: ecological intervention (Apter, 1982; Bronfenbrenner, 1979; Hobbs et al., 1984), parent empowerment (Dunst & Trivette, 1988; Dunst, Trivette, & Deal, 1988; Rappaport, 1984), family-focused intervention (Bailey et al., 1986), and family-centered services (McGonigel, Kaufmann, & Johnson, 1991a; Nelkin, 1987; Shelton, Jeppson, & Johnson, 1987). For clarity and consistency, the term *family-centered* will be used throughout this text.

Although "working with families" always has been an important part of most early intervention programs, a family-centered approach requires collaboration among professionals from every discipline and every system touching the lives of young children with disabilities and their families. Of equal if not greater significance, family-centered service also requires true collaboration between those professionals and families. The shift in thinking from professional-centered and service centered to family-centered demands a great deal of families and professionals as they assume new roles and new ways of thinking about the roles.

Traditionally, most professionals entered the field of early intervention with the desire to work with children. Professional training was "child-as-client" focused. Because a fundamental tenet of family-centered service delivery is family choice and responsiveness to family priorities, the concept of family-centered service challenges the long-standing role of the professional as the primary decision maker in the management of young children with disabilities (Bailey, 1987). The shift from a child focus to a family focus has come about because of concurrent activities occurring in the health care arena, as well as in special education. Since the early 1980s, visionary families and professionals have been involved in forums and task forces across the country, struggling to develop a different service direction for families and their children with disabilities or handicapping conditions.

At a joint meeting sponsored in 1986 by the National Institute on Disability and Rehabilitation Research (U.S. Department of Education) and the Division of Maternal and Child Health (U.S. Department of Health and Human Services), the participants laid out the principles and practices for family-centered health care for medically fragile children (Nelkin, 1987). During this period, the 99th Congress of the United States was engaged in heated debate, which ultimately resulted in a key piece of federal legislation, Public Law (PL) 99–457 (National Center for Clinical Infant Programs, 1989). That legislation, specifically Part H, has been the driving force behind implementation of the family-centered philosophy as well as cross-disciplinary and system collaboration in delivery of intervention services for children under 3 years of age and their families throughout the country. The vision of both the Maternal and Child Health efforts and Part H of PL 99–457 is that of a less complex, less fragmented service system, with families interacting with professionals in such a way as to maintain a sense of control over their lives.

This chapter explains the impact of the legislation and describes the changing practices that affect the ways in which "help" is delivered and collaboration can occur.

FEDERAL INITIATIVES AND MEDICAID WAIVERS

Since 1965, the federal Medicaid Program has been in existence as part of Title XIX of the Social Security Act (42 U.S.C. §1901, 1991) (Walker, 1991). In 1982, a federal Medicaid waiver known as the Katie Beckett waiver was developed by the Health Care Financing Administration (Brewer, McPherson, Magrab, & Hutchins, 1989). Prior to the waiver, a child who was dependent on medical equipment or who had severe disabilities could have the cost of their care paid for through Medicaid, only as long as the child remained hospitalized or in an institution providing skilled nursing care. This new waiver program provided states an option and incentive to allow children to return home to their families without the loss of these benefits. The waiver was named after Katie Beckett, the first child to receive this opportunity.

True pioneers, the families of such "technology dependent/medically fragile children" found ways to assume this responsibility because they believed that the best place for their child was at home within their family and their community. It soon became all too clear that best practice for delivery of services to children meant giving support to their families (Shoultz & Racino, 1988). The physical care of their children with complex medical needs seemed to cause far less stress than the difficulties encountered because of the lack of services, the fragmentation of services, and the unresponsiveness of systems to their needs in the service programs established to implement this waiver (Brewer, McPherson, Magrab, & Hutchins, 1989; Cardoso, 1991; Koop, 1987; Nelkin, 1987; Shelton, Jeppson, & Johnson, 1987).

In 1987, at a conference sponsored by the Bureau of Maternal and Child Health and Resource Development of the U.S. Department of Health and Human Services, and the American Academy of Pediatrics, parents and professionals alike articulated these issues and began to develop an action plan to address them. At the conclusion of the conference, then Surgeon General C. Everett Koop issued a report concerning children with special health care needs (Koop, 1987). Dr. Koop called for the establishment of a national agenda for families and professionals to work together through a system of family-centered, community-based, coordinated care (Brewer, McPherson, Magrab, & Hutchins, 1989). A set of principles was to serve as the philosophical base for such a system (Exhibit 21–1). Dr. Koop's report, along with publications disseminated by the Association for the Care of Children's Health and other organizations marked the beginning of a nationwide program to enhance the implementation of a family-centered approach to care for infants, children, and adolescents with special health care needs (Shelton, Jeppson, & Johnson, 1987).

Public Law 99–457

The principles of family-centered care were also the cornerstone of the federal law initiated by the Office of Special Education and Rehabilitative Services, U.S. Department of Education that was passed in October 1986. In essence, PL 99–457 amended the Education of the Handicapped Act by (1) mandating services to children with disabilities from the age of 3 years (Part B) and (2) establishing "a new Federal discretionary program to assist States in developing and implementing comprehensive, coordinated, interdisciplinary" systems of early intervention services for infants and toddlers with disabilities and their families (Part H). Final regulations for implementation of the Early Intervention Program promulgated in Part H of PL 99–457 were enacted in 1989 (Early Intervention Program for Infants

Exhibit 21–1 Key Elements of Family-Centered Care

- Recognizing that the family is the constant in a child's life, while the service systems and personnel within those systems change.
- Facilitating parent-professional collaboration at all levels of care
  —care of an individual child
  —program development, implementation, and evaluation
  —policy formation
- Honoring the racial, ethnic, cultural, and socioeconomic diversity of families.
- Recognizing family strengths and individuality and respecting different methods of coping.
- Sharing with parents, on a continuing basis and in a supportive manner, complete and unbiased information.
- Encouraging and facilitating family-to-family support and networking.
- Understanding and incorporating the developmental needs of infants, children, and adolescents and their families into care systems.
- Implementing comprehensive policies and programs that provide emotional and financial support to meet the needs of families.
- Designing accessible care systems that are flexible, culturally competent, and responsive to family-identified needs.

Source: Adapted from National Center for Family-Centered Care (1990). *What is family-centered care?* (brochure). Bethesda, MD: Association for the Care of Children's Health.

---

and Toddlers with Handicaps: Final Regulations, 1989; Education of the Handicapped Act Amendments of 1986). The 14 components of Part H are listed in Exhibit 21–2. In 1990, the 101st Congress reauthorized changing the name of the Education of the Handicapped Act to the Individuals with Disabilities Education Act (IDEA), and in 1991, Part H was also reauthorized as PL 102–119.

The fact that PL 99–457 passed at all was extraordinary. The climate of the times dictated less fiscal and programatic involvement of the federal government in education and other affairs of the states (Garwood & Sheehan, 1989). Nonetheless, powerful and energetic advocates, both within and outside Congress, were able to demonstrate effectively the compelling need for this legislation that would expand current special education law.

The discretionary Part H, with its sweeping changes in service delivery to the very youngest children with disabilities, has had the most far-reaching impact on current practices in early intervention. Silverstein, in a widely distributed document outlining the "intent and spirit" of PL 99–457, referred to the new federal initiative as a "window of opportunity" for policymakers, providers, and families (Silverstein, 1989). The stated goal of this legislation was to "enhance the capacity of families to meet the special needs of their infants and toddlers with handicaps" (PL 99–457, Part H). The law required collaboration and coordination at every

Exhibit 21–2 Minimum Components of a Statewide Comprehensive System for the Provision of Appropriate Early Intervention Services to Infants and Toddlers with Special Needs (PL 99–457, Part H)

- Definition of developmental delay

- Timetable for serving all in need in the state

- Comprehensive multidisciplinary evaluation of needs of children and families

- Individualized family service plan and case management services

- Child find and referral system

- Public awareness regarding access to and benefits of early intervention

- Central directory of services, resources, experts, and research and demonstration projects

- Comprehensive system of personnel development

- Single line of authority in a lead agency designated or established by the governor for implementation

- Policy pertaining to contractual arrangements with local service providers

- Procedures for timely reimbursement of funds

- Procedural safeguards

- Policies and procedures for personnel standards

- System for compiling data on early intervention programs

---

level of the system from the local early intervention program on up through the federal government. And most importantly, it required a shift in the roles of families on the continuum of power. They were to be central to the determination of services for their own children, and they were to have considerable and meaningful involvement in policy development and the implementation process as well. The intent was to nurture partnerships and collaboration between agencies and providers, as well as between families and professionals, so that an Individualized Family Service Plan (IFSP) could be funded and delivered using a multitude of resources pulled together by a single service coordinator. This blending and consolidating of resources and services was to be backed by interagency agreements at the state level. Through the development of the IFSP, families would become empowered, since historically everyone agreed that there were too many instances in which the family was without power or voice in deciding the types of services to be delivered to their child or themselves, where they would be delivered, and how often.

At a fundamental level, Part H has required governors, legislators, bureaucrats, early interventionists, and family members to examine their own personal values and priorities in order to reach some consensus as policy development has proceeded (Gallagher, 1992). Fifty-four states and jurisdictions either are currently implementing all components of Part H or are actively planning for implementation (Maroldo, 1992). Part H of PL 99–457 has been a tremendous impetus for change, and its full impact on the education and service delivery for all children with disabilities and their families is yet to be realized.

COLLABORATION FOR A FAMILY-CENTERED SYSTEM

The family eco-map presented in Figure 21–1 dramatically points out what life is like for a family with a severely disabled child. It is easy to understand the truth in this statement:

> Good intentions may be the paving stones on the road to hell. Despite the benevolence of donors, their attempts to improve the lot of unfortunate others may leave those others feeling out of control, incompetent and incapable of overcoming their problems. (Coates, Renzaglia, & Embree, 1983, p. 253)

Although the family is in the center of the eco-map and actually may even need or want all of the "helpers" surrounding them, the obvious question is: How much dignity or control can be left to this family? If it takes all these professionals and agencies to raise this child, what message is being delivered about the parents' basic parenting skills, the role of their extended family members and friends, and the ability to live a normal life as a family in the community? One is struck by the complexity and fragmentation of the service providers, the intrusion that such a system must create, and the potential for inordinate duplication. However, it is also true that no single professional or agency has all the necessary expertise to be able to develop and/or carry out the comprehensive intervention necessary for this family and child. Part H directly addresses these issues through a mandate for a collaborative effort embodied in the IFSP.

Pleas for collaboration reverberate through meetings of practitioners, legislative committees, and government agencies (Kagan, 1991, pp. x–xi). What exactly is meant by the term? *Collaboration* is defined as a process leading to a new structure "where resources, power and authority are shared and where people are brought together to achieve common goals that could not be accomplished by a single individual or organization independently" (Kagan, 1991, p. 3). Although collaboration is often confused with coordination or cooperation, the terms are not interchangeable, and the differences are more than semantic.

Cooperation between parties is the simplest of the three types of interaction to achieve, because it is based on informal relationships. The process can involve transferring information or agreeing to carry out certain activities determined by a third party (Kagan, 1991). Cooperation is a fairly superficial mode of interaction for agencies. Examples of cooperative efforts include sharing newsletters, dis-

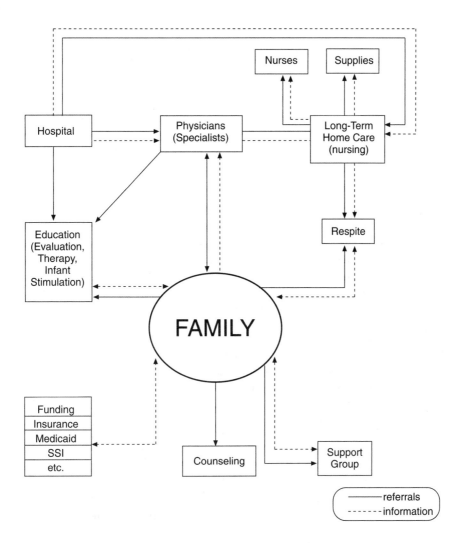

Figure 21–1 Eco-map for a family of an infant with severe disabilities

seminating information and agency brochures, and sending out invitations to staff development activities (Swan & Morgan, 1993). Swan and Morgan liken cooperation to "parallel play of children," demonstrating a "peaceful co-existence" that is "neither genuinely interactive nor interdependent" (p. 21).

Coordination is more complex because it can involve more formalized agreements and the sharing of resources. When agencies or disciplines coordinate, however, there are no expected changes in their previously defined roles or methods of conducting day-to-day operations. Some examples of coordinated efforts are joint budgeting or purchasing, collocation of staff, case conferences, and cross-referring of clients (Gans & Horton, 1975). Coordination is a prerequisite to collaboration.

Collaboration connotes the most durable and the most difficult relationship because previously separated organizations are merged into a new structure. Perhaps the most difficult aspect is that the power and authority must be shared or in some instances, transferred from one organization to another or given up by both (Kagan, 1991). The vision of Part H was that such system collaboration, with new structures and new ways of doing business, would be forged at the federal, state, and local levels of service delivery. In addition to system collaboration, Kagan also speaks of service collaboration, with a mission of improving direct services to children and families. In a recent report to the U.S. Senate, the Committee on Labor and Human Resources concluded that sweeping systemic changes have extremely limited success. According to this committee, service providers should focus their sights more narrowly on building a service package with and for *individual* families (GAO, 1992). The idea of early intervention through service collaboration, operationalized through the IFSP, is key to the Part H effort (McGonigal, Kaufmann, & Johnson, 1991a, 1991b).

Kjerland (1986) believes that a transdisciplinary team collaboration model best fits with family-centered service delivery. In such a team model, the parent is an "official" member of the team and each member is recognized as having equally important contributions. Implementation may be carried out by one member of the team, working in conjunction with the other members. "Teaming" is not easy, as each team member struggles to deal with issues such as conflict resolution, overt and implied hierarchies, and consolidating viewpoints that may be very different.

Incorporating families into the team, in truly meaningful and valued roles requires additional modifications (Bailey, 1987; Bailey, McWilliam, & Winton, 1992; Nash, 1990; Royu, Dunn, Hazel, & O'Brien, 1990). Meetings have to be held at a time and place convenient to the family. Value has to be placed on information that may not be based on "hard data." There has to be recognition that not all families want to be part of the team, at least in the beginning of their experience with early intervention (Nash, 1990).

Collaboration is designed as a means to an end, not an end in itself. Furthermore, there is debate as to whether the success of collaboration should be measured against child and family outcomes or system reform (Kagan, 1991). The vision of a collaborative system is to construct a service picture for each family, based on their needs and priorities. Access to services should be simpler and clearer, with a service coordinator to assist and *one* intake application form that the family can use to receive services from many providers and agencies. The persons involved with the child work as a unified team, cutting down the numbers of professionals necessary to carry out single activities and including the family members as part of that team. Funding streams should be merged or blended. Such a collaborative approach seems imperative if early intervention is to be truly helpful and not an additional stress factor for a family to deal with during a very confusing and vulnerable time. A service system based on collaboration can indeed be truly family-centered.

CHANGING CONCEPTIONS OF HELP-GIVING

Models of Help-Giving

One cannot begin to develop collaborative partnerships with families without understanding and "buying into" a very changed conception of help-giving. Brickman and colleagues (Brickman et al., 1983) have defined several *traditional models of helping,* with the beliefs each model presumes.

The *moral model* assumes that the help-seekers are responsible for creating their own problems and for solving them. This is the approach that "You made your bed, now lie in it." The judgmental or punitive overtones can lead to feelings of loneliness, guilt, and exhaustion on the part of the help-seeker.

The *medical model* assumes that the help-seekers are not responsible for their problems or for the solutions. Problems are illnesses, and only experts can fully understand and thus treat and correct them. Any movement toward solving these problems, as well as any change occurring, is attributed to the help-giver. Thus, this approach can lead to feelings of passivity, dependency, and helplessness on the part of the help-seeker.

The *enlightenment model* assumes the help-seekers are responsible for their problems, but they are viewed as not capable of reaching solutions, at least not alone. This model assumes that help-givers must guide and shape their behavior.

The *compensatory model* assumes that help-seekers are victims of prior experience and, thus, while they are not responsible for their problems, they are responsible for the solutions. Many of the self-help and poverty programs such as Head Start are based on this type of model.

Dunst and Trivette (1988) have developed a fifth model of helping that they call enabling. Based on the work of Brickman and colleagues (1983) and other researchers (Rappaport, 1984; Hobbs et al., 1984; Fisher, Nadler, & Whitcher-Alagna, 1983), Dunst and Trivette (1988) tell us that "The *enabling model* of helping de-emphasizes help-seeker responsibility for causing problems and emphasizes the ability to acquire the competencies necessary to solve problems, meet needs, and realize personal goals" (p. 351).

Enabling Relationships and Family-Centered Philosophy

This enabling model is the cornerstone of the family-centered philosophy that has so greatly influenced the delivery of early intervention services. It replaces what had been typical of early intervention helping relationships. Common practice had been for professionals to take control, telling the parent what was wrong, what needed to be done to correct the deficits, and where and how the intervention was to occur. The enabling approach focuses on the strengths and capabilities of the family so that they can apply their present abilities and acquire new ones, as necessary, to meet the needs of their child (Dunst, Trivette, & Deal, 1988). In the enabling-helping relationship, the help-seeker plays a major role in deciding what goals are important and what actions should be pursued to achieve those goals. With the support of the help-giver, competence emerges or develops. The help-seeker and the help-giver have joint responsibility for setting goals and carrying out activities to reach those goals and, therefore, there is less dependence on the help-giver (Rappaport, 1984). Dunst and Trivette (1988) outline several roles for help-givers that they consider to be enabling (Exhibit 21–3).

The rationale of the enabling approach is clear. When there is a mismatch between the help offered and the help needed, the assistance is usually not perceived as helpful. "Noncompliant parents" are often so labeled because they do not carry through on professionally designed and ordered interventions that too frequently have little or no relevance to them. Coates, Renzaglia, and Embree (1983) succinctly describe four other qualities of traditional helping relationships that can undermine competence and confidence.

- The help is so overwhelming that it reduces the control the recipients have over their lives.
- The helper is so competent that he or she undermines the acquisition of new skills or the emergence of current skill in the recipients.
- The help undermines perceived self-efficacy, leading to dependence and feelings of inferiority.
- The help creates confusion over who "gets the credit" or blame for changes or lack of change.

Early interventionists who embrace a family-centered philosophy enter into an enabling helping relationship with the families of the young children they serve, so that the family becomes empowered. Dunst and his colleagues state:

> Empowering families in early intervention does not mean giving or bestowing power on families—the power is theirs by right. Rather it

---

Exhibit 21–3 New Roles for Professionals

• Empathetic listener	• Resource person	• Mediator
• Teacher/therapist	• Enabler	• Advocate
• Consultant	• Mobilizer	

Source: From Dunst, Trivette, & Deal, 1988.

means interacting with families in such a way that they maintain or acquire a sense of control over their family life and attribute positive changes that result from early intervention to their own strengths, abilities and actions. (Dunst, Trivette, & Deal, 1988, p. 62)

Cautions about Partnerships

Brinker (1992) raises some cautions about accepting the ideas of collaboration and partnerships without question. In his conceptual critique of the effort to judge early intervention in terms of the extent to which it is family-centered, he states:

We should not revere terms such as family-centered without considering the very many different, potentially contradictory, value-laden meanings that are strongly determined by the unique characteristics of individual situations. (p. 309)

Brinker reminds us that a family enters the early intervention system because of concerns about their child. When clinicians and practitioners strive to define and enter into a partnership with a family, they may be stretching the boundaries of early intervention beyond the point at which the family is comfortable. Those who perform intervention need to be aware of their own knowledge of differing cultures and need to call to mind the uniqueness of each family entity. There must be recognition of the differing meanings applied to *disability, parenting, family structure and identity, communication styles, views of professionals,* and *early intervention goals,* which are inherent in every family and professional (Harry, 1992). Turnbull and Turnbull (1991), in their "ethical analysis" of family assessment and empowerment, state their belief that the "golden rule" should be applied to "helping" interactions with families, and they wonder how there can be true partnerships when the professional is doing all the asking and the parent is doing all the answering. Assessment of family need is presented as an exciting opportunity to broaden the target of intervention beyond the child. However, it can be "frightening and intimidating" when interventionists use sophisticated, impersonal instruments to pinpoint how the family functions, how the family might best be served, the quality of the home environment and of parent-child interaction, and what the family needs (Turnbull & Turnbull, 1991). The authors write:

Taking a family perspective, my first reaction is, you've got to be kidding! . . . disclose all of your family strengths and needs and have the scores summed up and entered into someone's computer? Will this assessment actually help our family or do more damage by invading privacy and creating more problems than it solves? (p. 486)

As the interventionist strives to collaborate with parents, what happens to professional expertise? What happens when the professional does know best or better than the family? The professional, in many instances, does have more experience or expertise than the family members. There is always a differential of power between client and professional, based on professional knowledge and client needs. Clients trust that a plan of treatment will be derived that is in their best interest (Brinker, 1992). So it is with families, especially at this time when they are most vulnerable and *are* often dependent on professional expertise and willing to be told what to do (Thomas, 1988). Early interventionists cannot incorporate family concerns without being given direction (i.e., training) regarding the process of negotiating family concerns versus professional concerns and family priorities versus professional knowledge. The dilemmas are clearly stated by Brinker (1992):

> How can we build on the important insight that families must be central to the service plans for their children, without overshadowing the fact that we know these families only because of their children's disabilities and our presumptive expertise about such disabilities? (p. 327)

It appears that these concerns have less to do with family-centered philosophy than with the methods used to implement that philosophy. No one can deny the intrinsic value of a system that is flexible and responsive, in which (1) the child is served in the context of the family and community, (2) parent skills and competence are developed and/or recognized, and (3) professional expertise can be tapped in meaningful ways. The tenets of family-centered philosophy can stand on their own merits as policy developers and service providers enter into collaboration with families. Empowerment is most likely to be found when there is true collaboration among professionals and the intended beneficiaries—families and children (Rappaport, 1984). If a family-centered system is to be fully realized, the collaboration must extend beyond parent-professional partnerships to include relationships among professionals and among agencies.

IMPLICATIONS FOR PRACTICE

It is clear from these considerations that collaboration is a new way of doing business that requires a change in the practices of a range of professionals in a wide variety of settings. Approaching service delivery in a collaborative manner impacts not only on relationships with families but also on the manner in which professionals relate to each other. Collaboration is based on shared decision making, with the understanding that the decisions made must match the priorities, strengths, and needs as defined by each individual family. The criteria on which success is measured also needs to be mutually defined by all parties to the collaborative process. This discussion brings us, in conclusion, to several implications for practice.

Collaboration Takes Time

"It was a good feeling to be listened to, without someone keeping notes, watching the clock or passing judgment" (Songer, 1993).

Administrative structure must recognize and provide for the time required to build trust and respect among all parties involved with a particular child. Time must be allowed for each team member to understand everyone's contributions and roles. There must be time to invite and respond to questions and time to present the information necessary so that decisions can be made. No longer can intervention time be defined only as direct contact with the client, or patient, or student.

The time element has special relevance in collaborating with families. For example, even in the intense and often crisis-oriented hospital setting, where time is not in abundance, medical professionals must be willing to work in partnership with families and must allocate the time to do so (Cardoso, 1991). It is also important to remember that parents may feel overwhelmed with the technical language, charts, and equipment of a medical environment and that family members need and deserve a firm handshake, a proper introduction, and information presented in a context and manner that is understandable to them. The fact is that, despite a potential reluctance of care providers to see parents as competent, the parents are often the only members of the team who have the complete knowledge of medical history, of the child's emotional tolerance, and of each professional's view of their child (Cardoso, 1991). The time committed to communicating with the family, teaching care to family, and affirming family competence is a necessity in helping families shift from the role of grateful recipient to partner in the health care process. Along with the obvious medical care to the child, this should be a primary goal of hospital staff (Thomas, 1988). The time committed to collaborating with families has similar benefits for all early intervention efforts.

Collaboration Must Demonstrate Respect

> I felt very involved in the process, yet not as a full team member. I continued to experience that now familiar feeling that my observations and reports were not as valid as everyone else's. After the evaluation team had administered their tests I asked what their perspectives were. Was I surprised when they informed me that they would need to meet together to discuss their findings and to develop recommendations, and then they would contact us to have a meeting. I felt like I'd been left empty. I imagined the team wasn't sharing their findings because they were so bad. I also wondered what they would be saying about my baby in their private meeting, or even about my family, that I couldn't or shouldn't hear. (Songer, 1993)

The forming of a team is difficult. Team members, including families, must come to respect each member's contribution and value to the collaborative effort. This is difficult enough when team members know each other or work for a single agency. It requires extraordinary skill when this is not the case and team members bring entirely different perspectives to the collaboration. Respect is demonstrated by holding meetings that are mutually convenient to all, *including families,* even if this means rotating location and time. Respect is demonstrated by ensuring that all team members, *including families,* are privy to the same information, so that everyone can contribute to the discussion in meaningful ways. Respect is demonstrated by the incorporation of the differing viewpoints at all times. For example, families should be present during diagnostic and evaluation procedures so that their comments and suggestions are incorporated into the testing process itself (Rogers, 1982). Although parents may not have test results or hard data to present during goal setting and implementation meetings, their views must be perceived as equally valuable and their contributions must be met with more than a polite nod. Their comments should be acknowledged during the discussion, not merely as an afterthought.

It is easier to respect some people than others. It is easier to collaborate with those who have similar values, parenting style, or cultural beliefs (Harry, 1992). This is especially true in relationships with families. When a "good" family freely chooses an intervention program and then decides to quit, move on, or switch to another program, the staff is likely to examine what went wrong and what they could have done differently to keep the family engaged. When a "bad" family quits or does not participate, professional concern is often expressed in terms of noncompliance, with the onus of blame for not continuing placed on the family (Brinker, 1992). Professionals may presume that they know best and may demonstrate a lack of respect for the differing priorities and values of the family. The skills of negotiation, communication, and facilitation need to be part of every professional training endeavor (Brinker, 1992).

Collaboration Requires a Shift in Power and Control

Communication and control were major issues for my husband and me. We were constantly dealing with multiple helpers and the messages we were given were different, depending on who was delivering them. We acutely felt that we had little control. Information wasn't always easy to obtain and we often felt that Jonathan wasn't really ours. We didn't possess the skills necessary to provide the care that Jonathan needed; we couldn't always hold him when we wanted to and we couldn't make decisions concerning his care because we were not really qualified. It was difficult for both of us because we desperately needed to reclaim our child. (Songer, 1993)

Collaboration means that power and control must be shared or even relinquished. As team members strive for consensus and the development of integrated service plans, issues of control are almost always present. Some members of the team may be used to always having control, some may be accustomed to relinquishing control, and some may be willing to do so temporarily. Some members may passively fight control (smile willingly, then proceed to do the opposite), and still others may fight for control (the "pushy parent" or the "autocratic physician"). Collaboration implies that no one has all the answers and that anyone may have contributions to make to the effort. Collaboration implies balance and give and take.

Any team member may be anywhere on the control continuum at any point in time. For example, during brain surgery, the surgeon has control, but during the rehabilitation planning meeting, the physical therapist may be the team leader. During the intensive care nursery stay, the neonatologist calls the shots because he or she manages the baby's critical care, but at the discharge planning meeting, the parents may assume control as they make known their needs for help in caring for their baby.

Most importantly, however, in the special circumstance of collaborating with families, no one can ever forget that, in most cases, the family is and will be the constant for that child. Any relationship that increases the feeling of control and competence in family members is bound to have lasting impact.

As new collaborations are developed, all participants must come to believe that what results for themselves and/or their patients/clients is something better

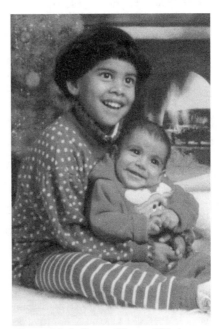

Figure 21–2 Sisters, Kim and Lindsey

than what would have resulted if the collaboration had not occurred. Collaboration, especially parent-professional collaboration, is the spirit of family-centered care. This change in orientation must be reflected at all levels of care, in work with individuals, families, the development of new services, and the formation of new policy.

BIBLIOGRAPHY

Apter, S. (1982). *Troubled children/troubled systems*. New York: Pergamon Press.

Bailey, D.B. (1987). Collaborative goal-setting with families: Resolving differences in values and priorities for services. *Topics in Early Childhood Special Education, 7*(2), 59–71.

Bailey, D.B., McWilliam, P.J., & Winton, P.J. (1992). Building family-centered practices in early intervention: A team-based model for change. *Infants and Young Children, 5*(1), 73–82.

Bailey, D.B., Simeonsson, R.J., Winton, P.J., Huntington, G.S., Comfort, M., Isbell, P., O'Donnell, K.J., & Helm, J.M. (1986). Family-focused intervention: A functional model for planning, implementing, and evaluating individualized family services in early intervention. *Journal of the Division for Early Childhood, 10*, 156–171.

Brewer, E.J., McPherson, M., Magrab, P.R., & Hutchins, V.L. (1989). Family-centered, community-based, coordinated care for children with special health care needs. *Pediatrics, 83*(6), 1055–1060.

Brickman, P., Kidder, L.H., Coates, D., Rabinowitz, V., Cohn, E., & Karuza, J. (1983). The dilemmas of helping: Making aid fair and effective. In J. Fisher, A. Nadler, & B.M. DePaulo (Eds.), *New directions in helping* (Vol. 1) (pp. 17–49). New York: Academic Press.

Brinker, R.P. (1992). Family involvement in early intervention: Accepting the unchangeable, changing the changeable, and knowing the difference. *Topics in Early Childhood Special Education, 12*(3), 307–332.

Bronfenbrenner, U. (1979). *The ecology of human development: Experiments by nature and design*. Cambridge: Harvard University Press.

Cardoso, P. (1991). A parent's perspective: Family-centered care. *Children's Health Care, 20*(4), 258–260.

Coates, D., Renzaglia, G.J., & Embree, M.C. (1983). When helping backfires: Help and helplessness. In J. Fisher, A. Nadler, & B.M. DePaulo (Eds.), *New directions in helping* (Vol. 1) (pp. 251–279). New York: Academic Press.

Dunst, C., & Trivette, C. (1988). Helping, helplessness and harm. In J. Witt, S. Elliott, & F. Gresham (Eds.), *Handbook of behavior therapy* (pp. 343–375). New York: Plenum Press.

Dunst, C.J., Trivette, C.M, & Deal, A.G. (1988). *Enabling and empowering families: Principles and guidelines for practice*. Cambridge, MA: Brookline Books.

Early intervention program for infants and toddlers with handicaps: Final regulations, 34 CFR 303. (1989). *Federal Register, 54*(119), 26306–26348.

Education of the Handicapped Act Amendments of 1986 (P.L. 99–457), (1986).

Fisher, J.D., Nadler, A., & Whitcher-Alagna, S. (1983). Four conceptualizations of reactions to aid. In J. Fisher, A. Nader, B.M. DePaulo (Eds.), *New directions in helping* (Vol. 1) (pp. 51–84). New York: Academic Press.

Gallagher, J. (1992). The role of values and facts in policy development for infants and toddlers with disabilities and their families. *Journal of Early Intervention, 16*(1) 1–11.

Gans, S.P., & Horton, G.T. (1975). *Integration of human services: The state and municipal levels*. New York: Praeger.

Garwood, S.G., & Sheehan, R. (1989). *Designing a comprehensive early intervention system: The challenge of Public Law* (PL 99–457). Austin, TX: Pro-Ed.

General Accounting Office. (1992). *Integrating human services: Linking at-risk families with services more successful than system reform efforts*. Report to the Chairman, Subcommittee on Children, Family, Drugs, and Alcoholism, Committee on Labor and Human Resources, U.S. Senate. Washington, DC: Author.

Harry, B. (1992). Developing cultural self-awareness: The first step in values clarification for early interventionists. *Topics in Early Childhood Special Education, 12*(3), 333–350.

Hobbs, N.V., Dokecki, P.R., Hoover-Dempsey, K.V., Moroney, R.M., Shayne, M.W., & Weeks, K.H. (1984). *Strengthening families.* San Francisco: Jossey Bass.

Individuals with Disabilities Education Act (P.L. 100–476), 20 U.S.C. §§1400–14895 (1990).

Kagan, S.L. (1991). *United we stand: Collaboration for child care and early education services.* New York: Teachers College Press.

Kjerland, L. (1986). *Early intervention tailor made.* Eagan, MN: Project Dakota, Inc.

Koop, C.E. (1987). *Surgeon General's report: Children with special health care needs—campaign 87—commitment to family-centered, coordinated care for children with special health care needs.* Washington, DC: U.S. Government Printing Office.

Maroldo, R. (Ed.) (1992). *Early childhood report: Children with special needs and their families.* LRP Publication, 3(10).

McGonigal, M.H., Kaufmann, R.K., & Johnson, B.H. (1991a). A family-centered process for the Individualized Family Service Plan. *Journal of Early Intervention, 15*(1), 46–56.

McGonigal, M.J., Kaufmann, R.K., & Johnson, B.H. (1991b). *Guidelines and recommended practices for the Individualized Family Service Plan* (2nd ed). Bethesda, MD: Association for the Care of Children's Health.

Nash, J.K. (1990). Public Law 99–457: Facilitating family participation on the multidisciplinary team. *Journal of Early Intervention, 14*(4), 318–326.

National Center for Clinical Infant Programs (1989). *The intent and spirit of P.L. 99–457: A sourcebook.* Washington, DC: Project Zero to Three.

National Center for Family Centered Care (1990). *What is family centered care?* Bethesda, MD: Association for the Care of Children's Health.

Nelkin, V. (1987). *Family-centered health care for medically fragile children: Principles and practices.* Washington, DC: Georgetown University Child Development Center, National Center for Networking Community Based Services.

Rappaport, J. (1984). Studies in empowerment: Introduction to the issues. In J. Rappaport, C. Swift, & R. Hess (Eds.), *Studies in empowerment: Steps toward understanding and action* (pp. 1–37). New York: Haworth Press.

Rogers, S. (1982). A child's evaluation: It's a family affair. In S. Brown & M.S. Moersch (Eds.), *Parents on the team* (pp. 69–75). Ann Arbor, MI: University of Michigan Press.

Royu, C., Dunn, W., Hazel, R., & O'Brien, M. (1990). Collaborative teams. *Transitions Newsletter of the Kansas Early Childhood Research Institute, 2*(1), 1–3.

Shelton, T.L., Jeppson, E.S., & Johnson, B.H. (1987). *Family-centered care for children with special health care needs.* Washington, DC: Association for the Care of Children's Health.

Shoultz, B., & Racino, J. (1988). *Supporting people with medical and physical needs in the community.* Syracuse, NY: Center on Human Policy.

Silverstein, R. (1989). A window of opportunity. *The intent and spirit of P.L. 99–457: A sourcebook.* Washington, DC: Project Zero to Three (pp. A1–A7).

Songer, N. (1993). Personal communication.

Swan, W.W., & Morgan, J.L. (1993). *Collaborating for comprehensive services for young children and their families.* Baltimore: Paul H. Brookes.

Thomas, R.B. (1988). The struggles for control between families and health care providers when a child has a complex health care need. *Zero to Three: Bulletin of the National Center on Clinical Infant Programs, VIII* (3), 15–18.

Trohanis, P. (1989). An introduction to P.L. 99–457 and the national policy agenda for serving young children with special needs and their families. In J.J. Gallagher (Ed.), *Policy, implementation and P.L. 99–457* (pp. 1–17). Baltimore: Paul H. Brookes.

Turnbull, A.L., & Turnbull, H.R. (1991). Family assessment and family empowerment: An ethical analysis. In L. Meyer, C. Peck, & L. Brown (Eds.), *Critical issues in the lives of people with severe disabilities* (pp. 485–488). Baltimore: Paul H. Brookes.

Report to U.S. House of Representatives. (Report No. 99–860) Project Zero to Three (1986). *Education of Handicapped Act amendments.* Washington, DC: Author.

Walker, P. (1991). Where there is a way, there is not always a will: Technology, public policy, and the school integration of children who are technology-assisted. *Children's Health Care, 20*(2), 68–74.

Index